FETAL
ECHOCARDIOGRAPHY

FETAL ECHOCARDIOGRAPHY

SECOND EDITION

Julia A. Drose, BA, RDMS, RDCS, RVT

Associate Professor
Department of Radiology
Chief Sonographer
Divisions of Diagnostic Ultrasound and Prenatal Diagnosis & Genetics
University of Colorado Hospital
Denver, Colorado

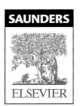

SAUNDERS

ELSEVIER

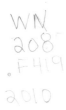

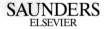

SAUNDERS
ELSEVIER

11830 Westline Industrial Drive
St. Louis, Missouri 63146

FETAL ECHOCARDIOGRAPHY, SECOND EDITION   ISBN: 978-1-4160-5669-0

Notice

Neither the Publisher nor the Author assumes any responsibility for any loss or injury and/ or damage to persons or property arising out of or related to any use of the material contained in this book. It is the responsibility of the treating practitioner, relying on independent expertise and knowledge of the patient, to determine the best treatment and method of application for the patient.

The Publisher

Library of Congress Cataloging-in-Publication Data

Fetal echocardiography / [edited by] Julia A. Drose. — 2nd ed.
    p. ; cm.
  Includes bibliographical references and index.
  ISBN 978-1-4160-5669-0 (hardcover : alk. paper) 1. Fetal heart—Ultrasonic imaging.
I. Drose, Julia A.
  [DNLM: 1. Fetal Heart—ultrasonography. 2. Heart Defects, Congenital—ultrasonography.
3. Echocardiography. 4. Ultrasonography, Prenatal. WQ 210.5 F4192 2010]
  RG628.3.E34F48 2010
  618.3'26107543—dc22

                                                                        2008045320

ISBN: 978-1-4160-5669-0

Vice President and Publisher: Andrew Allen
Publisher: Jeanne Olson
Associate Developmental Editor: Luke Held
Publishing Services Manager: Patricia Tannian
Project Manager: Claire Kramer
Designer: Charles Seibel

Printed in China

Last digit is the print number: 9 8 7 6 5 4 3 2

Working together to grow
libraries in developing countries

www.elsevier.com | www.bookaid.org | www.sabre.org

ELSEVIER   BOOK AID International   Sabre Foundation

For **Mackenzie, Caroline, Brady,** *and* **Taylor**

You are fearless, powerful, and utterly amazing.
You are the loves of my life.

Contributors

Amanda K. Auckland, BS, RDMS, RDCS, RVT
Sonographer
Division of Ultrasound
University of Colorado Hospital
Aurora, Colorado

Tina M. Bachman, BS, RDMS, RDCS, RVT
Sonographer
Division of Ultrasound
University of Colorado Hospital
Aurora, Colorado

Heidi S. Barrett, RDMS, RVT
Sonographer
Division of Ultrasound
University of Colorado Hospital
Aurora, Colorado

Teresa M. Bieker, MBA-H, RDMS, RDCS, RVT
Lead Sonographer
Division of Ultrasound
University of Colorado Hospital
Aurora, Colorado

Danielle M. Bolger, RDMS, RVT
Sonographer
Division of Ultrasound
University of Colorado Hospital
Aurora, Colorado

Julia A. Drose, BA, RDMS, RDCS, RVT
Associate Professor
Department of Radiology
Chief Sonographer
Divisions of Diagnostic Ultrasound and Prenatal
    Diagnosis & Genetics
University of Colorado Hospital
Denver, Colorado

Marisa R. Lydia, RDMS, RDCS, RVT
Sonographer
Obstetrix Medical Group
Lone Tree, Colorado

Sarah H. Martinez, BS, RDMS, RDCS, RVT
Clinical Applications Specialist
GE Healthcare
Denver, Colorado

Kristin E. McKinney, MD
Assistant Professor of Radiology
Division of Ultrasound
University of Colorado Hospital
Aurora, Colorado

Cynthia L. Rapp, BS, RDMS, RDCS
Vice President of Clinical Program Development
The Medipattern Corporation
Toronto, Ontario, Canada

Paul D. Russ, MD
Professor of Radiology
University of Colorado Hospital
Aurora, Colorado

Elizabeth M. Shaffer, MD
Associate Professor of Pediatrics
The Children's Hospital
Denver, Colorado

Britt C. Smyth, BA, RDMS, RDCS, RVT
Sonographer
Division of Ultrasound
University of Colorado Hospital
Aurora, Colorado

Elizabeth R. Stamm, MD
Associate Professor of Radiology
University of Colorado Hospital
Aurora, Colorado

Karrie L. Villavicencio, MD
Assistant Professor of Pediatric Cardiology
University of Colorado Hospital
Denver, Colorado

Marsha Wheeler, MD
Associate Professor of Obstetrics and Gynecology
University of Colorado Hospital
Denver, Colorado

Adel K. Younoszai, MD
Assistant Professor of Pediatrics
Director of Cardiac Imaging
The Children's Hospital
Denver, Colorado

Reviewers

Beth Anderhub, MEd, RDMS, RSDMS
Professor and Program Director of Diagnostic
    Medical Sonography
St. Louis Community College
St. Louis, Missouri

Marcia Cooper, MSRS, RT(R)(M)(CT)(QM), RDMS,
RVT
Clinical Coordinator and Associate of Imaging
    Sciences
Morehead State University
Morehead, Kentucky

Janice Dolk, MA, RT(R), RDMS
Sonography Consultant and Lab Instructor
Palm Beach Community College
Port St. Lucie, Florida

Charlotte Henningsen, MS, RT, RDMS, RVT,
FSDMS
Chair and Professor
Department of Diagnostic Medical Sonography
Florida Hospital College of Health Sciences
Orlando, Florida

Cheryl Morrow, RT(R), RDMS, RDCS, RUT
Staff Sonographer
Sonowave
Tyler, Texas

Susanna Ovel, RT, RDMS, RVT
Sonographer III
Radiological Associates of Sacramento
Sacramento, California

David Rands, BA, RDMS, RDCS, RVT, ARRT(R)
Instructor
University of Arkansas Medical Sciences
Little Rock, Arkansas

Anthony Swartz, BS, RT(R), RDMS
Lead Sonography and Manager
Maternal-Fetal Medicine Department
WakeMed Health and Hospitals
Raleigh, North Carolina

Kerry Weinberg, MPS, RT(R), RDMS, RDCS
Program Director
Diagnostic Medical Sonography
New York University
New York, New York

Preface

The Prenatal Diagnosis and Genetics Center at the University of Colorado Hospital provides a multidisciplinary approach to diagnosing fetal cardiac disease that involves sonography, perinatology, pediatric cardiology, radiology, and genetic counseling. This combination of specialties provides the skills and different perspectives necessary to diagnose and manage the complex problems presented by the fetus with cardiac abnormalities.

The purpose of this book is to extend this approach to all those involved in fetal echocardiography by providing a description of sonographic technique and diagnosis, as well as insight into the management of these children, both before and after birth. Each chapter has been written and critiqued by practitioners with expertise in this field. All contributors are currently or were previously associated with our fetal cardiovascular center.

New to This Edition

The second edition of *Fetal Echocardiography* provides the most current information available on performing and interpreting fetal echocardiograms. It also acts as a study guide for those just entering the field.

Important New Features Have Been Added

- Color Images
  - All of the line art has been redrawn in full color.
  - Color Doppler images are included throughout the book.
- Chapter Outlines
  - Outlines are now included at the beginning of each chapter, providing readers with an at-a-glance view of chapter contents.

New Chapters Have Been Added On

- Prenatal Intervention in the Fetus with Cardiac Disease
- First-Trimester Fetal Echocardiography
- Three-Dimensional Fetal Echocardiography

Ancillaries

A companion CD in the back of the book has been developed for the second edition and contains valuable resources to enhance knowledge and reinforce learning.

- Multimedia
  - Video clips show scanning planes that are necessary to perform a fetal echocardiogram.
- Study Questions
  - More than 250 multiple-choice questions help readers reinforce information presented in the book and are sorted by chapter.

I would like to acknowledge the contributors to this book for their willingness to share their knowledge and their dedication to our profession.

It is hoped that obstetricians, pediatric cardiologists, radiologists, sonographers, and others involved in the investigation of fetal heart disease will find this a useful reference.

JULIA A. DROSE, BA, RDMS, RDCS, RVT

Acknowledgments

First and foremost, to my family: Donna Patterson, Lou Patterson, Jack Drose, Greg Drose, Lora Drose, Emily Patterson, Mackenzie Patterson, Caroline Patterson, Brady Drose, Taylor Drose, Kate Huisken, Brice Huisken, and Avery Huisken. Thank you all for your continued love and support.

Thank you also to all of the sonographers, genetic counselors, nurses, and staff involved with fetal echocardiography at the University of Colorado Hospital: June Altman, Liana Amarillas, Sonia Archibeque, Amanda Auckland, Tina Bachman, Heidi Barrett, Danielle Bolger, Tracy Bieker, Stella Bizzarro, Sandy Buckley, James Cacari, Tyra Cade, Kathleen Digiulio, Juan Gamez, George Kennedy, Cheryl Kurth, Tyanne Rosie, Britt Smyth, Emily Todd, and Michele Winslow. We succeed because of your dedication to the field of fetal echocardiography and your understanding of how important it is to provide the best possible care to our patients.

I would also like to thank the physicians that make our program a collaborative effort: Jill Davies, Lorraine Dugoff, Henry Galan, John Hobbins, Michael Manco-Johnson, Kristin McKinney, Melissa Palmer, Nayana Patel, Paul Russ, Elizabeth Shaffer, Elizabeth Stamm, Karrie Villavicencio, Marsha Wheeler, Virginia Winn, and Adel Younoszai.

Finally, thank you to the individuals at Elsevier who helped with the production of this edition: Jeanne Olson, Publisher; Luke Held, Associate Developmental Editor; Jeanne Robertson, freelance artist; Patricia Tannian, Publishing Services Manager, Claire Kramer, Project Manager; and Charles Seibel, Designer.

Contents

FETAL
ECHOCARDIOGRAPHY

CHAPTER 1

Embryology and Physiology of the Fetal Heart

Julia A. Drose

Congenital heart disease is the most common severe congenital abnormality found among live births.[1–13]

Because development of the heart is an interaction of genes, environment, and chance, approximately 70% to 85% of cases of congenital heart disease have multifactorial causes.[14–17]

To delineate the etiology and pathogenesis of congenital heart disease requires an understanding of both normal and abnormal cardiac development.

Embryology

All major organ systems are formed between the fourth and eighth weeks of development (Table 1–1). This is called the period of *organogenesis*. It is during this time that the embryo is most susceptible to factors that interfere with development.

The cardiovascular system, including the heart, blood vessels, and blood cells, originates from the mesodermal germ layer.[18] Cardiovascular morphogenesis is controlled by mechanisms that are common to all developmental processes: cell growth, cell migration, cell death, differentiation, and adhesion.

The heart initially consists of paired tubular structures that by the twenty-second day of development (the embryo is approximately 2.5 to 3 mm in length) form a single, slightly bent heart tube (Fig. 1–1). This heart tube consists of an inner endocardial tube and a surrounding myoepicardial mantle. At this stage, the heart tube connects with the developing arch system and with the vitelline and umbilical veins.[19]

The second stage of cardiac development begins with the formation of the atrioventriculobulbar loop. The cephalic portion of the heart tube bends ventrally and to the right, whereas the caudal atrial portion begins to bend in a dorsocranial

TABLE 1-1	Timing of Embryologic Heart Formation
Timing	**Event**
Days 21–22	Umbilical veins, vitelline veins, cardinal veins form
	Single heart tube forms
	Pericardial cavity forms
Day 23	Heart tube grows rapidly, forcing it to fold on itself
Days 25–28	Atrioventriculobulbar loop forms
	Common atrium forms
	Atrioventricular canal forms connecting common atrium to early embryonic ventricles
	Septum primum appears
Days 27–37	Endocardial cushions appear
Day 28	Heart begins to beat
	Ventricular septum appears as a small ridge in common ventricle
	Ventricles begin to dilate
Days 28–35	Absorption of bulbous cordis and sinus venosus
	Four-chambered heart forms
Day 29	Pulmonary veins form
Days 31–35	Placental circulation begins
	Atrioventricular node develops
	Ostium secundum is formed
	Sinoatrial node develops
Day 33	Tricuspid and mitral valves form
Days 35–42	Coronary arteries form
Days 36–42	Inferior vena cava forms
Days 43–49	Superior vena cava forms
	Coronary sinus forms
Day 49	Formation of muscular interventricular septum
Day 56	Aorta and pulmonary arteries form
	Aortic and pulmonic valves form

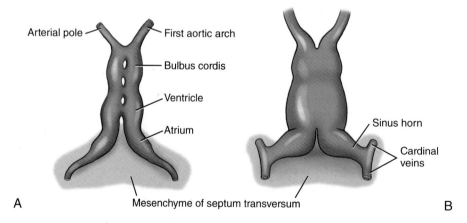

Figure 1–1 Formation of a single heart tube from two paired tubular structures. **A,** Ventral view at approximately 21 days showing beginning of fusion. **B,** At 22 days fusion is almost complete.

direction and to the left, thus forming a loop (Fig. 1–2).[18]

As this heart loop continues to bend, a common atrium is formed and enters the pericardial cavity, carrying along the right and left segments of the sinus venosus. From here the atrioventricular canal forms, which connects the common atrium to the early embryonic ventricles.

It is at this time (approximately 28 days) that contractions are thought to begin in the ventricu-

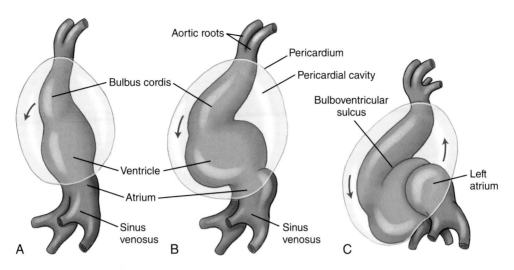

Figure 1–2   Formation of the atrioventriculobulbar loop at approximately 22 days **(A)**, at approximately 23 days **(B),** and at approximately 24 days **(C)**. As this loop is formed, a common atrium is formed and enters the pericardial cavity.

lobulbar portion of the heart, and the heart beat is initiated.[20] Circulation occurs from the sinus venosus into the right atrium, into the left atrium, and then into the atrioventricular canal and the ventricles.

Stage three in the development of the heart consists of absorption of the bulbus cordis and sinus venosus. At this stage, the atrioventriculobulbar loop begins to untwist and the cardiac septa develop, forming a four-chambered heart.[19]

Formation of the septa within the heart results from the development of endocardial cushion tissue in the atrioventricular canal and the truncoconal region. This occurs between the twenty-seventh and thirty-seventh days of development, when the embryo is 4 to 14 mm in length (Fig. 1–3).

In the atrium, the septum primum—a sickle-shaped crest descending from the roof of the atrium—does not completely divide the atrium in two, but leaves an open ostium primum for communication between the two chambers. When the ostium primum is obliterated owing to fusion of the septum primum with the endocardial cushions, the ostium secundum forms within the septum primum.

Last, a septum secundum is formed, but an interatrial opening, the foramen ovale, remains until birth when pressure in the left atrium increases, causing the two septa to press against each other and close this communication.[20]

Septum formation within the atrioventricular canal occurs when two large endocardial cushions fuse, resulting in a right (tricuspid) and left (mitral) atrioventricular orifice (Fig. 1–4). This usually occurs by day 33 of development.[18]

The interventricular septum is formed by the end of the seventh week of development (Fig. 1–5). It results from the dilation of the two primitive ventricles (right and left conus swellings), which causes the medial walls to become apposed and fuse together. This forms the muscular portion of the interventricular septum. Formation of the membranous portion follows.

During the eighth week of development, the truncus swellings or cushions of the primitive heart grow and twist around each other to form the aorticopulmonary septum (Fig. 1–6). This septum divides the truncus arteriosus into an aortic channel and a pulmonary channel.

The cushions of the conus cordis develop simultaneously. These conus cushions unite with the aorticopulmonary septum. After this fusion occurs, the septum divides the conus into an anterolateral portion (the right ventricular outflow tract) and a posteromedial portion (the left ventricular outflow tract).

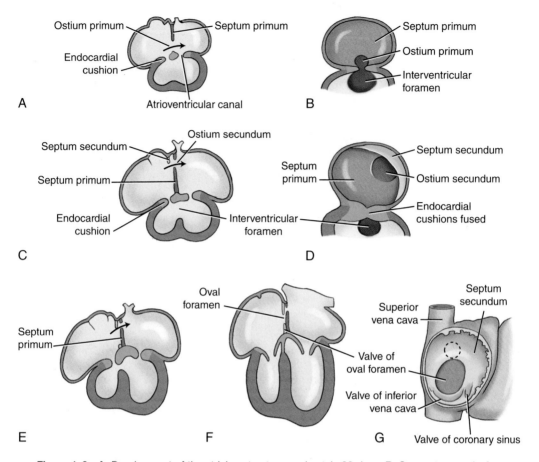

Figure 1–3 **A,** Development of the atrial septa at approximately 30 days. **B,** Same stage as in **A** but seen from the right. **C,** Development at approximately 33 days. **D,** Same stage as in **C** but seen from the right. **E,** Development at approximately 37 days. **F,** Newborn heart. **G,** View of the atrial septum seen from the right, same stage as in **F.**

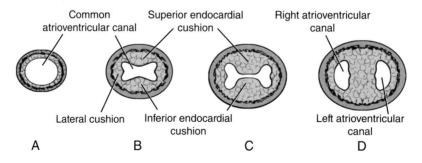

Figure 1–4 Formation of the septum in the atrioventricular canal. **A,** Approximately 28 days. **B,** Approximately 30 days. **C,** Approximately 33 days. **D,** Approximately 35 days. The initial circular opening gradually becomes elongated in the transverse direction, resulting in a right (tricuspid) and left (mitral) atrioventricular orifice.

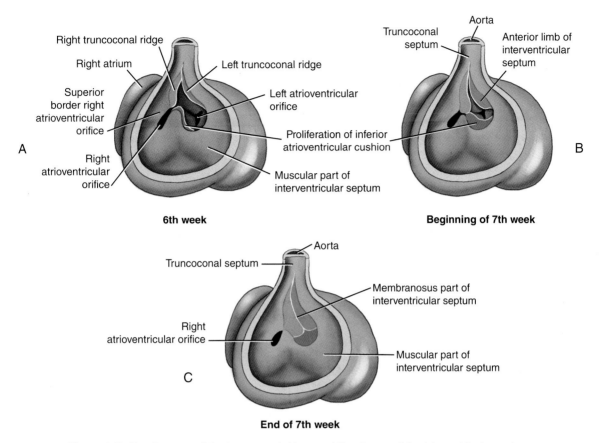

Figure 1–5 Development of the truncoconal ridges and the closure of the interventricular septum. The proliferation of the right and left conus swellings, combined with the proliferation of the inferior atrioventricular cushion, eventually closes the interventricular foramen and forms the membranous portion of the interventricular septum. **A,** At 6 weeks. **B,** Beginning of the seventh week. **C,** End of the seventh week.

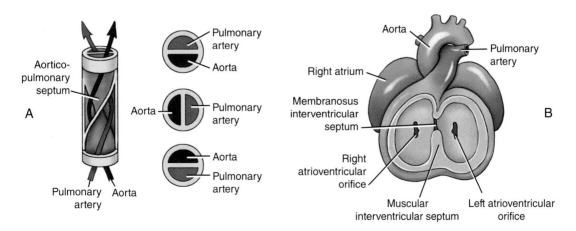

Figure 1–6 A, Formation of the aorticopulmonary septum. **B,** Division of the aorta and pulmonary artery at the eighth week of development. This is accomplished by the aorta and pulmonary artery twisting around each other.

Next, the opening that remained between the two ventricles closes as a result of the conus septum fusing with tissue from the inferior endocardial cushions along the top of the muscular interventricular septum (see Fig. 1–5). This becomes the membranous part of the interventricular septum.[18,19]

Between 5 and 7 weeks of development, the semilunar valves (aortic and pulmonic valves) are formed.

Aortic Arches

During the fourth and fifth weeks of development, six pairs of arteries arising from the most distal portion of the truncus arteriosus are formed (Table 1–2). They are known as aortic arches (Fig. 1–7). These arches form communications between the aortic sac and the two dorsal aortas.

The first pair of arches is formed when the embryo is approximately 1.3 mm in length (day 19 to day 20), and the second pair is formed when the length of the embryo is 3 mm (day 20 to day 23). These first and second arch pairs disappear as the third pair is formed when the embryo is approximately 4 mm in length (day 24 to day 25).

The dorsal aortas beyond the dorsal ends of the third pair of arches persist as the internal carotid arteries. This third pair of arches form the stems of the internal carotid arteries. The external carotid arteries arise from these arches, which connect with the aortic sac to form the common carotid arteries.

The fourth pair of arches appear when the embryo reaches 5 to 6 mm in length (day 26 to day 30). When the embryo is about 14 mm long (day 36 to day 42), the dorsal aorta between the third and fourth arches atrophies. This is also the stage at which the right dorsal aorta between the subclavian artery and the common dorsal aorta disappears. Thus, the fourth left arch and the common dorsal aorta become the definitive aorta, and the fourth right arch becomes the proximal part of the right subclavian artery. Also at this time (when the embryo is between 14 and 16 mm long), the right limb of the aortic sac elongates to form the innominate artery.

The distal segment of both subclavian arteries and the proximal portion of the left subclavian artery develop from the seventh intersegmental artery. The fifth aortic arch pair never fully develops.

Finally, the right sixth aortic arch, which first appears when the embryo is 6 mm in length (approximately day 30), becomes the right pulmonary artery, whereas the left sixth aortic arch persists as the left pulmonary artery and, during intrauterine life, as the ductus arteriosus.[18,19]

Coronary Arteries

The coronary arteries arise as thickenings of the aortic endothelium when the embryo approaches 10 to 12 mm in length (day 35 to day 42). This occurs at the same time that the truncus arteriosus divides into aortic and pulmonary segments. Both coronary arteries pass to the sides of the truncus arteriosus, and the anterior descending coronary artery begins to be laid down. Both circumflex arteries have developed by the time the embryo is 14 mm long (day 42), and by the time the length of the embryo is 20 mm (day 43 to day 49) all larger branches have formed.[19]

Pulmonary Veins

The pulmonary veins are thought to originate from two sources: a presplanchnic source consisting of a channel formed from the confluence of the vascular plexus of the lung, which extends to the middle part of the sinus venosus without opening into it, and from the main pulmonary stem, which is an outgrowth of the heart tube.[19]

TABLE 1–2   Timing of Aortic Arch Formation

Timing	Event
Days 19–20	First pair of aortic arches form
Days 20–23	Second pair of aortic arches form
Days 24–25	Third pair of aortic arches form
	First and second pairs of aortic arches disappear
	Third pair of aortic arches becomes the internal carotid arteries
Days 26–30	Fourth pair of aortic arches form
	Fourth left arch becomes the definitive aorta
	Fourth right arch becomes the right subclavian artery
	Fifth pair of aortic arches never fully develop
Day 30	Sixth pair of aortic arches form
	Sixth right arch becomes right pulmonary artery
	Sixth left arch becomes left pulmonary artery (ductus arteriosus)

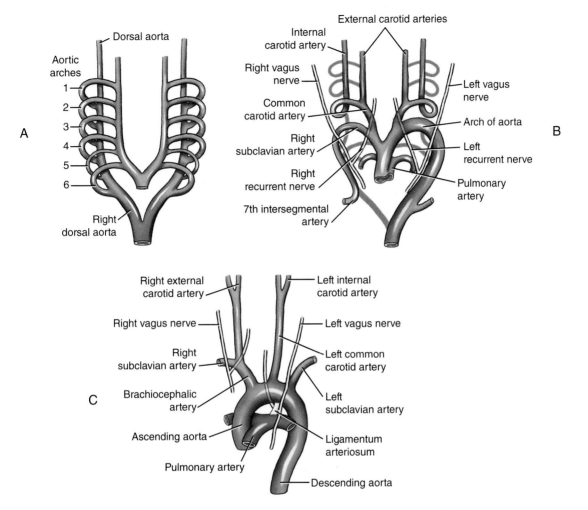

Figure 1–7 A, Diagram of the aortic arches and dorsal aortas before transformation into the definitive vascular pattern. **B,** Diagram of the aortic arches and dorsal aortas after the transformation. The obliterated components are indicated by purple lines. **C,** The great arteries in the adult. After the disappearance of the distal part of the sixth aortic arch and the fifth arch on the right, the right recurrent laryngeal nerve hooks around the right subclavian artery. On the left, the nerve remains in place and hooks around the ligamentum arteriosum.

The common pulmonary vein develops when the embryo is about 5 mm in length (day 29). This common pulmonary vein is eventually absorbed into the left atrium. Next, the right and left pulmonary veins are absorbed, resulting in four separate pulmonary veins entering the left atrium, two superior and two inferior.

Systemic Veins

When the embryo reaches 3 mm in length (day 21 to day 23), it contains three series of veins: the umbilical veins draining the chorion, the vitelline veins draining the yolk sac, and the cardinal veins, which are responsible for draining the embryo itself.[18,19]

As the liver develops (usually when the embryo is 4 to 9 mm in length), the vitelline veins are converted to the portal and hepatic veins.

The umbilical veins are rerouted through the hepatic sinusoids. At this time, the right and proximal parts of the left umbilical veins disappear. This results in a passage through the hepatic sinusoids, which forms the ductus venosus.

By the time the embryo reaches 9 mm in length (day 31 to day 35), the circulation proceeds from the placenta, through the umbilical vein, through the ductus venosus, and into the sinus venosus.

When the embryo is between 4 and 22 mm, the differentiation of the cardinal system and the development of the superior and inferior vena cavae occur. The precardinal, postcardinal, and subcardinal veins develop when the embryo is 4 mm long (day 26 to day 30).

By the time the embryo is 11 mm in length (day 36 to day 42), the hepatic portion of the inferior vena cava (IVC) develops from the vitelline veins. The supracardinal veins then develop, whereas the postcardinal veins begin to atrophy. When the embryo is 22 mm long (day 50 to day 56), the IVC has fully developed from the vitelline, subcardinal, and supracardinal veins.

At an embryo length of approximately 20 mm (day 43 to day 49), the superior vena cava has developed from the precardinal veins, whereas the azygos and hemiazygos veins form from the supracardinal veins.[19]

Conduction System

Two theories exist concerning the development of the sinoatrial node. The first is that it is derived from the sinus venosus musculature when the embryo reaches 7 to 10 mm in length (day 31 to day 35). The second theory is that the sinoatrial node appears as a new formation on the ventrolateral surface of the superior vena cava.[20,21]

The atrioventricular node appears when the embryo is approximately 8 to 9 mm in length. Controversy also exists as to its origin. The accepted theory is that the proximal part of the atrioventricular node develops from the sinus venosus and the distal portion arises from the atrial canal.[22]

There is a difference of opinion as to whether both the atrioventricular node and the atrioventricular bundle originate in situ or whether the atrioventricular bundle originates from proliferation of atrioventricular node tissue.[19]

There is also debate as to whether the bundle branches originate in situ from the ventricular trabeculae,[23,24] originate from the proliferation of tissue from the atrioventricular bundle,[24] or originate in situ from the junction of the anterior and posterior parts of the ventricular septum.[22]

The atrioventricular bundle and the left bundle branch appear when the embryo is 10 to 11 mm long, whereas the right bundle branch develops when the embryo is about 13 mm in length.

Fetal Circulation

Several important physiological and structural differences exist between the fetal and adult cardiovascular systems (Fig. 1–8).

Unlike in the adult, fetal gas exchange (oxygen and carbon dioxide) takes place in the placenta. For oxygenated blood to reach the systemic circulation and deoxygenated blood to return to the placenta for oxygenation, the fetus has several sites of intercommunication: the ductus venosus, the foramen ovale, and the ductus arteriosus. Additionally, in the fetal heart both the right and the left ventricles eject in parallel, rather than in series, into the systemic circulation.[25-27]

In utero, oxygenated blood travels from the placenta to the fetus through the umbilical vein at an average rate of about 175 ml/kg fetal weight per minute. The oxygen saturation of this blood is about 85%. On entering the fetus, the majority of this blood flows through the ductus venosus, bypassing the liver and entering the IVC. The remainder of this oxygenated blood enters the liver sinusoids and mixes with the portal circulation.

The ductus venosus contains a sphincter mechanism located at the level of the umbilical vein, which regulates the flow of umbilical blood through the liver sinusoids. It is presumed that this sphincter closes as a result of a uterine contraction when the venous return is too high, thus preventing sudden overloading of the heart.[28]

The blood that has entered the IVC mixes with the deoxygenated blood returning from the fetal lower limbs. It then enters the right atrium of the fetal heart. The majority of the blood that enters the IVC through the ductus venosus is shunted directly into the left atrium by way of the foramen ovale. This is thought to occur because the narrow caliber of the ductus venosus causes this blood volume to travel at a faster velocity then that entering from the hepatic veins. A small amount

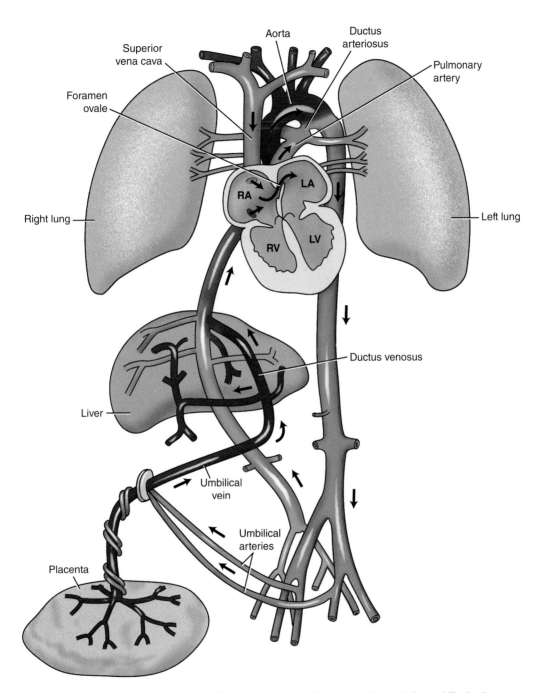

Figure 1–8 Fetal circulatory system. Blood courses from the placenta through the umbilical vein and into the ductus venosus. From here it enters the right atrium *(RA)* by way of the inferior vena cava. Blood from the superior vena cava also enters the right atrium. Most of this blood traverses the foramen ovale, entering the left atrium *(LA)* and then the left ventricle *(LV)*. It then enters the aorta and eventually returns to the placenta by way of the umbilical arteries. The blood in the right atrium that does not cross the foramen ovale enters the right ventricle *(RV)* and then moves through the pulmonary artery and into the descending aorta through the ductus arteriosus, virtually bypassing the lungs.

of blood is prevented from entering the left atrium by the lower edge of the septum secundum, the crista dividens, which overrides the orifice of the inferior vena cava. This blood mixes with the desaturated blood returning from the fetal head and arms by way of the superior vena cava and with the slower moving blood in the IVC coming from the hepatic veins. It then enters into the right ventricle and on into the pulmonary artery.

Because the resistance in the pulmonary vessels is high in utero, the main portion of the blood that enters the pulmonary artery passes directly through the ductus arteriosus to the descending aorta. The blood that has been shunted from the right atrium into the left atrium mixes with a small amount of desaturated blood, which is returned from the lungs by the pulmonary veins.

This left atrial blood enters the left ventricle and thus the ascending aorta. Most of this blood supplies the head and upper extremities of the fetus through the vessels arising from the aortic arch (bracheocephalic artery, left common carotid artery, left subclavian artery). The remainder continues down the descending aorta, mixing with the blood that has been shunted through the ductus arteriosus. From this point, it flows out of the fetus by way of the two umbilical arteries and returns to the placenta. This returning blood has an oxygen saturation of approximately 58%.[29]

At birth, many changes occur in the cardiovascular system. These changes occur as a result of the cessation of placental blood flow and the beginning of pulmonary respiration.

The ductus arteriosus closes almost immediately after birth. This is caused by bradykinin, a vasoactive peptide that is released from the lungs after initial inflation, and results in the contraction of the muscular wall of the ductus arteriosus.[30,31] Once obliterated, the ductus arteriosus forms the ligamentum arteriosum.

Closure of the ductus arteriosus results in increased pressure within the left atrium. This increase in pressure, combined with a decrease in pressure within the right atrium resulting from interruption of placental blood flow, causes the septum primum and septum secundum to appose each other. This results in a functional closing of the foramen ovale. Complete fusion of the foramen ovale is usually complete by 1 year of age.[32]

The umbilical arteries close immediately after birth. Closure occurs because of contraction of the smooth musculature within their walls and is thought to be caused by thermal and mechanical stimuli and a change in oxygen tension.[30] Total obliteration of the umbilical arteries is accomplished by 2 to 3 months of age and results in the distal portions of the arteries forming the medial umbilical ligaments. The proximal portions of the umbilical arteries remain open and become the superior vesicle arteries.

Closure of the umbilical vein and the ductus venosus occurs shortly after closure of the umbilical arteries. The umbilical vein forms the ligamentum teres in the lower segment of the falciform ligament within the liver. The ductus venosus, which courses from the ligamentum teres to the inferior vena cava, is also obliterated and forms the ligamentum venosum.

Cardiac Output

Because the right and left sides of the fetal heart function as parallel circulations, it is not possible to completely separate their cardiac output.

The right ventricle ejects about two thirds of the total ventricular output—approximately 300 ml/kg fetal weight per minute. The left ventricle ejects about 150 ml/kg fetal weight per minute.[33] As would be expected, cardiac output increases with gestational age.[34]

Only about 8% of the total ventricular output flows through the pulmonary arteries. The remainder of the output from the right ventricle (about 57% of the combined ventricular output) enters the descending aorta from the ductus arteriosus. Because the right ventricular output is composed of all blood entering from the superior vena cava and all coronary sinus return, this allows preferential distribution of this unoxygenated blood to the placenta.

Approximately 21% of the cardiac output from the left ventricle perfuses the brain, head, upper limbs, and upper thorax by way of the aortic arch. The remaining 10% that is ejected from the left ventricle traverses the aortic isthmus and joins with the blood flowing across the ductus arteriosus and entering the descending aorta.

Congenital Heart Disease

Pathogenesis

Heart development occurs as a result of an interaction of genes, environment, and chance. An abnormal interaction of any of these processes may lead to a congenital heart defect. Congenital heart disease is usually defined as a gross structural abnormality of the heart or intrathoracic great vessels that is actually or potentially of functional significance.[2] To understand the etiology of congenital heart defects, classification on the basis of groups with similar pathogenetic mechanisms is often used.[35]

Tissue Migration Abnormalities. The tissue that forms the outflow tracts of the heart originates in the neural crest and branchial arch mesenchyme. These cells migrate along an undefined pathway to specific locations in the conotruncus and conotruncal septum.

Interference with this migration results in a spectrum of conotruncal malformations, including the following[35-37]:

- Conotruncal septation defects
- Ventricular septal defects
- Double-outlet right ventricle
- Tetralogy of Fallot
- Pulmonary atresia with ventricular septal defect
- Aorticopulmonary window
- Truncus arteriosus
- Complete transposition (d-transposition) of the great arteries

Abnormal Intracardiac Blood Flow. Another group of congenital cardiac abnormalities are thought to result from abnormal blood flow patterns.[38,39] From the early stages of cardiogenesis, the force of cardiac contraction and the volume of blood pumping through and by the heart chambers are essential elements in the growth and development of all heart structures. A reduction in the volume distribution of intracardiac blood flow is thought to be a mechanism in the pathogenesis of both right- and left-sided heart defects.

Manipulation studies of the intracardiac blood flow in chicks has been shown to affect heart morphogenesis.[35] For example, a decrease in left atrial blood flow may result in a variety of left-sided heart defects, such as hypoplastic left heart syndrome, mitral atresia, and aortic atresia. This is because tissues and structures will not grow without a sufficient blood supply.

Atkins et al[40] described a foramen ovale area–to–atrial septum area ratio as an index of transatrial blood flow. They reported an inverse correlation between the ratio and the size of the left side of the heart. In the normal heart, the ratio

is about 0.20. In left-sided heart defects such as coarctation of the aorta and aortic valve stenosis, the ratio was found to be 0.14 and 0.11, respectively. In fetal hearts with an obligatory right-to-left shunt, as in pulmonary atresia with intact ventricular septum, the ratio increased to 0.40. In perimembranous ventricular septal defects, the foramen ovale to atrial septum ratio was reported to be greater than normal, suggesting that the ventricular septal defect may remain patent because of an in utero left-to-right shunt.[41]

Defects thought to be caused by abnormal intracardiac blood flow include the following:

- Perimembranous ventricular septal defect
- Left-sided heart defects
  - Hypoplastic left heart
  - Aortic atresia
  - Mitral atresia
  - Bicuspid aortic valve
  - Aortic valve stenosis
  - Coarctation of the aorta
  - Interrupted aortic arch
- Right-sided heart defects
  - Bicuspid pulmonary valve
  - Secundum atrial septal defect
  - Pulmonary valve stenosis
  - Pulmonary valve atresia with intact ventricular septum
  - Hypoplastic right heart

Left- and right-sided heart defects tend to cluster in families, suggesting a single gene abnormality with variable phenotypic expression as opposed to a multifactorial pattern of inheritance.[35,38,42]

Cell Death Abnormalities. Selective reabsorption of regions of the ventricular myocardium is thought to be one of the mechanisms involved in the formation of the atrioventricular valves.[43] Cell death impedes this process and results in malformations such as the following:

- Muscular ventricular septal defect
- Ebstein anomaly

Extracellular Matrix Abnormalities. Extracellular matrix abnormalities affect the endocardial cushions of the heart. Embryologically, the endocardial cushions fuse to form the mitral and tricuspid orifices at the atrioventricular level and the aortic and pulmonary orifices in the outflow tracts. These fusions occur as endocardial cells are transformed into mesenchymal cells that migrate into the cushion tissue and cause them to adhere to each other. If this transformation does not occur or the process is delayed, endocardial cushion defects occur, including the following[35]:

- Ostium primum atrial septal defect
- Inflow ventricular septal defect
- Atrioventricular septal defect

Abnormal Targeted Growth. Abnormalities of targeted growth all involve impedance of the mechanism by which the pulmonary veins connect to the left atrium. As described previously, this connection results from the common pulmonary vein being absorbed into the left atrium, resulting in four remaining veins.[35,44] Failure of this process to occur or be completed results in abnormalities such as the following:

- Partial anomalous pulmonary venous return
- Total anomalous pulmonary venous return
- Cor triatriatum

These types of congenital abnormalities are often associated with abnormalities of visceral situs.

By definition, total anomalous pulmonary venous return will always be present in a fetus with right atrial isomerism (asplenia syndrome) because both chambers are morphologically right. In the setting of left atrial isomerism (polysplenia syndrome), total anomalous pulmonary venous return will be identified in 6% to 8% of cases.[45,46]

Looping and Situs Defects. The final classification of congenital cardiac defects consists of those resulting from abnormal looping of the heart tube.[47] If the heart tube, which normally bends to the right, instead bends to the left, ventricular inversion and corrected transposition (l-transposition) of the great arteries occurs.

Situs abnormalities have been associated with the absence of a control gene mapped to chromosome 12.[48] In the absence of this control gene, there is a random chance of situs solitus, situs inversus, bilateral left-sidedness, or bilateral right-sidedness occurring.

In summary, understanding normal fetal cardiovascular physiology and cardiogenesis and the different types of abnormalities that can occur in the fetal heart may contribute to a better understanding and more accurate diagnosis of cardiac anomalies encountered in utero.

References

1. Benacerraf BR, Sanders SP: Fetal echocardiography. Radiol Clin North Am 1990; 8:131–147.
2. Mitchell SC, Korones SB, Berendes HW: Congenital heart disease in 56,109 births: Incidence and natural history. Circulation 1971; 43:323–332.
3. DeVore GR: The prenatal diagnosis of congenital heart disease—a practical approach for the fetal sonographer. J Clin Ultrasound 1985; 13:229–245.
4. Taussig HB: World survey of common cardiac malformations: Developmental error or genetic variant? In: Engle MA, Perloff J (eds): Congenital Heart Disease After Surgery. New York, Yorke Medical, 1983, pp 1–42.
5. McCurdy CM, Reed KL: Basic technique of fetal echocardiography. Semin Ultrasound CT MRI 1993; 14:267–276.
6. Hoffman JIE, Christianson R: Congenital heart disease in a cohort of 19,502 births with long-term follow-up. Am J Cardiol 1978; 42:641–647.
7. Fyfe DA, Kline CH: Fetal echocardiographic diagnosis of congenital heart disease. Pediatr Clin North Am 1990; 37:45–67.
8. Oberhaensli I, Extermann P, Friedli B, et al. Ultrasound screening for congenital cardiac malformations in the fetus. Pediatr Radiol 1989; 19:94–99.
9. Copel JA, Kleinman CS: The impact of fetal echocardiography on perinatal outcome. Ultrasound Med Biol 1986; 12:327–335.
10. Veille JC, Mahowald MB, Sivakoff M: Ethical dilemmas in fetal echocardiography. Obstet Gynecol 1989; 73:710–714.
11. Ianniruberto A: Management of fetal cardiac structural abnormalities. Fetal Ther 1986; 1:89–91.
12. Ferencz C, Rubin JD, McCarter RJ, et al: Congenital heart disease: Prevalence at livebirth. Am J Epidemiol 1985; 121:31–36.
13. Chinn A, Fitzsimmons J, Shepart TH, et al: Congenital heart disease among spontaneous abortuses and stillborn fetuses: Prevalence and associations. Teratology 1989; 40:475–482.
14. Jones KL: Smith's Recognizable Patterns of Human Malformation, 5th ed. Philadelphia, WB Saunders, 1997, pp 1–746.
15. Nora JJ, Fraser FC: Cardiovascular disease. In: Nora JJ, Fraser FC (eds): Medical Genetics: Principles and Practice, 3rd ed. Philadelphia, Lea & Febiger, 1989, pp 321–337.
16. Stamm ER, Drose AI, Thickman D: The fetal heart. In: Nyberg DA, Mahony BS, Pretorius DH (eds):

Diagnostic Ultrasound of Fetal Anomalies: Text and Atlas, vol 2. Chicago, Year Book Medical, 1991, pp 800–827.

17. Romero R, Pilu G, Jeanty P, et al: The heart. In: Romero R, Pilu G, Jeanty P, et al. (eds): Prenatal Diagnosis of Congenital Anomalies. Norwalk, CT, Appleton & Lange, 1988, pp 125–194.

18. Sadler TW: Langman's Medical Embryology, 6th ed. Baltimore, Williams & Wilkins, 1990, pp 179–227.

19. Bharati S, Lev M: Embryology of the heart and great vessels. In: Mavroudis C, Backer CL (eds): Pediatric Cardiac Surgery. St Louis, CV Mosby, 1994, pp 1–13.

20. Gow RM, Hamilton RM: Developmental biology of specialized conduction tissue. In: Freedom RM, Benson LN, Smallhorn JF (eds): Neonatal Heart Disease. London, Springer-Verlag, 1992, pp 65–81.

21. Walls EW: The development of the specialized conducting tissue of the human heart. J Anat 1947; 81:93–100.

22. Anderson RH, Taylor IM: Development of atrioventricular specialized tissue in human heart. Br Heart J 1972; 34:1205–1210.

23. Sanabria T: Recherches sur la differenciation du tissu nodal et connecteur du coeur des mammiferes. Arch Biol 1936; 47:1–70.

24. Fields EF: The development of the conducting system in the heart of sheep. Br Heart J 1951; 13:129–147.

25. De Smedt MCH, Visser GHA, Meijboom EJ: Fetal cardiac output estimated by Doppler echocardiography during mid- and late gestation. Am J Cardiol 1987; 60:338–342.

26. Van Der Mooren K, Barendregt LG, Wladimiroff JW: Flow velocity wave forms in the human fetal ductus arteriosus during the normal second half of pregnancy. Pediatr Res 1991; 30:487–490.

27. Kleinman CS, Donnerstein RL: Ultrasonic assessment of cardiac function in the intact human fetus. J Am Coll Cardiol 1985; 5:84S–94S.

28. Gribbe G, Hirvonen L, Lind J, et al: Cineangiocardiographic recording of the cyclic changes in volume of the left ventricle. Cardiology 1959; 34:348–350.

29. Tobin JR, Wetzel RC: Cardiovascular physiology and shock. In: Mavroudis C, Backer CL: Pediatric Cardiac Surgery. St Louis, CV Mosby, 1994, pp 17–35.

30. Adams FH, Lind J: Physiologic studies on the cardiovascular status of normal newborn infants with special reference to the ductus arteriosus. Pediatrics 1957; 19:431–437.

31. Lind J, Boesen T, Wegelius C: Selective angiocardiography in congenital heart disease. Prog Cardiovasc Dis 1959–1960; 2:293–314.

32. Patten BM: The development of the heart. In: Gould SE (ed): Pathology of the Heart and Blood Vessels, 3rd ed. Springfield, Mass, Thomas, 1968, pp 20–90.

33. Heymann MA, Hanley FL: Physiology of circulation. In: Mavroudis C, Backer CL (eds): Pediatric Cardiac Surgery. St Louis, CV Mosby, 1994, pp 14–23.

34. Veille JC, Sivakoff M, Nemeth M: Evaluation of the human fetal cardiac size and function. Am J Perinatol 1990; 7:54–59.

35. Rose V, Clark E: Etiology of congenital heart disease. In: Freedom RM, Benson LN, Smallhorn JF (eds): Neonatal Heart Disease. London, Springer-Verlag, 1992, pp 3–17.

36. Kirby ML, Gale TF, Stewart DR: Neural crest cells contribute to normal aorticopulmonary septation. Science 1983; 22:659–1061.

37. Kirby ML, Turenage KL, Hays BM: Characterization of conotruncal malformations following ablation of "cardiac" neural crest. Anat Rec 1985; 213:87–93.

38. Brenner JI, Berg KA, Schneider DS, et al: Congenital cardiovascular malformations in first degree relatives of infants with hypoplastic left heart syndrome. Arch Pediatr Adolesc Med 1989; 143:1492–1494.

39. Burn J: The aetiology of congenital heart disease. In: Anderson RH, Macartney FJ, Shinebourne RA, et al (eds): Pediatric Cardiology. Edinburgh, Churchill Livingstone, 1987, pp 15–63.

40. Atkins DL, Chark EB, Marvin WJ: Foramen ovale/atrial septum ratio: a marker of transatrial blood flow. Circulation 1982; 66:281–283.

41. Hawkins JA, Clark EB, Marvin WJ, et al: Foramen ovale atrial septal ratio: Evidence for different pathogenic mechanisms in congenital heart defects [abstract]. Pediatr Res 1987; 19:326A.

42. Boughman JA, Berg KA, Astemborski JA, et al: Familial risks of congenital heart defect assessed in a population based epidemiological study. Am J Med Genet 1987; 26:839–849.

43. Pexieder T: Cell death in the morphogenesis and teratogenesis of the heart. Adv Anat Embryol Cell Biol 1975; 51:1–100.

44. Neill CA: Development of the pulmonary veins. Pediatrics 1956; 18:880–887.

45. Yildirim SV, Tokel K, Varan B, et al: Clinical investigations over 13 years to establish the nature of the cardiac defects in patients having abnormalities of lateralization. Cardiol Young 2007; 17:275–282.

46. Valsangiacomo ER, Hornberger LK, Barrea C, et al: Partial and total anomalous pulmonary venous connection in the fetus: Two-dimensional and Doppler echocardiographic findings. Ultrasound Obstet Gynecol 2003; 22:257–263.

47. Nakamura A, Kullkowski R, Lacktis J, et al: Heart looping: A regulated response to deforming forces. In: VanPraagh R, Takao A (eds): Etiology and Morphogenesis of Congenital Heart Disease. Mt Kisko, Futura, 1980, pp 81–98.

48. Layton WM Jr: The biology of asymmetry and the development of the cardiac loop. In: Ferrans VJ, Rosenquist GC, Weinstein C (eds): Cardiac Morphogenesis. New York, Elsevier, 1985, pp 134–140.

CHAPTER 2

Scanning: Indications and Technique

Julia A. Drose

Prenatal diagnosis of congenital heart disease is important in optimizing obstetrical and neonatal care. Congenital heart disease has been reported to occur in approximately 8 per 1000 live births.[1-8] These incidence rates, which are based on live-born infants, underestimate, perhaps considerably, the true incidence of congenital heart disease in the fetus.[1,2,4,9] Early fetal loss and stillbirths are often the result of complex heart defects or of

TABLE 2–1 Frequency of Congenital Heart Lesions Among Affected Abortuses and Stillborn Infants	
Defect	**Frequency (%)**
Ventricular septal defect	35.7
Coarctation of the aorta	8.9
Atrial septal defect	8.2
Atrioventricular septal defect	6.7
Tetralogy of Fallot	6.2
Single ventricle	4.8
Truncus arteriosus	4.8
Hypoplastic left heart syndrome	4.6
Complete transposition of the great arteries	4.3
Double-outlet right ventricle	2.4
Hypoplasia of the right ventricle	1.7
Single atrium	1.2
Pulmonic stenosis	0.7
Aortic stenosis	0.5
Miscellaneous	10.6

Modified from Hoffman JIE: Incidence of congenital heart disease. II: Prenatal incidence. Pediatr Cardiol 1995; 16:155–165.

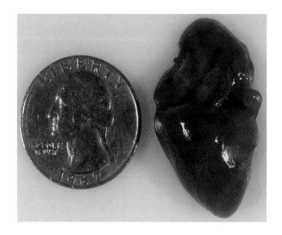

Figure 2–1 The small size of the heart in a 20-week fetus is shown in relationship to a quarter.

chromosomal defects that have an associated heart defect. For this reason, the total congenital heart disease incidence in the fetus has been reported to be as much as five times that found in live-born children.[1,9–14] The pooled reported frequency of congenital heart lesions among affected abortuses and stillborn infants shows that ventricular septal defects occur most often (Table 2–1). Coarctation of the aorta and atrial septal defects were also frequently mentioned.[15]

In utero identification of congenital heart disease allows a variety of treatment options to be considered, including delivery at an appropriate facility, termination, and in some cases in utero therapy.[5,16–18] Conversely, a normal fetal echocardiogram in the setting of an increased risk factor provides reassurance for both patient and physician.

Timing

The American Institute of Ultrasound in Medicine Technical Bulletin for Performance of the Fetal Cardiac Ultrasound Examination recommends that fetal echocardiographic examinations be performed between 18 and 22 weeks' gestation.[19] It is at this time that optimal image quality, and therefore diagnostic accuracy, is achieved. It should be

borne in mind that, even at 18 weeks' gestation, the fetal heart is a very small structure, and a thorough evaluation may be challenging (Fig. 2–1).

Fetal echocardiography performed earlier in pregnancy is feasible in some cases and may be reasonable in a population at risk for a heart defect.[7] However, alterations in chamber size, myocardial thickening, and size of the great arteries may occur later in pregnancy.[20–22] Therefore a normal appearance of the fetal heart at any time in pregnancy does not exclude congenital heart disease.[23]

Later in gestation, the echocardiographic examination may be compromised by increased attenuation from the fetal skull, ribs, spine, and limbs and a decrease in amniotic fluid as pregnancy progresses.[20,21]

Optimally, fetal echocardiography should be performed sufficiently late in gestation so as not to miss late developing lesions and early enough to provide a full cohort of options. This may vary depending on the indication or type of lesion being evaluated.

Equipment

Fetal echocardiography requires the use of high-resolution ultrasound equipment.[24] Acceptable transducer frequencies range from 5 to 7 MHz, depending on gestational age, maternal body habitus, and the amount of amniotic fluid present. Adequate transducer penetration is also necessary. All equipment used for fetal echocardiography should have M-mode and pulsed Doppler imaging capabilities to provide physiological assessment and color Doppler imaging capabilities to assess spatial and directional information. All these modalities are vital for performing a complete and accurate examination. Additionally, ultrasound equipment with compound imaging capabilities, which allows for off-axis beam steering, can be an asset.

Compound imaging allows additional lines of information to be added to an image without affecting frame rate. This helps suppress many of the artifacts inherent in conventional imaging.

Indications

The most common indication for performing a fetal echocardiogram is a *family history of congenital heart disease* (Box 2–1). The risk of occurrence for a fetus varies depending on the type of lesion and the relationship of the fetus to the affected relative. The risk of congenital heart disease in a fetus with an affected sibling is approximately 2% to 4%.[25-29] If two or more siblings are affected, this risk increases to about 10% (Table 2–2). When the mother of the fetus is the affected relative, the risk of a heart defect is also approximately 10% to 12%.[28,30,31] If the affected relative is the father, the risk is lower (Table 2–3).[25-27] If congenital heart disease does recur in families, it is not limited to the same type of defect.

Exposure to known cardiac teratogens also increases fetal risk for a heart defect.[5,32] The list of substances considered teratogenic is extensive (Table 2–4).

The specific risk of occurrence varies with the length and types of exposure and with the specific substance involved. Referrals for fetal echocardiography due to teratogen exposure have decreased over the past decade.[8] This most likely

TABLE 2–2 Risk of Occurrence for Any Congenital Heart Defect in Siblings

	Suggested Risk	
Defect	If One Sibling Affected	If Two Siblings Affected
Aortic stenosis	2	6
Atrial septal defect	2.5	8
Atrioventricular septal defect	3	10
Coarctation of the aorta	2	6
Ebstein anomaly	1	3
Endocardial fibroelastosis	4	12
Hypoplastic left heart syndrome	2	6
Pulmonary atresia	1	3
Pulmonary stenosis	2	6
Tetralogy of Fallot	2.5	8
Transposition of the great arteries	1.5	5
Tricuspid atresia	1	3
Truncus arteriosus	1	3
Ventricular septal defect	3	10

Modified from Nora JJ, Fraser FC, Bear J, et al: Medical Genetics: Principles and Practice, 4th ed. Philadelphia, Lea & Febiger, 1994, p 371.

TABLE 2–3 Suggested Offspring Occurrence Risk for Congenital Heart Defects Given One Affected Parent (%)

	Suggested Risk (%)	
Defect	Father Affected	Mother Affected
Aortic stenosis	3	13–18
Atrial septal defect	1.5	4–4.5
Atrioventricular septal defect	1	14
Coarctation of the aorta	2	4
Pulmonary stenosis	2	4–6.5
Tetralogy of Fallot	1.5	2.5
Ventricular septal defect	2	6–10

Modified from Nora JJ, Fraser FC, Bear J, et al: Medical Genetics: Principles and Practice, 4th ed. Philadelphia, Lea & Febiger, 1994, p 371.

BOX 2–1

Indications for Fetal Echocardiography in Order of Frequency of Referral

Family history of congenital heart disease
Maternal diabetes mellitus
Suspicion of congenital heart disease on obstetrical ultrasonography
Arrhythmia
Extracardiac congenital anomalies
Systemic lupus erythematosus
Chromosome anomaly
Teratogen exposure
Other

Modified from: Friedberg MK, Silverman NH: Changing indications for fetal echocardiography in a university center population. Prenat Diagn 2004; 24:781–786.

TABLE 2–4   Substances Associated with Congenital Heart Disease

Substance	Associated Congenital Heart Disease
Alcohol	Atrial septal defect, ventricular septal defect, interrupted aortic arch, coarctation, tetralogy of Fallot, pulmonary stenosis, double-outlet right ventricle, dextrocardia
Amantadine	Single ventricle, pulmonary atresia
Amphetamine	Ventricular septal defect, atrial septal defect, transposition of the great arteries
Azathioprine	Pulmonary stenosis
Barbiturates	Interrupted aortic arch, coarctation
Cannabis	Ventricular septal defect
Carbamazepine	Atrial septal defect
Chlordiazepoxide	Congenital heart disease (unspecified)
Codeine	Congenital heart disease (unspecified)
Cortisone	Ventricular septal defect, coarctation
Cyclophosphamide	Tetralogy of Fallot
Cytarabine	Tetralogy of Fallot
Daunorubicin	Tetralogy of Fallot
Dextroamphetamine	Atrial septal defect
Diazepam	Congenital heart disease (unspecified)
Dilantin (hydantoin)	Atrial septal defect, ventricular septal defect, interrupted aortic arch, coarctation, pulmonary stenosis, aortic stenosis
Indomethacin	Ductal constriction
Lithium	Ebstein anomaly, tricuspid atresia, atrial septal defect, mitral atresia, dextrocardia
Methotrexate	Dextrocardia
Oral contraceptives	Congenital heart disease (unspecified)
Paramethadione	Tetralogy of Fallot
Penicillamine	Ventricular septal defect
Primidone	Ventricular septal defect, interrupted aortic arch, coarctation
Progesterone	Ventricular septal defect, tetralogy of Fallot, truncus arteriosus
Quinine	Congenital heart disease (unspecified)
Retinoic acid (Accutane)	Ventricular septal defect, interrupted aortic arch, coarctation, tetralogy of Fallot, truncus arteriosus, double-outlet right ventricle, pulmonary atresia
Thalidomide	Ventricular septal defect, transposition of the great arteries, truncus arteriosus, tetralogy of Fallot, double-outlet right ventricle, pulmonary atresia, atrial septal defect
Trifluoperazine	Transposition of the great arteries
Trimethadione	Ventricular septal defect, transposition of the great arteries, tetralogy of Fallot, hypoplastic left heart syndrome, double-outlet right ventricle, pulmonary atresia, truncus arteriosus, atrial septal defect, aortic stenosis, pulmonary stenosis
Valproic acid	Ventricular septal defect, coarctation, interrupted aortic arch, tetralogy of Fallot, hypoplastic left heart syndrome, aortic stenosis, atrial septal defect, pulmonary stenosis
Warfarin (Coumadin)	Congenital heart disease (unspecified)

Data from Sandor GGS, Smith DF, MacLeod PM: Cardiac malformations in the fetal alcohol syndrome. J Pediat 1981; 98:771–773; Nora JJ, Nora AH: Maternal transmission of congenital heart diseases: New recurrence risk figures and question of cytoplasmic inheritance and vulnerability to teratogens. Am J Cardiol 1987; 60:460–463; Stamm ER, Drose JA, Thickman D: The fetal heart. In: Rumack CM, Wilson SR, Charboneau JW (eds): Diagnostic Ultrasound, vol II. St. Louis, Mosby–Year Book, 1991, p 801; Jones KL: Smith's Recognizable Patterns of Human Malformation, 3rd ed. Philadelphia, WB Saunders, 1988; Nora J, Fraser FC, Bear J, et al: Medical Genetics: Principles and Practice. Philadelphia, Lea & Febiger, 1994; Romero R, Pilu G, Jeanty P, et al: The heart. In: Romero R, Pilu G, Jeanty P, et al. (eds): Prenatal Diagnosis of Congenital Anomalies. Norwalk, CT, Appleton & Lange, 1988; Taybi H: Radiology of Syndromes and Metabolic Disorders. Chicago, Year Book Medical, 1983; Briggs GG, Freman RK, Yaffe SJ: Drugs in Pregnancy and Lactation. Baltimore, Williams & Wilkins, 1990, pp 1–686; Okuda H, Nagao T: Cardiovascular malformations induced by prenatal exposure to phenobarbital in rats. Congenital Anomalies 2006; 46:97–104; Samren EB, van Duijn CM, Lieve-Christiaens GCM, et al: Antiepileptic drug regimens and major congenital abnormalities in the offspring. Ann Neurol 1999; 46:739–746; Miller LC, Chan W, Litvinova A, et al: Fetal alcohol spectrum disorders in children residing in Russian orphanages: A phenotypic survey. Alcohol Clin Exp Res 2006; 30:531–538; Williams LJ, Correa A, Rasmussen S. Maternal lifestyle factors and risk for ventricular septal defects. Birth Defects Res 2004; 70:59–64.

represents an increase in awareness of minimizing teratogen exposure in women of reproductive age.

Chromosomal abnormalities have been reported to occur in 13% of live-born infants with congenital heart defects.[33–36] The incidence of an abnormal karyotype in the fetus with a congenital heart abnormality is approximately 35%.[2,37] A study by Nicolaides et al[38] in 1993 found chromosomal abnormalities in 101 of 156 (65%) fetuses they identified as having a heart defect.

Again, the specific type and occurrence risk of a congenital heart defect varies depending on the chromosomal abnormality. Some abnormal karyotypes have a relatively low association with heart defects, whereas others, such as trisomy 21, are associated with a 40% to 50% occurrence.[36–39] The most striking relationship is apparent with trisomy 13 and trisomy 18, in which the association with congenital heart abnormalities is almost 100%.[38] Recent literature has reported live-born infants with trisomy 13 and trisomy 18 to have congenital heart disease in 38% and 45%, respectively.[40] The discrepancy in these data is probably due to the more recent data consisting only of live births, excluding spontaneous miscarriages or terminated pregnancies. As with teratogenic agents, the list of abnormal karyotypes and syndromes associated with heart defects is extensive (Table 2–5).

Several *maternal conditions* also carry an inherent risk to the fetus. Fetuses of diabetic mothers have a reported fivefold to eighteenfold increased risk of congenital heart disease compared with control subjects.[41,42] Diabetes, as an indication for fetal echocardiography, has undergone a marked increase over the last decade.

Text continued on p. 26

TABLE 2–5 Chromosome Abnormalities and Syndromes Associated with Congenital Heart Disease

Syndrome	Associated Congenital Heart Disease	Risk (%)
Aase-Smith syndrome	Ventricular septal defect	
Achondroplasia	Interrupted aortic arch, coarctation	
Acrocephalosyndactyly, type I	Interrupted aortic arch, coarctation	
Acrocephalopolysyndactyly, type IV	Congenital heart disease (unspecified)	
Acromicric dysplasia	Atrial septal defect	
Acyl-CoA	Cardiomegaly	
Adams Oliver syndrome	Congenital heart disease (unspecified)	
Alacrima-aptyalism syndrome	Dextrocardia	
Alagille syndrome	Atrial septal defect, ventricular septal defect, pulmonary stenosis	
Antley-Bixler syndrome	Atrial septal defect	33
Apert syndrome	Ventricular septal defect, coarctation, tetralogy of Fallot	10
Arachnodactyly	Congenital heart disease (unspecified)	
Arthrochalasis multiplex congenita	Atrial septal defect, interrupted aortic arch, coarctation, ventricular septal defect, tetralogy of Fallot, bicuspid aorta, bicuspid tricuspid valve, dextrocardia, coarctation	
Arthrogryposis multiplex congenita	Ventricular septal defect, coarctation, aortic stenosis	
Asymmetric crying face	Tetralogy of Fallot, ventricular septal defect	
Bardet-Biedl syndrome (Laurence-Moon)	Ventricular septal defect, total anomalous pulmonary venous connection	
Beckwith-Wiedeman syndrome	Atrial septal defect, ventricular septal defect, cardiomegaly	
Beemer lethal malformation syndrome	Tetralogy of Fallot, double-outlet right ventricle	
Bernheim syndrome	Cardiomegaly, hypoplastic left heart syndrome, aortic stenosis, interrupted aortic arch, coarctation	
Berry-Treacher Collins syndrome	Congenital heart disease (unspecified)	
Bixler syndrome	Congenital heart disease (unspecified)	
Bourneville-Pringle syndrome	Rhabdomyoma, interrupted aortic arch, coarctation	
Bowen-Conradi-Hutterite syndrome	Congenital heart disease (unspecified)	
C syndrome	Atrioventricular septal defect	
Campomelic dysplasia	Congenital heart disease (unspecified)	

Continued

TABLE 2–5   Chromosome Abnormalities and Syndromes Associated with Congenital Heart Disease—cont'd

Syndrome	Associated Congenital Heart Disease	Risk (%)
Cardiac-limb syndrome	Atrial septal defect, ventricular septal defect	85
Cardiofacial syndrome–asymmetric facies	Atrial septal defect, atrioventricular septal defect, interrupted aortic arch, coarctation, ventricular septal defect, pulmonary stenosis, tetralogy of Fallot	
Cardiomelic syndrome	Atrial septal defect, ventricular septal defect	85
Carpenter syndrome	Ventricular septal defect, pulmonary stenosis, transposition of the great arteries	3
Cat-eye syndrome (partial trisomy 22)	Total anomalous pulmonary venous connection, ventricular septal defect, atrial septal defect, tetralogy of Fallot, pulmonary stenosis	40
Cayler syndrome	Atrial septal defect, atrioventricular septal defect, interrupted aortic arch, coarctation, ventricular septal defect, tetralogy of Fallot, right aortic arch, pulmonary stenosis, atrial stenosis	
CHARGE (coloboma of the eye, heart anomaly, choanal atresia, retardation, and genital and ear anomalies) syndrome	Atrioventricular septal defect, coarctation, ventricular septal defect, atrial septal defect, truncus arteriosus, double-outlet right ventricle, tetralogy of Fallot, right aortic arch	50
CHILD (congenital hemidysplasia with ichthyosiform erythroderma and limb defects) syndrome	Ventricular septal defect, atrial septal defect	
CHIME (colobomas, heart defects, ichthyosiform dermatosis, mental retardation, and ear defects or epilepsy) syndrome	Tetralogy of Fallot, transposition of the great arteries	
Chondroectodermal dysplasia	Atrial septal defect, single atrium	50
Coffin-Siris (Coffin-Laury) syndrome	Congenital heart disease (unspecified)	
Cohen syndrome	Congenital heart disease (unspecified)	29
Congenital abducens–facial paralysis	Dextrocardia	
Congenital facial diplegia	Dextrocardia	
Congenital oculofacial paralysis	Dextrocardia	
Conradi-Hunermann syndrome (chondrodysplasia punctata)	Ventricular septal defect	
Crouzon syndrome	Coarctation	
Cryptophthalmos syndrome	Atrial septal defect, truncus arteriosus, ventricular septal defect, transposition of the great arteries, right aortic arch	
Cryptophthalmos–syndactyly syndrome	Atrial septal defect, truncus arteriosus, transposition of the great arteries, ventricular septal defect, right aortic arch	
DeLange syndrome	Ventricular septal defect, tetralogy of Fallot, double-outlet right ventricle, interrupted aortic arch, coarctation	29
Dermal faciocardial skeletal syndrome	Atrial septal defect, pulmonary stenosis	
Diastrophic dysplasia	Congenital heart disease (unspecified)	
DiGeorge syndrome (22q)	Ventricular septal defect, coarctation, truncus arteriosus, transposition of the great arteries, tetralogy of Fallot, interrupted aortic arch, double-outlet right ventricle	95
Distichiasis–lymphedema	Truncus arteriosus	95
Duane syndrome	Atrial septal defect	
Dysencephalia syndrome	Atrial septal defect	
Dyssegmental dysplasia	Congenital heart disease (unspecified)	
Eagle-Barrett syndrome	Atrial septal defect, ventricular septal defect, pulmonary stenosis	
Ehlers-Danlos syndrome	Interrupted aortic arch, coarctation, atrial septal defect, ventricular septal defect, dextrocardia, tetralogy of Fallot, bicuspid aortic valve, bicuspid tricuspid valve	

TABLE 2–5 Chromosome Abnormalities and Syndromes Associated with Congenital Heart Disease—cont'd		
Syndrome	**Associated Congenital Heart Disease**	**Risk (%)**
Elfin facies syndrome	Atrial septal defect, interrupted aortic arch, coarctation, aortic stenosis, mitral regurgitation, ventricular septal defect, tetralogy of Fallot	100
Ellis–van Creveld syndrome (chondrodysplasia punctata)	Atrial septal defect, single atrium	
Emery-Dreifuss syndrome	Cardiomyopathy	
Facioneuro syndrome	Cardiomegaly	
Factor V deficiency	Atrial septal defect, ventricular septal defect	
Ferrell-Okihiro-Halel syndrome (Ferrell-Okihiro-Halal syndrome)	Atrial septal defect	
Fanconi pancytopenia	Atrial septal defect	14
Femoral-facial syndrome	Truncus arteriosus, pulmonary stenosis	
Franceschetti-Klein syndrome	Ventricular septal defect, atrial septal defect	
Franceschetti-Zwahler-Klein syndrome	Ventricular septal defect, atrial septal defect	
Fraser syndrome	Atrial septal defect, ventricular septal defect, truncus arteriosus, transposition of the great arteries, right aortic arch	
Friedreich ataxia	Pulmonary stenosis, asymmetrical septal hypertrophy	
Gardner-Silengo-Wachtel syndrome	Congenital heart disease (unspecified)	
Geleophysic dwarfism	Atrial septal defect, hypertrophic cardiomyopathy, aortic insufficiency, pulmonary stenosis, mitral stenosis	
Golabi-Ito-Hall (X-linked mental retardation)	Atrial septal defect	
Goldenhar syndrome	Tetralogy of Fallot, atrial septal defect, ventricular septal defect, coarctation, interrupted aortic arch, right aortic arch	
Goodman syndrome	Congenital heart disease (unspecified)	
Halarz syndrome	Atrial septal defect, interrupted aortic arch, coarctation, dextroposition, ventricular septal defect, tetralogy of Fallot, absent right pulmonary artery	
Hand-heart syndrome	Atrial septal defect, ventricular septal defect	85
Heart-hand syndrome, type IV	Ventricular septal defect, pulmonary stenosis, single atrium	
Hirschsprung disease	Interrupted aortic arch, coarctation, ventricular septal defect, mitral stenosis	
Holt-Oram syndrome	Atrial septal defect, ventricular septal defect	85
Hydrolethalus syndrome	Truncus arteriosus, ventricular septal defect, atrioventricular septal defect, hypoplastic left heart syndrome, double aortic arch	
Hypogonadotropic syndrome	Atrial septal defect	
Hypertelorism-hypospadias syndrome	Congenital heart disease (unspecified)	25
Hypertelorism-microtia-facial clefting	Congenital heart disease (unspecified)	
Hypertrichosis osteochondrodysplasia	Aortic stenosis	
Ivemark syndrome	Atrial isomerism, atrioventricular septal defect, complete heart block	
Johanson-Blizzard syndrome	Truncus arteriosus, atrial septal defect, transposition of the great arteries, single atrium, total anomalous pulmonary venous connection	
Kabuki make-up syndrome	Congenital heart disease (unspecified)	32
Kallman syndrome	Atrial septal defect, Ebstein anomaly, right aortic arch	
Kallman–deMorsier syndrome	Atrial septal defect, Ebstein anomaly, right aortic arch	
Kartagener syndrome	Dextrocardia	
Keutel syndrome	Ventricular septal defect, pulmonary stenosis	
Klippel-Feil syndrome	Ventricular septal defect, transposition of the great arteries, total anomalous pulmonary venous connection	

Continued

TABLE 2–5 **Chromosome Abnormalities and Syndromes Associated with Congenital Heart Disease—cont'd**

Syndrome	Associated Congenital Heart Disease	Risk (%)
Klippel-Trenaunay-Weber syndrome	Cardiomegaly	
Kneist-like dysplasia	Atrial septal defect	
Larsen syndrome	Congenital heart disease (unspecified)	
Laurence-Moon syndrome (Bardet-Biedl)	Ventricular septal defect, total anomalous pulmonary venous connection	
Leopard syndrome	Pulmonary stenosis, complete heart block, cardiomyopathy	
Lethal facial-cardiomelic dysplasia	Dilated right heart, single atrium, interrupted aortic arch, transposition of the great arteries, ventricular septal defect, mitral atresia	
Locking digits–growth defect	Atrial septal defect	
Lutembacher syndrome	Atrial septal defect, mitral stenosis, cardiomegaly	
Majewski syndrome	Atrial septal defect	
Marfan syndrome	Dilated aortic root	95
Marshall-Smith syndrome	Atrial septal defect	
McDonough syndrome	Atrial septal defect, ventricular septal defect, aortic stenosis, pulmonary stenosis	
Meckel syndrome	Atrial septal defect, ventricular septal defect	
Meckel-Gruber syndrome	Ventricular septal defect, atrial septal defect, coarctation, pulmonary stenosis	
Mesomelic dysplasia	Congenital heart disease (unspecified)	
Miller-Dieker syndrome	Congenital heart disease (unspecified)	
Mobius syndrome	Dextrocardia	
Mutchinick syndrome	Atrial septal defect, pulmonary stenosis	
Myhre syndrome	Congenital heart disease (unspecified)	
Nakago syndrome	Cardiomegaly, hypertrophic hypoplastic left heart syndrome	
Neurofibromatosis	Atrial septal defect, pulmonary stenosis, coarctation, interrupted aortic arch, ventricular septal defect, complete heart block, hypertrophic cardiomyopathy	
Noonan syndrome	Pulmonary stenosis, ventricular septal defect, atrial septal defect, interrupted aortic arch, coarctation, total anomalous pulmonary venous connection, hypertrophic cardiomyopathy, atrial stenosis, tetralogy of Fallot	65
Oculoauriculovertebral anomaly	Interrupted aortic arch, coarctation, ventricular septal defect, tetralogy of Fallot, right aortic arch	
Okihiro syndrome	Atrial septal defect	
Opitz syndrome	Congenital heart disease (unspecified)	
Opitz-Kaveggia FG syndrome	Ventricular septal defect, hypoplastic left heart syndrome	
Oropalatal-digital syndrome	Interrupted aortic arch, coarctation	
Pallister-Hall syndrome	Atrioventricular septal defect	
Pena-Shokeir syndrome	Interrupted aortic arch, coarctation, transposition of the great arteries, right ventricular hypertrophy	
Pentalogy of Cantrell	Atrial septal defect, ventricular septal defect, total anomalous pulmonary venous connection, pulmonary stenosis, tetralogy of Fallot, ectopia cordis	
Pierre Robin syndrome	Atrial septal defect	9
Poland syndrome	Tetralogy of Fallot, atrial septal defect, ventricular septal defect, interrupted aortic arch, coarctation	
Polydactyly chondrodystrophy, types 1 and 2	Transposition of the great arteries, truncus arteriosus, transposition of the great arteries, double-outlet right ventricle	
Polysyndactyly–cardiac malformations	Atrial septal defect, ventricular septal defect, atrioventricular septal defect, single ventricle	
Potter syndrome	Congenital heart disease (unspecified)	
Prune-belly syndrome	Atrial septal defect, ventricular septal defect, pulmonary stenosis	

TABLE 2–5 Chromosome Abnormalities and Syndromes Associated with Congenital Heart Disease—cont'd		
Syndrome	**Associated Congenital Heart Disease**	**Risk (%)**
Pulmonary venolobar syndrome	Atrial septal defect, interrupted aortic arch, coarctation, dextroposition, ventricular septal defect, tetralogy of Fallot, absent right pulmonary artery	
Radial-renal syndrome	Ventricular septal defect	
Radial-renal-ocular syndrome	Atrial septal defect	
Rolland-Desbuquois syndrome	Congenital heart disease (unspecified)	
Rubinstein-Taybi syndrome	Atrial septal defect, ventricular septal defect	25
Rubinstein-Taylor syndrome	Congenital heart disease (unspecified)	36
Saldino-Noonan syndrome	Congenital heart disease (unspecified)	
Salonen-Herva-Norio syndrome	Ventricular septal defect, atrioventricular septal defect, truncus arteriosus, hypoplasia of left ventricle, double aortic arch	
Schinzel-Giedion syndrome	Atrial septal defect	
Scimitar syndrome	Atrial septal defect, interrupted aortic arch, coarctation, dextroposition, ventricular septal defect, tetralogy of Fallot, absent right pulmonary artery	
Seckel syndrome	Ventricular septal defect	
Shone syndrome	Interrupted aortic arch, coarctation	
Short rib polydactyly syndrome, type II	Atrial septal defect	
Short rib polydactyly syndrome (non-Majewski type)	Transposition of the great arteries, double-outlet left ventricle, double-outlet right ventricle, atrioventricular defect, hypoplasia of right ventricle	
Siegler syndrome	Ventricular septal defect	
Silverman-Handmaker-type dwarfism	Congenital heart disease (unspecified)	
Situs inversus viscerum	Atrial septal defect	
Silver syndrome	Tetralogy of Fallot, ventricular septal defect	
Smith-Lemli-Opitz syndrome	Ventricular septal defect, atrioventricular septal defect	
Sofer syndrome	Ventricular septal defect	
Sternal-cardiac malformations association	Atrial septal defect	
Stevenson syndrome	Congenital heart disease (unspecified)	40
Sturge-Weber anomaly	Coarctation	
Thanatophoric dysplasia	Interrupted aortic arch, coarctation	
Thalassemia major	Cardiomyopathy	
Thrombocytopenia–absent radius	Atrial septal defect, tetralogy of Fallot, dextrocardia	33
Treacher Collins syndrome	Ventricular septal defect, atrial septal defect	
Tuberous sclerosis	Rhabdomyoma, angioma, coarctation, interrupted aortic arch	
VACTERL (vertebral abnormalities, anal atresia, cardiac abnormalities, tracheoesophageal fistula or esophageal atresia, renal agenesis and dysplasia, and limb defects) syndrome	Hypoplastic left heart syndrome, ventricular septal defect	50
Varadi syndrome	Interrupted aortic arch, coarctation	
Venolobar syndrome	Atrial septal defect, interrupted aortic arch, coarctation, dextroposition, ventricular septal defect, tetralogy of Fallot, absent right pulmonary artery	
Velocardiofacial syndrome	Ventricular septal defect, tetralogy of Fallot, right aortic arch	80
Verma-Naumoff syndrome	Congenital heart disease (unspecified)	
Waardenburg syndrome	Ventricular septal defect	
Weaver syndrome	Ventricular septal defect	
Weill-Marchesani syndrome	Pulmonary stenosis, ventricular septal defect	
William syndrome	Aortic stenosis, pulmonary stenosis, ventricular septal defect, atrial septal defect, interrupted aortic arch, mitral regurgitation, tetralogy of Fallot, coarctation	100

Continued

TABLE 2–5 Chromosome Abnormalities and Syndromes Associated with Congenital Heart Disease—cont'd

Syndrome	Associated Congenital Heart Disease	Risk (%)
Williams-Beuren syndrome	Interrupted aortic arch, coarctation, aortic stenosis, pulmonary stenosis, ventricular septal defect, atrial septal defect, mural regurgitation, tetralogy of Fallot	100
Zellweger syndrome	Ventricular septal defect, atrial septal defect	
Chromosome Abnormalities		
Monosomy 1q	Ventricular septal defect	
Monosomy 1q4	Ventricular septal defect, truncus arteriosus, pulmonary atresia, pulmonary stenosis	
Monosomy 2q	Atrial septal defect, coarctation, interrupted aortic arch, ventricular septal defect	
Monosomy distal 4q	Congenital heart disease (unspecified)	
Monosomy 5p	Congenital heart disease (unspecified)	
Monosomy 5q (interstitial)	Coarctation, interrupted aortic arch	
Monosomy 6q (proximal)	Congenital heart disease (unspecified)	
Monosomy 7p2	Ventricular septal defect, hypoplastic left heart syndrome	
Monosomy 7q1	Coarctation	
Monosomy 8p2	Ventricular septal defect, pulmonary stenosis	
Monosomy 9 (mosaic)	Coarctation, interrupted aortic arch	
Monosomy 10q2	Ventricular septal defect, pulmonary stenosis	
Monosomy 11q	Ventricular septal defect, truncus arteriosus	50
Monosomy 13q	Congenital heart disease (unspecified)	55
Monosomy 14q	Atrial septal defect	
Monosomy 14q	Atrial septal defect	
Monosomy 16q	Ventricular septal defect	
Monosomy 18q	Congenital heart disease (unspecified)	25
Monosomy 22	Congenital heart disease (unspecified)	
Monosomy 22q (DiGeorge syndrome)	Ventricular septal defect, coarctation, truncus arteriosus, transposition of the great arteries, tetralogy of Fallot, interrupted aortic arch, double-outlet right ventricle	95
Partial monosomy 9p	Congenital heart disease (unspecified)	
Partial monosomy 11p	Tetralogy of Fallot, cardiomyopathy	
Partial trisomy 10q	Congenital heart disease (unspecified)	50
Partial trisomy 14q	Congenital heart disease (unspecified)	
Partial trisomy 22 (Cat-eye syndrome)	Total anomalous pulmonary venous connection, ventricular septal defect, atrial septal defect	40
T 20p syndrome	Ventricular septal defect, tetralogy of Fallot	
Tetrasomy 9p	Congenital heart disease (unspecified)	
Trisomy 1q25-1q32	Congenital heart disease (unspecified)	
Trisomy 1q32-QTER	Truncus arteriosus	
Trisomy 2q	Ventricular septal defect, aortic stenosis	
Trisomy 3q2	Congenital heart disease (unspecified)	33
Trisomy distal 4q	Congenital heart disease (unspecified)	
Trisomy 4p	Congenital heart disease (unspecified)	
Trisomy 5p	Congenital heart disease (unspecified)	
Trisomy 5p3	Ventricular septal defect	
Trisomy 5q3	Congenital heart disease (unspecified)	
Trisomy 6p2	Ventricular septal defect	
Trisomy 7p2	Ventricular septal defect	
Trisomy 7q2-3	Congenital heart disease (unspecified)	
Trisomy 8 (mosaic)	Ventricular septal defect, atrial septal defect	50
Trisomy 9 (mosaic)	Ventricular septal defect, coarctation, double-outlet right ventricle, atrial septal defect	50
Trisomy 9p	Ventricular septal defect	26
Trisomy 10p	Congenital heart disease (unspecified)	
Trisomy 11p	Congenital heart disease (unspecified)	
Trisomy 12p	Ventricular septal defect	

TABLE 2–5 Chromosome Abnormalities and Syndromes Associated with Congenital Heart Disease—cont'd

Syndrome	Associated Congenital Heart Disease	Risk (%)
Trisomy 13 (Patau syndrome)	Ventricular septal defect, atrial septal defect, dextroposition, hypoplastic left heart syndrome, atrioventricular septal defect, tetralogy of Fallot, coarctation, interrupted aortic arch	90+
Trisomy 13q	Congenital heart disease (unspecified)	
Trisomy 14p	Ventricular septal defect	
Trisomy 14 (mosaic)	Tetralogy of Fallot	90
Trisomy 15q2	Ventricular septal defect	
Trisomy 16p	Atrial septal defect, tetralogy of Fallot	
Trisomy 16q	Congenital heart disease (unspecified)	
Trisomy 18 (Edwards syndrome)	Bicuspid aortic valve, pulmonary stenosis, ventricular septal defect, atrial septal defect, atrioventricular septal defect, double-outlet right ventricle, coarctation, interrupted aortic arch	99+
Trisomy 18p	Coarctation, interrupted aortic arch	
Trisomy 19q	Congenital heart disease (unspecified)	
Trisomy 20p	Congenital heart disease (unspecified)	
Trisomy 20ptr ≈ q11	Ventricular septal defect	
Trisomy 21 (Down syndrome)	Atrioventricular septal defect, ventricular septal defect, atrial septal defect, tetralogy of Fallot, coarctation, interrupted aortic arch, pulmonary atresia	50
Trisomy 22	Atrial septal defect, ventricular septal defect	67
Triploidy	Atrial septal defect, ventricular septal defect	
Turner syndrome (45X)	Bicuspid aortic valve, aortic stenosis, coarctation, ventricular septal defect, atrial septal defect, atrioventricular septal defect, pulmonary stenosis, interrupted aortic arch, total anomalous pulmonary venous connection	20+
4p– (Wolf syndrome)	Atrial septal defect, ventricular septal defect	40
5p– (cri-du-chat syndrome)	Ventricular septal defect	30
9p–	Ventricular septal defect, pulmonary stenosis	
13q–	Ventricular septal defect	25
+14q–	Ventricular septal defect, atrial septal defect, tetralogy of Fallot	50
18q–	Ventricular septal defect	50
22q–	Interrupted aortic arch, tetralogy of Fallot, truncus arteriosus, transposition of the great arteries, double-outlet right ventricle, coarctation	95
Interstitial deletion 17p	Congenital heart disease (unspecified)	
Ring 14	Pulmonary stenosis, aortic stenosis	
Ring 15	Congenital heart disease (unspecified)	
Ring 22	Congenital heart disease (unspecified)	
XXXY	Atrial septal defect	14

Data from Paladini D, Calabro R, Palmieri S, et al: Prenatal diagnosis of congenital heart disease and fetal karyotyping. Obstet Gynecol 1993; 81:679–682; Ropel DA: The heart. In: Stevenson RE, Hall JG, Goodman RM (eds): Human Malformations and Related Anomalies, vol II. New York, Oxford University Press, 1993, p 238; Copel JA, Pilu G, Kleinman CS: Congenital heart disease and extracardiac anomalies: Associations and indications for fetal echocardiography. Am J Obstet Gynecol 1986; 154:1121–1132; Respondek ML, Binotto CN, Donnenfeld A, et al: Extracardiac anomalies, aneuploidy and growth retardation in 100 consecutive fetal congenital heart defects. Ultrasound Obstet Gynecol 1994; 4:272–278; Stamm ER, Drose JA, Thickman D: The fetal heart. In: Rumack CM, Wilson SR, Charboneau JW (eds): Diagnostic Ultrasound, vol 2. St. Louis, Mosby–Year Book, 1991, p 801; Jones KL: Smith's Recognizable Patterns of Human Malformation, 3rd ed. Philadelphia, WB Saunders, 1988; Nora J, Fraser FC, Bear J, et al: Medical Genetics: Principles and Practice. Philadelphia, Lea & Febiger, 1994; Romero R, Pilu G, Jeanty P, et al: The heart. In: Prenatal Diagnosis of Congenital and Metabolic Anomalies. Norwalk, CT, Appleton & Lange, 1988; Taybi H: Radiology of Syndromes and Metabolic Disorders. Chicago, Year Book Medical, 1983; Nyberg DA, Emerson DS: Cardiac malformations. In: Nybert DA, Mahony BS, Pretorius DH (eds): Diagnostic Ultrasound of Fetal Anomalies: Text and Atlas. Chicago, Year Book Medical, 1990, pp 300–341; Buyse ML: Birth Defects Encyclopedia. Dover, Center for Birth Defects Information Services, 1990, pp 1–1805.

TABLE 2–6   Incidence (%) of Associated Congenital Heart Defects Occurring with Extracardiac Malformations in Infants

System or Lesion	Frequency of Congenital Heart Disease (%)
Central Nervous System	
Hydrocephalus	4.5–14.8
Dandy-Walker malformation	2.5–4.3
Agenesis of the corpus callosum	14.9
Meckel-Gruber syndrome	13.8
Gastrointestinal	
Tracheoesophageal fistula	14.7–39.2
Duodenal atresia	17.1
Jejunal atresia	5.2
Anorectal anomalies	22
Imperforate anus	11.7
Ventral Wall	
Omphalocele	19.5–32
Gastroschisis	0–7.7
Diaphragmatic Hernia	9.6–22.9
Genitourinary	
Renal agenesis (bilateral)	42.8
Renal agenesis (unilateral)	16.9
Horseshoe kidney	38.8
Renal dysplasia	5.4
Ureteral obstruction	2.1

Modified from Copel JA, Pilu G, Kleinman CS: Congenital heart disease and extracardiac anomalies: Associations and indications for fetal echocardiography. Am J Obstet Gynecol 1986; 154:1121–1132.

This is thought to be the result of an overall increase in type 2 diabetes secondary to an increase in obesity and other medical problems.[41,43] Congenital cardiac defects most often associated with diabetes are transposition of the great arteries, truncus arteriosus, and tetralogy of Fallot.[44]

Maternal phenylketonuria has a reported risk of 12% to 16% to the fetus of having a congenital heart defect.[5,32,45,46]

Complete heart block in the fetus is associated with maternal collagen vascular disease (systemic lupus erythematosus). In these patients, circulating antinuclear antibodies of the SSA or SSB type appear to damage the developing conduction tissue.[14] These fetuses may also be at risk for premature closure of the ductus arteriosus as a result of maternal steroid treatment.

Maternal infection has also been reported to be associated with heart defects in the fetus. Commonly these are either dilated or hypertrophic cardiomyopathies.[47,48]

The presence of *extracardiac anomalies* found in a fetus during an obstetrical sonographic examination also warrants a fetal echocardiogram.[49] Some extracardiac malformations carry a low risk of associated congenital heart disease, whereas for others the risk is high. The overall incidence of extracardiac malformations in children identified as having congenital heart disease ranges from 25% to 45% (Table 2–6).[49,50] Heart abnormalities such as atrioventricular (AV) septal defects are associated with extracardiac defects in more than 50% of cases, whereas atrial septal defects, ventricular septal defects, tetralogy of Fallot, and cardiac malposition are associated with extracardiac malformations in about 30% of cases.[50]

A suspicion of a *structural or rhythm abnormality* seen in the fetal heart on a routine obstetrical examination is another indication for a formal fetal echocardiogram. Up to 90% of congenital heart disease occurs in unselected "normal" obstetric patients.[6,18,43] Therefore routine obstetrical scanning should identify the majority of fetuses with heart lesions needing a formal fetal echocardiogram.

The identification of *nonimmune hydrops fetalis* is also considered an indication for fetal echocardiography. In some cases it may reflect structural heart disease, whereas in others it can be the result of an arrhythmia.[29] Hydrops fetalis has been reported to be associated with structural heart disease in 13.7% of cases and cardiac rhythm abnormalities in 10.4%.[51]

Polyhydramnios is a recognized indication for fetal echocardiography.[52,53] An increase in amniotic fluid may not be caused directly by the heart defect but is more likely related to associated defects in the fetus, such as those that cause difficulty in swallowing or compression of the esophagus. Fetal echocardiogram referrals for fetuses with polyhydramnios have also decreased over years past.[8] It is usually only cases of significant polyhydramnios that are associated with a cardiac cause and that warrant a formal fetal echocardiogram.

Finally, in fetuses with an increased nuchal translucency identified in the first trimester, the frequency of congenital heart disease is increased compared with that of the general population.[43,54,55] In a fetus with an increased nuchal translucency and a confirmed chromosome anomaly, the percent risk is that associated with the specific anomaly. As an isolated finding, an increased nuchal translucency carries a risk of an associated heart defect of approximately 2% to 5%.[43,54-57] This risk increases exponentially with an increase in nuchal translucency thickness.[57]

Many, although not all, congenital heart defects found in chromosomally normal fetuses with an increased nuchal translucency are left-sided defects such as hypoplastic left heart syndrome, coarctation of the aorta, aortic stenosis, or aortic atresia. Interestingly, pathological examination of the heart and great vessels in these fetuses after termination has shown a greater degree of narrowing of the aortic isthmus than seen in normal fetuses. It is hypothesized that this narrowing could result in greater perfusion of the head and neck, which in turn results in a transient increase in subcutaneous neck edema, thus the increased nuchal translucency. However, it should be kept in mind that a variety of heart defects are seen in the setting of increased nuchal translucency with normal chromosomes, so this does not explain this finding in all affected fetuses.[54]

Position

The first step in any fetal echocardiographic examination is to establish fetal position. Unlike pediatric or adult patients, the fetus cannot be placed in a standard position, nor can the heart be approached consistently from routine angles. Although the fetus may move throughout the examination, establishing a basic position allows the examiner to identify various heart structures quickly.[20] Once fetal position is understood, the location and orientation of the heart should be established. In a cross-sectional transverse view of the fetal chest, the correct orientation for the fetal heart is with the apex pointing to the left and the bulk of the heart occupying the left side of the chest (Fig. 2–2). The angle of the fetal heart relative to midline is normally 45 degrees plus or minus 20 degrees. In other words, a line traversing the interventricular septum will fall between 25 and 65 degrees leftward from a line extending between the spine and the mid anterior chest wall.[58] In this correct orientation, the left atrium will be located closest to the fetal spine and the

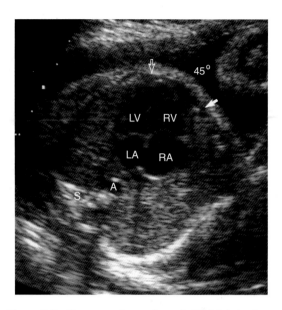

Figure 2–2 Transverse image through the fetal chest showing the normal orientation of the fetal heart, with the apex *(open arrow)* pointing to the left. The angle between the arrows demonstrates normal cardiac axis at 45 degrees. *A,* Aorta; *LA,* left atrium; *LV,* left ventricle; *RA,* right atrium; *RV,* right ventricle; *S,* spine.

right ventricle will be nearest the anterior chest wall. This normal orientation is termed *levocardia.* Abnormal positions of the fetal heart include the following:

- Dextrocardia: The heart is located in the right side of the chest with the apex pointing to the right.
- Dextroposition: The heart is located in the right side of the chest with the apex pointing to the left.
- Mesocardia: The heart is located in the mid chest with the apex pointing directly midline.

All these types of cardiac malposition are associated with structural abnormalities and are discussed in Chapter 3. Extreme levocardia has also been associated with congenital heart defects. Shipp et al[59] reported that 44% of fetal heart defects were associated with levocardia greater than 57 degrees. In another study[60] levocardia greater than 75 degrees correlated with a positive predictive value of 76% for a heart defect in fetuses.

The fetal heart normally occupies approximately one third of the fetal thorax.[22,61-65] Fetal

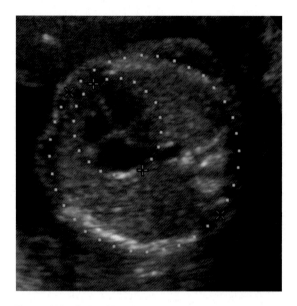

Figure 2–3 Calculating fetal heart size by measuring the circumference of the fetal heart and comparing it with the circumference of the fetal chest. Both measurements should be acquired from the same image.

heart size can be calculated by measuring the diameter or the circumference of the heart and comparing it with the diameter or circumference of the fetal chest, respectively. When this ratio is calculated, both measurements must be obtained from the same image (Fig. 2–3).

The echocardiographic views necessary to perform a complete evaluation of the fetal cardiac system include the following:*

- Four-chamber view
  - Apical
  - Subcostal
- Long-axis view of the aorta
- Long-axis view of the pulmonary artery
- Short-axis view of the ventricles
- Short-axis view of the great vessels
- View of the aortic arch
- View of the ductal arch
- View of the superior vena cava and inferior vena cava
- Three-vessel view

Four-Chamber Views

The first view to obtain when beginning a fetal echocardiographic examination is the four-

*References 6, 12, 28, 31, 32, 61, 66-72.

BOX 2–2

Uses for the Apical Four-Chamber View

Evaluate heart position
Evaluate heart axis
Evaluate heart size
Evaluate chamber size
Identify moderator band in right ventricle
Doppler imaging of mitral valve and tricuspid valve above and below valves
Identify superior pulmonary veins entering left atrium
Identify foraminal flap entering left atrium
Angle transducer posteriorly to obtain five-chamber view
Doppler imaging of aortic valve above and below valve

---

chamber view. Obstetrical ultrasound guidelines include the four-chamber view of the fetal heart as a standard part of every examination.[73] The four-chamber view has been reported to have a detection rate for congenital heart disease of between 40% and 57%.[74,75] Detection rates are usually higher for complex lesions and lower for isolated lesions. The four-chamber view alone is specifically suboptimal in identifying conotruncal abnormalities such as truncus arteriosus or tetralogy of Fallot. Therefore evaluation of the aortic and pulmonary outflow tracts should also be part of every routine obstetrical examination.[15,76-81]

There are two different four-chamber views: the apical four-chamber view and the subcostal four-chamber view. In the following sections the techniques for obtaining these views are discussed.

Apical Four-Chamber View

The apical four-chamber view is obtained via a transverse view of the fetal chest, with the apex of the heart pointing directly toward or away from the transducer. In the apical four-chamber view, the interventricular and interatrial septa are parallel to the transducer (Fig. 2–4). From this projection, all four heart chambers can be visualized. In this view, the following structures should be identified (Box 2–2):

- Two atrial chambers of approximately equal size. The left atrium should be closest to the fetal spine.
- Two ventricular chambers of approximately equal size and thickness, with the right ven-

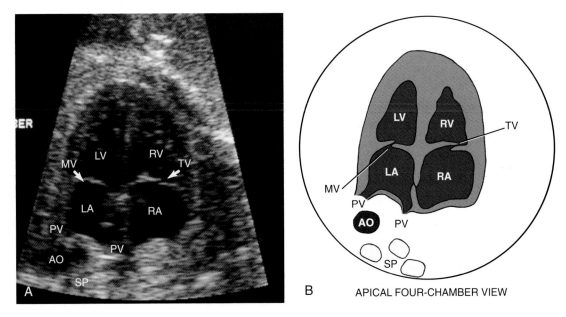

Figure 2–4 Sonogram of an apical four-chamber view **(A)** and schematic of an apical four-chamber view **(B)**. *LV,* Left ventricle; *RV,* right ventricle; *LA,* left atrium; *RA,* right atrium; *MV,* mitral valve; *TV,* tricuspid valve; *PV,* pulmonary veins; *SP,* spine; *AO,* aorta.

tricle becoming slightly larger than the left ventricle as pregnancy progresses.[61] The right ventricle should lie closer to the anterior chest wall (opposite the spine) than does the left ventricle. Additionally, the moderator band of the trabecula septomarginalis should be identified in the right ventricle, coursing from the interventricular septum to the lower free wall of the ventricle.[72] Discrepancy in ventricular size has been associated with a variety of heart defects, and in some cases may be the first or only indication that a problem exists.[82,83]

- The AV valves (mitral and tricuspid) should be located between the atria and ventricles, with the septal leaflet of the tricuspid valve inserting slightly more apically than that of the mitral valve.
- The interventricular septum should be located between the right and left ventricles, and the interatrial septum should be located between the right and left atria. A normal opening in the atrial septum, the foramen ovale, should be visualized with the foraminal flap opening into the left atrium (Fig. 2–5).

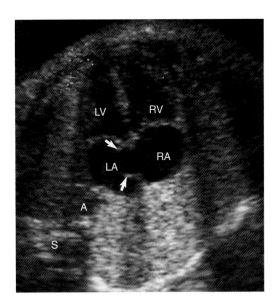

Figure 2–5 Sonogram of an apical four-chamber view showing the foraminal flap *(arrows)* opening into the left atrium *(LA)*. *RA,* Right atrium; *LV,* left ventricle; *RV,* right ventricle; *S,* spine; *A,* aorta.

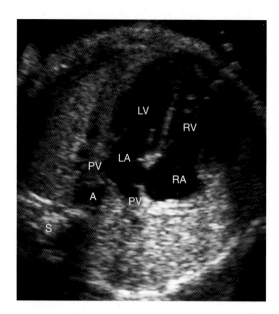

Figure 2–6   Sonogram of an apical four-chamber view showing the superior pulmonary veins *(PV)* entering the left atrium *(LA)*. *RA,* Right atrium; *LV,* left ventricle; *RV,* right ventricle; *S,* spine; *A,* aorta.

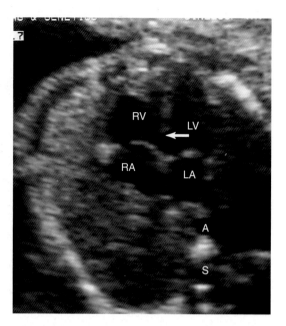

Figure 2–7   Sonogram of an apical four-chamber view showing a "pseudo" ventricular septal defect *(arrow)* caused by the ultrasound beam insonating the interventricular septum at a parallel angle. *S,* Spine; *A,* aorta; *LA,* left atrium; *RA,* right atrium; *LV,* left ventricle; *RV,* right ventricle.

- A slight angulation of the transducer usually allows identification of the two superior pulmonary veins entering the left atrium (Fig. 2–6).[84]

The apical four-chamber view is not optimal for interrogating the interventricular septum. In this view, the angle of incidence of the sound beam is parallel to the interventricular septum and may result in an artifactual dropout of echoes at the level of the membranous interventricular septum, simulating a "pseudo" septal defect (Fig. 2–7).[71]

The mitral and tricuspid valves are evaluated optimally in the apical four-chamber view because the angle of incidence of the sound beam is perpendicular to the AV valves. Additionally, Doppler interrogation of the mitral and tricuspid valves to look for stenosis or valvular insufficiency is most accurate in this projection because a Doppler interrogation angle of near 0 degrees can be obtained. The pulsed Doppler sample gate should be placed in the left atrium (just proximal to the mitral valve) to evaluate for mitral insufficiency (Fig. 2–8) and in the right atrium (just proximal to the tricuspid valve) to evaluate for tricuspid insufficiency (Fig. 2–9).

Color Doppler imaging may be advantageous in searching for insufficiency (Fig. 2–10) because the entire atrium can usually be evaluated simultaneously, as opposed to using the pulsed Doppler sample gate, which must be moved throughout the chamber to identify small jets of insufficiency. If an area of significant valvular insufficiency is identified by Doppler imaging, it will appear during systole as retrograde flow that is sometimes so high that it results in aliasing (Fig. 2–11).

By placing the Doppler sample volume distal to the mitral valve in the left ventricle (Fig. 2–12) or distal to the tricuspid valve in the right ventricle (Fig. 2–13), AV valve velocities can be obtained. Normal values for both peak and mean flow velocities across the mitral and tricuspid valves have been reported (Table 2–7). These velocities seem to remain constant throughout gestation.

No detectable flow may indicate valvular atresia, whereas an increase in velocity to greater than normal ranges is often indicative of valvular stenosis. Again, color Doppler imaging may expedite locating a stenotic jet.

TABLE 2–7 Mitral and Tricuspid Valve Velocities in the Normal Fetus		
Valve	Maximum Velocity (cm/sec)	Mean Velocity (cm/sec)
Mitral	47 ± 1.1 (range 20.8–67.6)	11.2 ± 0.3 (range 6.6–16.5)
Tricuspid	51 ± 1.2 (range 34.1–78.2)	11.8 ± 0.4 (range 7.2–16.9)

Modified from Reed KL, Meijboom EJ, Sahn D, et al: Cardiac Doppler flow velocities in human fetuses. Circulation 1986; 73:41–46.

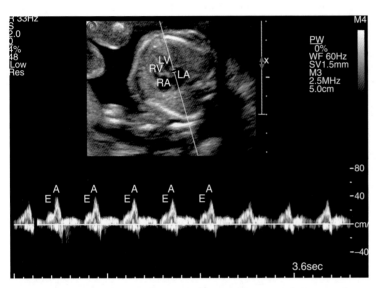

Figure 2–8 Normal pulsed Doppler tracing of the mitral valve with the sample volume placed within the left atrium (*LA*) to interrogate for mitral valve insufficiency. Inflow is seen above the baseline with the normal E point–A point relationship of the mitral waveform. If regurgitation was present, it would appear as reversed flow into the atrium (below the baseline) during systole. *LV,* Left ventricle; *RA,* right atrium; *RV,* right ventricle.

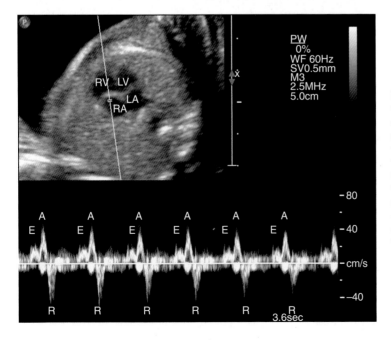

Figure 2–9 Normal pulsed Doppler tracing of the tricuspid valve with the sample volume placed within the right atrium (*RA*) to interrogate for tricuspid valve insufficiency. Inflow is seen above the baseline with the normal E point–A point relationship of the tricuspid waveform. A normal amount of tricuspid regurgitation (*R*) is seen as reversed flow below the baseline during the beginning of systole. *LA,* Left atrium; *LV,* left ventricle; *RV,* right ventricle.

A posterior angulation of the transducer from the apical four-chamber view will allow visualization of the aortic outflow tract within the four chambers. This projection is often referred to as the *apical five-chamber view* (Fig. 2–14). The five-chamber view is useful for confirming the presence and proper orientation of the aorta and for evaluating the aortic valve for insufficiency or stenosis with color or pulsed Doppler imaging.

Subcostal Four-Chamber View

The subcostal four-chamber view is obtained by imaging the fetal chest in a transverse projection from the anterior chest wall and angling the transducer slightly cephalad (Fig. 2–15). As with the apical four-chamber view, this view also allows identification and comparison of both atria and ventricles (Box 2–3). M-mode measurements of the ventricles can be obtained in this view by placing the M-mode cursor perpendicular to the septum at the level of the AV valves (Fig. 2–16).[61] Several nomograms for normal ventricular dimensions throughout gestation have been developed (Figs. 2–17 to 2–19).

Most of these nomograms reflect the maximal diameter of the ventricle that would be obtained in the end-diastolic phase of the cardiac cycle. However, both systolic and diastolic ventricular dimensions are necessary for calculating ventricular function.

• End-diastolic measurements of the ventricles are obtained at the point at which the mitral (left ventricle) or tricuspid (right ventricle) valve leaflets close. Measurements should be made from the endocardial surface of the ventricular wall to the interventricular septum (see Fig. 2–16).

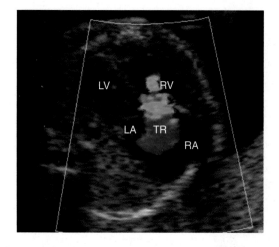

Figure 2–10 Four-chamber view in a fetus with Ebstein anomaly showing massive tricuspid regurgitation *(TR)* by color Doppler imaging. The regurgitant jet occupies most of the right atrium *(RA)*. *LA,* Left atrium; *LV,* left ventricle; *RV,* right ventricle.

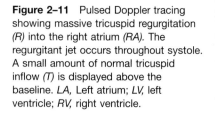
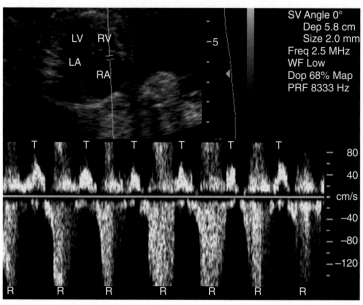

Figure 2–11 Pulsed Doppler tracing showing massive tricuspid regurgitation *(R)* into the right atrium *(RA)*. The regurgitant jet occurs throughout systole. A small amount of normal tricuspid inflow *(T)* is displayed above the baseline. *LA,* Left atrium; *LV,* left ventricle; *RV,* right ventricle.

- End-systolic measurements of the ventricles are obtained at the point of maximal inward excursion of the right and left ventricular walls, again measuring from the endocardial surface of either ventricular wall to the interventricular septum. It is important to exclude the chordae tendinae in this measurement.

- Ventricular free wall thickness (see Figs. 2–16, 2–20, and 2–21) and thickness of the interventricular septum (see Figs. 2–16 and 2–22) can

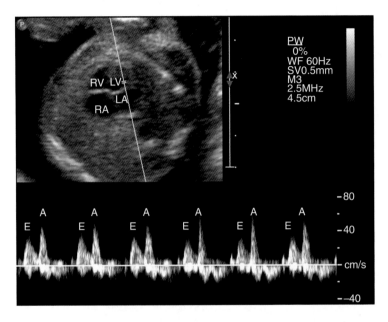

Figure 2–12   Pulsed Doppler cursor placement distal to the mitral valve, in the left ventricle *(LV)*, to access mitral outflow. The normal E-point, A-point relationship is displayed above the baseline. *LA,* Left atrium; *RA,* right atrium; *RV,* right ventricle.

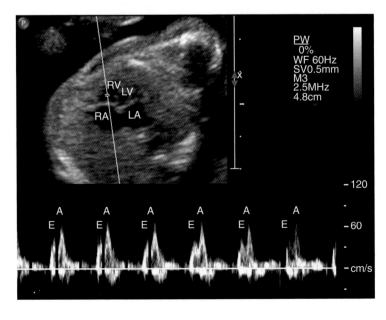

Figure 2–13   Pulsed Doppler cursor placement distal to the tricuspid valve, in the right ventricle *(RV)*, to access tricuspid outflow. The normal E-point, A-point relationship is displayed above the baseline. *LA,* Left atrium; *LV,* left ventricle; *RA,* right atrium.

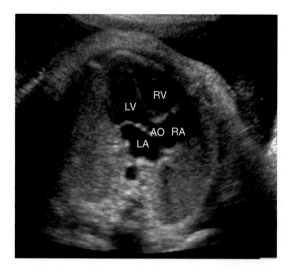

Figure 2–14 Apical five-chamber view showing the aorta *(AO)* arising form the left ventricle *(LV). LA,* Left atrium; *RA,* right atrium; *RV,* right ventricle.

BOX 2–3

Uses for Subcostal Four-Chamber View

Evaluate heart position
Evaluate heart axis
Evaluate heart size
Evaluate chamber size
Identify moderator band in right ventricle
Identify superior pulmonary veins entering left atrium
Identify foraminal flap entering left atrium
Evaluate interventricular septum for ventricular septal defect
Measure atria or ventricular size with calipers or M-mode
Measure interventricular septum and heart walls with calipers or M-mode
Evaluate heart wall contractility with M-mode

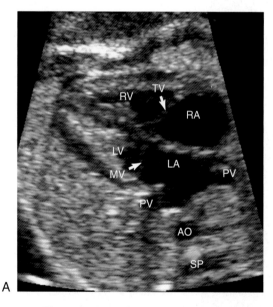

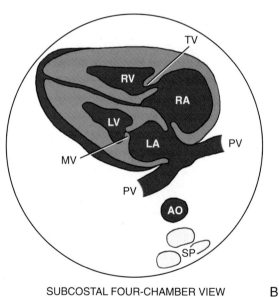

SUBCOSTAL FOUR-CHAMBER VIEW   B

Figure 2–15 A, Sonogram of a subcostal four-chamber view. **B,** Schematic of a subcostal four-chamber view. *AO,* Aorta; *LA,* left atrium; *LV,* left ventricle; *MV,* mitral valve; *PV,* pulmonary veins; *RA,* right atrium; *RV,* right ventricle; *SP,* spine; *TV,* tricuspid valve.

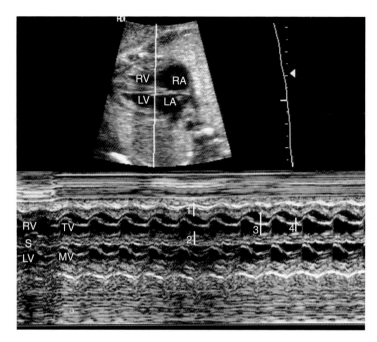

Figure 2–16 M-mode tracing of normal fetal cardiac ventricles from a subcostal four-chamber view. The M-mode cursor should be placed through the left ventricle *(LV)* and right ventricle *(RV)* at the level of the mitral *(MV)* and tricuspid *(TV)* valves. Ventricular measurements from this projection include heart wall thickness *(1)*, interventricular septal thickness *(2)*, end-diastolic ventricular dimension *(3)*, and end-systolic ventricular dimension *(4)*. *LA,* Left atrium; *RA,* right atrium; *S,* interventricular septum.

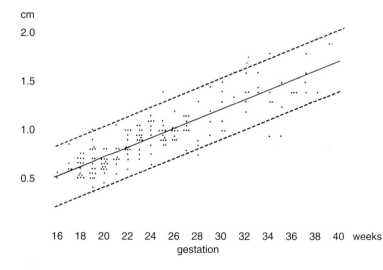

Left Ventricular Internal Dimension

Figure 2–17 Left ventricular internal dimension plotted against gestational age (n = 175). $Y = 0.049 \times -0.262$, $r = 0.876$, $t = 23.944$, $P < 0.001$, standard error of estimate $y \times 2 = 0.3$. (From Allan LD, Joseph MC, Boyd EG, et al: M-mode echocardiography in the developing human fetus. Br Heart J 1982; 47:573–583.)

also be measured at this level. Allan et al[85] reported that normally the interventricular septum thickness remains less than 5 mm throughout gestation. These measurements are also acquired at end-diastole.

- Atrial measurements are performed by moving the M-mode cursor so that it courses through both atria at the largest diameter (Fig. 2–23). Measurements are taken from either the left or the right atrial wall, depending on which atrium is being investigated, to the interatrial septum. The atrial walls do not exhibit significant contraction; therefore systolic and diastolic measurements are usually similar (Fig. 2–24).

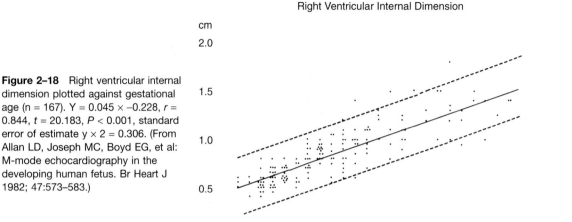

Right Ventricular Internal Dimension

Figure 2–18 Right ventricular internal dimension plotted against gestational age (n = 167). Y = 0.045 × –0.228, r = 0.844, t = 20.183, P < 0.001, standard error of estimate y × 2 = 0.306. (From Allan LD, Joseph MC, Boyd EG, et al: M-mode echocardiography in the developing human fetus. Br Heart J 1982; 47:573–583.)

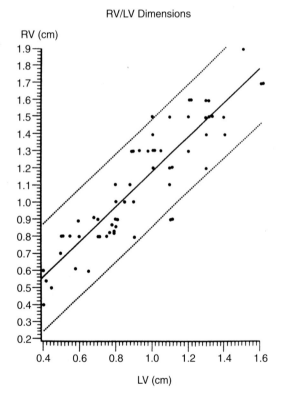

RV/LV Dimensions

Figure 2–19 Maximal right ventricular internal dimension *(RV)* plotted against maximal left ventricular internal dimension *(LV)* (n = 62). Y = 1.03x + 0.144, r = 0.899, P = 0.0001. (From Shime J, Gresser CD, Rakowski H: Quantitative two-dimensional echocardiographic assessment of fetal cardiac growth. Am J Obstet Gynecol 1986; 154:294–300.)

It is also possible to evaluate an arrhythmia in this projection by placing the M-mode cursor through an atrial wall and a ventricular wall simultaneously (Fig. 2–25). This allows visualization of the timing of arrhythmic events and may aid in making a definitive diagnosis.

Either pulsed Doppler (Fig. 2–26) or color Doppler (Fig. 2–27) imaging can be used in this projection to evaluate the foramen ovale. The documentation of flow by either modality rules out restriction of the foraminal flap. A spectral Doppler tracing will display normal foraminal flow into the left atrium as being twice the fetal heart rate.

The interventricular septum is best evaluated for the presence of a septal defect in the subcostal four-chamber view. Color Doppler imaging is the best means of achieving this, again because it allows a large area to be evaluated at one time (Fig. 2–28). Pulsed Doppler imaging alone may not detect flow across the septum if the sample volume is not positioned precisely.

Although some larger ventricular septal defects may be detected with gray-scale imaging alone, many remain undetected by any means. Even if a ventricular septal defect is present, the pressures in the fetal heart are relatively equal; therefore flow may not be appreciated across the interventricular septum.

The superior pulmonary veins can also be visualized entering the left atrium in the subcostal four-chamber view (Fig. 2–29). Pulsed Doppler

Posterior Left Ventricular Wall Thickness

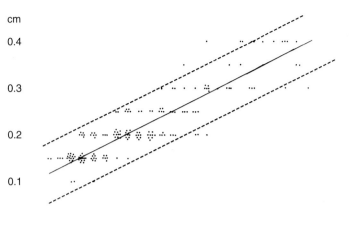

Figure 2–20 Posterior left ventricular wall thickness plotted against gestational age (n = 175). Y = 0.012 × −0.063, r = 0.884, t = 24.929, P < 0.001, standard error of estimate y × 2 = 0.66. (From Allan LD, Joseph MC, Boyd EG, et al: M-mode echocardiography in the developing human fetus. Br Heart J 1982; 47:573–583.)

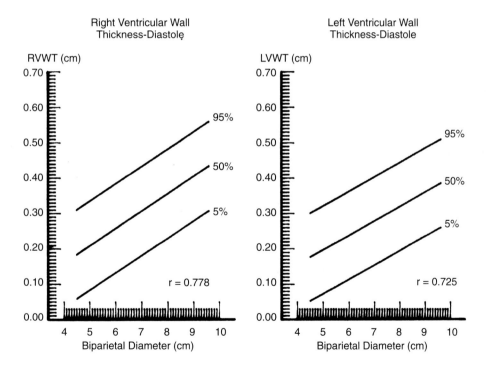

Figure 2–21 Right ventricular wall thickness and left ventricular wall thickness plotted against biparietal diameter. (From Devore GR, Siassi B, Platt LD: Fetal echocardiography. IV. M-mode assessment of ventricular size and contractility during the second and third trimesters of pregnancy in the normal fetus. Am J Obstet Gynecol 1984; 150:981–988.)

SEPTAL THICKNESS

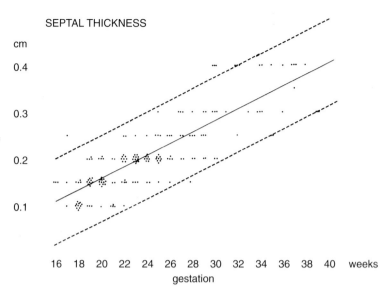

Figure 2–22 Septal thickness plotted against gestational age (n = 178). The 95% confidence limits represent twice the standard error of the mean in each graph. $Y = 0.012 \times -0.088$, $r = 0.836$, $t = 20.183$, $P < 0.001$, standard error of estimate $y \times 2 = 0.088$. (From Allan LD, Joseph MC, Boyd EG, et al: M-mode echocardiography in the developing human fetus. Br Heart J 1982; 47:573–583.)

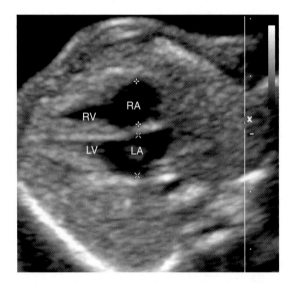

Figure 2–23 Measurement of the atria by placing the cursors through the largest dimension of the right atrium *(RA)* and left atrium *(LA)*. The cursors should be placed from the atrial wall to the interatrial septum. *RV,* Right ventricle; *LV,* left ventricle.

imaging may be helpful in confirming the presence and direction of venous flow (Fig. 2–30).

Obtaining a subcostal four-chamber view is essential when a complete fetal echocardiogram is performed. Most of the remaining fetal heart views are obtained by angling the transducer systematically toward the fetal right shoulder from this view (Fig. 2–31).

Long-Axis View of the Aorta

A slight angulation from the subcostal four-chamber view toward the fetal right shoulder will result in visualization of a long-axis view of the proximal aorta. In this view, continuity of the anterior wall of the aorta with the interventricular septum and the posterior wall of the aorta with the anterior leaflet of the mitral valve can be ascertained (Fig. 2–32) (Box 2–4).

The aorta at this level normally courses anteriorly. The aortic root, which normally is approximately 9% smaller than the pulmonary root between 14 and 42 weeks' gestation, can be measured in this view at the level of the valve (Fig. 2–33).[86] Nomograms plotting aortic root diameter against gestational age have been established (Fig. 2–34). The aortic valve can be interrogated with pulsed Doppler imaging in this view, if the angle is appropriate, both proximally (Fig. 2–35) looking for aortic insufficiency and distally (Fig. 2–36) to detect stenosis. Normal mean and peak velocities through the fetal aorta have been established (Table 2–8), and similar to the other heart valves, these velocities do not change

BOX 2–4

Uses for Long-Axis View of the Aorta

Evaluate continuity of anterior aortic root with interventricular septum
Evaluate continuity of posterior aortic root with anterior leaflet of mitral valve
Evaluate interventricular septum for ventricular septal defect
Evaluate aortic valve above and below valve (if Doppler angle is appropriate)
Place pulsed Doppler sample volume between aortic valve and mitral valve to evaluate arrhythmias
Place M-mode cursor through right ventricle and left atrium to evaluate arrhythmia

LEFT ATRIAL
cm INTERNAL DIMENSION

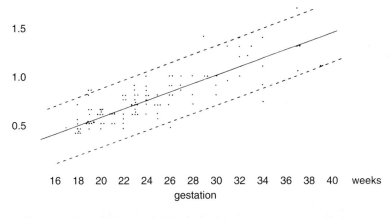

Figure 2–24 Left atrial internal dimension plotted against gestational age (n = 107). Y = 0.0400 × –0.214, r = 0.823, t = 14.968, P < 0.001, standard error of estimate y × 2 = 0.296. (From Allan LD, Joseph MC, Boyd EG, et al: M-mode echocardiography in the developing human fetus. Br Heart J 1982; 47:573–583.)

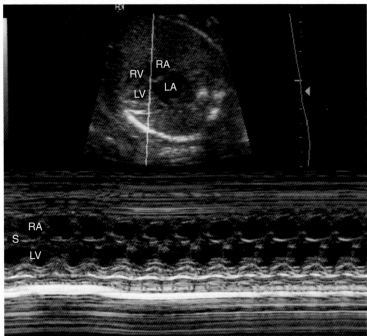

Figure 2–25 Proper M-mode cursor placement to evaluate an arrhythmia from a subcostal four-chamber view. M-mode cursor must traverse an atrial and ventricular wall at the same time. *LA,* Left atrium; *LV,* left ventricle; *RA,* right atrium; *RV,* right ventricle; *S,* spine.

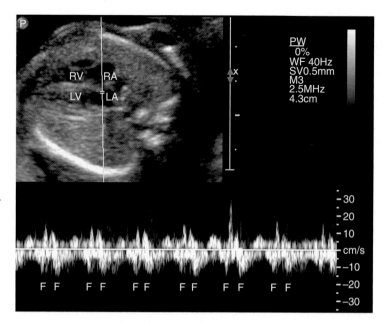

Figure 2–26 Normal pulsed Doppler tracing of flow traversing the foramen ovale from the right atrium *(RA)* into the left atrium *(LA)*. Foraminal flow *(FF)* normally occurs at twice the fetal heart rate. *LV,* Left ventricle; *RV,* right ventricle.

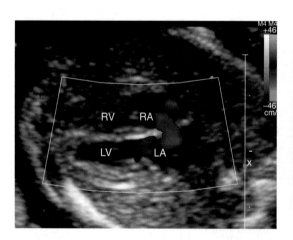

Figure 2–27 Confirming the presence of normal flow through the foramen ovale, from the right atrium *(RA)* to the left atrium *(LA)* with color Doppler imaging. *RV,* Right ventricle; *LV,* left ventricle.

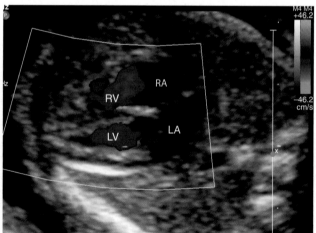

Figure 2–28 Using color Doppler imaging to evaluate the interventricular septum. If a large enough ventricular septal defect is present, color can often be seen traversing the septum. *LA,* Left atrium; *LV,* left ventricle; *RA,* right atrium; *RV,* right ventricle.

significantly throughout gestation. Color Doppler imaging through the aortic valve may also be useful in identifying anomalous jets.

The long-axis view of the aorta provides another useful means of evaluating an arrhythmia. By using a wide sample gate and placing the pulsed Doppler cursor between the mitral and aortic valves (Fig. 2–37), left ventricular inflow and outflow can be evaluated simultaneously. The inflow through the mitral valve reflects rhythm disturbances occurring in the atria, whereas the left ventricular outflow through the aorta reflects the ventricular response. Being able to visualize both events simultaneously may help in differentiating arrhythmias.

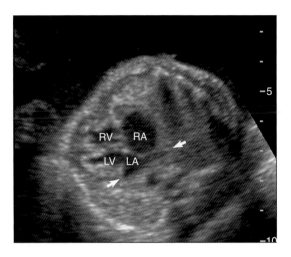

Figure 2–29 Identifying the two superior pulmonary veins *(arrows)* entering the left atrium in a subcostal four-chamber view. *LA,* Left atrium; *LV,* left ventricle; *RA,* right ventricle; *RV,* right ventricle.

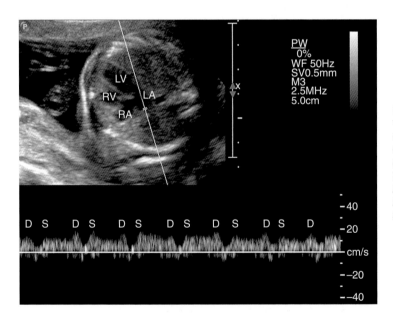

Figure 2–30 Evaluating the pulmonary veins with pulsed Doppler imaging to confirm the presence and normal direction of blood flow into the left atrium *(LA).* Normal pulmonary vein waveform is displayed above the baseline. *D,* Diastolic peak; *LV,* left ventricle; *RA,* right atrium; *RV,* right ventricle; *S,* systolic peak.

TABLE 2–8 Aortic and Pulmonary Valve Velocities in the Normal Fetus		
Valve	**Maximum Velocity (cm/sec)**	**Mean Velocity (cm/sec)**
Aorta	70 ± 2.6 (range 56–94)	18 ± 0.7 (range 13.7–22.5)
Pulmonary	60 ± 1.9 (range 42.1–81.6)	16 ± 0.6 (range 9.2–25.7)

Modified from Reed KL, Meijboom E, Sahn D, et al: Cardiac Doppler flow velocities in human fetuses. Circulation 1986; 73:41–46.

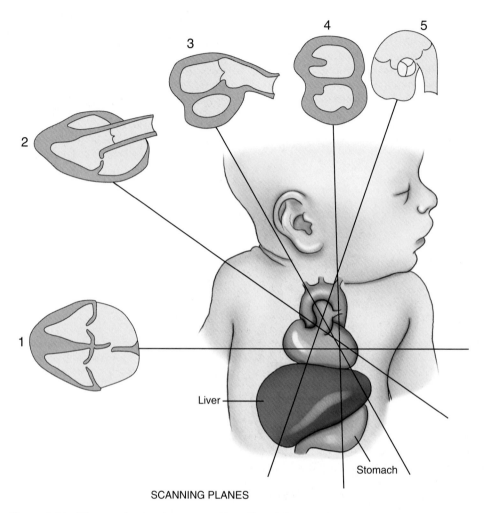

SCANNING PLANES

Figure 2–31   Diagram showing the systematic angling of the transducer necessary to obtain several fetal echocardiographic views. From a subcostal four-chamber view *(1)*, the transducer is angled toward the fetus' right shoulder to obtain a long-axis view of the aorta *(2)*, a long-axis view of the pulmonary artery *(3)*, a short-axis view of the ventricles *(4)*, and a short-axis view of the great vessels *(5)*. (Modified from Romero R, Pilu G, Jeanty P, et al: The heart. In: Romero R, Pilu G, Jeanty P, et al [eds]: Prenatal Diagnosis of Congenital Anomalies. Norwalk, CT, Appleton & Lange, 1988.)

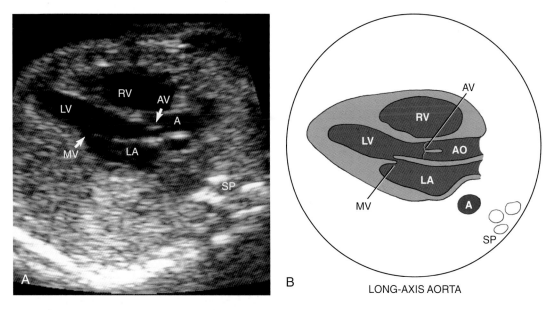

Figure 2–32 Sonogram of a long-axis view of the aorta **(A)** and schematic of a long-axis view of the aorta **(B)**. *A,* Descending aorta; *AO,* aorta; *AV,* aortic valve; *LA,* left atrium; *LV,* left ventricle; *MV,* mitral valve; *RV,* right ventricle; *SP,* spine.

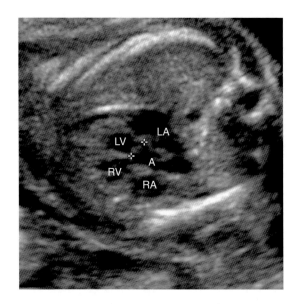

Figure 2–33 Measurement (calipers) of the aorta *(A)* at the level of the valve from a long-axis view. *LA,* Left atrium; *LV,* left ventricle; *RA,* right atrium; *RV,* right ventricle.

Uses for Long-Axis View of the Pulmonary Artery

Evaluate continuity of pulmonary artery with right ventricle

Doppler imaging of pulmonic valve above and below valve

Long-Axis View of the Pulmonary Artery

The right ventricular outflow tract can be visualized by rotating the transducer further in the direction of the fetal right shoulder. In the normal fetus, this view demonstrates the pulmonary artery coursing cephalad, leftward, and posteriorly from the right ventricle (Fig. 2–38) (Box 2–5). The course of the pulmonary artery should cross that of the aorta in the normal fetus. In other words, by angling the transducer from the long-axis view of

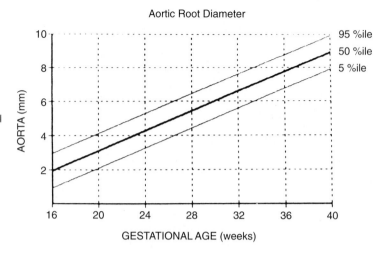

Figure 2–34 Normal aortic root diameter plotted against gestational age. (From Cartier MS, Davidoff A, Warneke LA, et al: The normal diameter of the fetal aorta and pulmonary artery: Echocardiographic evaluation in utero. AJR Am J Roentgenol 1987; 149:1003–1007.)

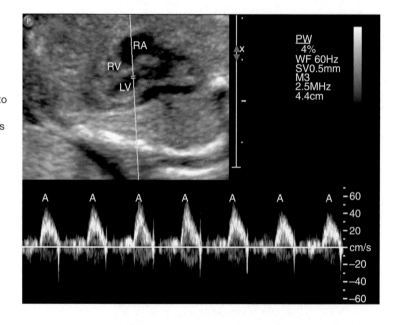

Figure 2–35 Pulsed Doppler imaging to interrogate the aortic valve for valvular insufficiency. Proper cursor placement is proximal to the aortic valve, in the left ventricle *(LV)*. Aortic inflow *(A)* is seen above the baseline. If valvular insufficiency was present, it would be displayed as retrograde flow below the baseline in diastole. *RA,* Right atrium; *RV,* right ventricle.

the aorta to the long-axis view of the pulmonary artery, the great vessels should "criss-cross" directions if they are oriented correctly.

The pulmonary artery can be measured in this view at the level of the pulmonic valve and correlated with gestational age (Fig. 2–39). Color Doppler or pulsed Doppler imaging, or both, are again used in this projection to evaluate the valve proximally (Fig. 2–40) for pulmonic insufficiency and distally (Fig. 2–41) for pulmonic stenosis.

Normal pulmonic velocities have also been established (Fig. 2–42).

Short-Axis View of the Ventricles

A further rightward rotation of the transducer results in a sagittal view of the fetal thorax and a short-axis view through the ventricles (Fig. 2–43). The more echogenic moderator band should be apparent near the apex to help identify the right ventricle.

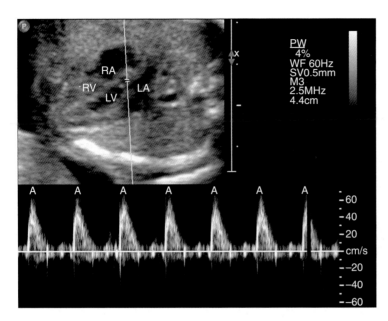

Figure 2–36 Pulsed Doppler imaging to interrogate the aortic valve for stenosis. Proper cursor placement is distal to the aortic valve, in the ascending aorta. Aortic outflow *(A)* is seen above the baseline. *LA,* Left atrium; *LV,* left ventricle; *RA,* right atrium; *RV,* right ventricle.

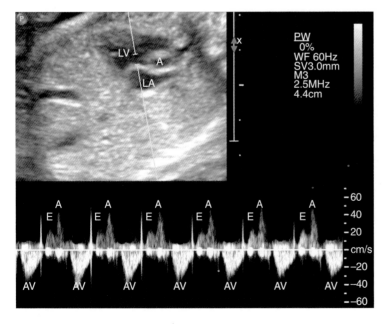

Figure 2–37 Pulsed Doppler imaging is used in a long-axis view of the aorta to evaluate fetal arrhythmias. The sample volume should be placed in the left ventricular outflow tract, with the sample gate opened wide enough to receive mitral inflow (normal E point–A point relationship displayed above the baseline) and aortic outflow *(AV)* simultaneously. *A,* Aorta; *LA,* left atrium; *LV,* left ventricle.

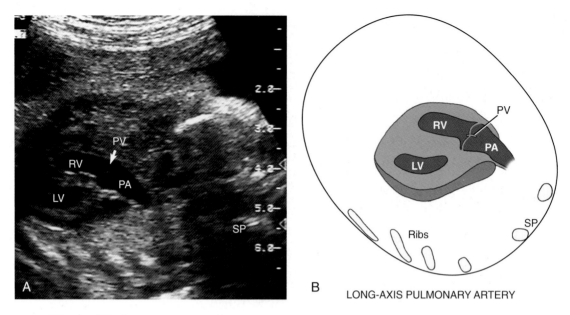

Figure 2–38 Sonogram of a long-axis view of the pulmonary artery **(A)** and schematic of a long-axis view of the pulmonary artery **(B).** *LV,* Left ventricle; *PA,* pulmonary artery; *PV,* pulmonic valve; *RV,* right ventricle; *SP,* spine.

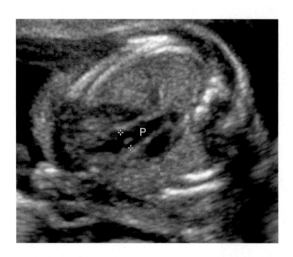

Figure 2–39 Measurement of the pulmonary artery *(P)* (cursors) at the level of the pulmonic valve in a long-axis view.

The short-axis view of the ventricles is useful for obtaining measurements of the ventricular free walls, interventricular septum, and chamber size (Fig. 2–44) (Box 2–6). Color Doppler imaging should again be used in this view to evaluate the interventricular septum for defects. With the color turned on, the ventricles should be scanned from the apex to the level of the AV valves (Fig. 2–45). If color is seen crossing the septum, pulsed Doppler imaging can be used to confirm the presence of a septal defect.

Short-Axis View of the Great Vessels

From the short-axis view of the ventricles, a short-axis view of the great vessels can be obtained by angling the transducer slightly toward the fetal left shoulder (Fig. 2–46). In this view, the aorta appears as a circular structure with the pulmonary artery coursing over it. The aortic, pulmonic, and tricuspid valves are usually well visualized in this projection. With appropriate resolution, the three valve leaflets of the aorta can often be appreciated (Fig. 2–47). The main pulmonary artery can be seen bifurcating into the ductus arteriosus and the right pulmonary artery (Box 2–7).[87]

Measurements of the proximal aorta and the pulmonary artery at the level of the valves can be obtained from this projection (Fig. 2–48). This is also an ideal view from which to interrogate the pulmonary and tricuspid valves for insufficiency

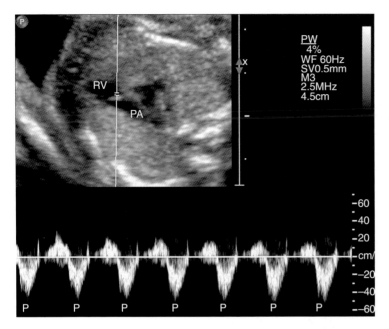

Figure 2–40 Pulsed Doppler imaging to evaluate the pulmonic valve for insufficiency. Proper cursor placement is proximal to the valve, in the right ventricle *(RV)*. Normal pulmonary inflow *(P)* is displayed below the baseline. If valvular insufficiency was present, retrograde flow would be seen in the right ventricle (above the baseline) during diastole. *PA,* Pulmonary artery.

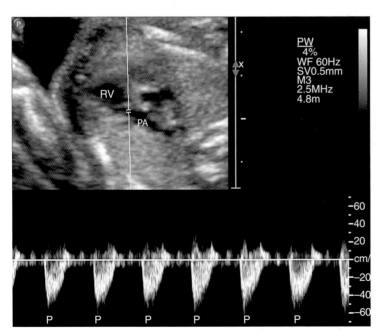

Figure 2–41 Pulsed Doppler imaging to evaluate the pulmonic valve for stenosis. Proper cursor placement is distal to the valve, in the pulmonary artery *(PA)*. Normal pulmonic outflow *(P)* is seen below the baseline. *RV,* Right ventricle.

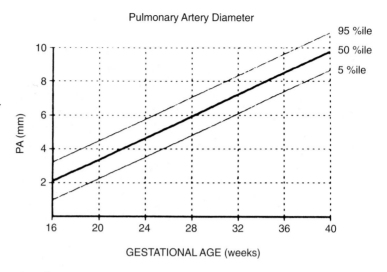

Figure 2–42 Normal pulmonary artery diameter plotted against gestational age. (From Cartier MS, Davidoff A, Warneke LA, et al: The normal diameter of the fetal aorta and pulmonary artery: Echocardiographic evaluation in utero. AJR Am J Roentgenol 1987; 149:1003–1007.)

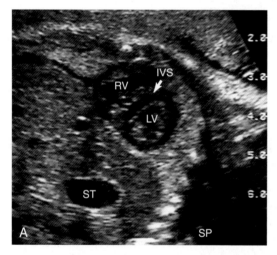
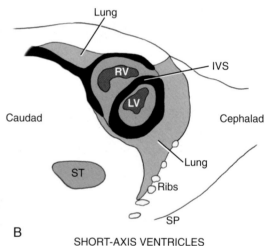

Figure 2–43 Sonogram of a short-axis view of the ventricles **(A)** and schematic of a short-axis view of the ventricles **(B)**. *IVS,* Interventricular septum; *LV,* left ventricle; *RV,* right ventricle; *SP,* spine; *ST,* stomach.

BOX 2–6

Uses for Short-Axis View of the Ventricles

Evaluate interventricular septum for ventricular septal defect from apex to level of atrioventricular valves
Measure ventricular size with M-mode or calipers
Measure interventricular septum and left ventricular and right ventricular heart walls with M-mode or calipers
Evaluate heart wall contractility with M-mode

BOX 2–7

Uses for Short-Axis View of the Great Vessels

Evaluate relationship of aorta to pulmonary artery
Measure size of aortic valve and pulmonic valve with calipers
Doppler imaging of pulmonic valve above and below valve
Doppler imaging of tricuspid valve above and below valve
Place M-mode cursor through aorta and left atrium to evaluate arrhythmia

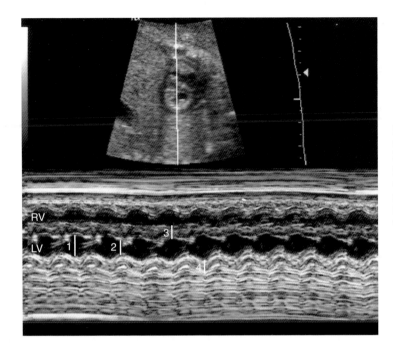

Figure 2–44   M-mode cursor placed through the right ventricle *(RV)* and the left ventricle *(LV)* in a short-axis projection. Measurements can be obtained of the ventricles in end-diastole *(1)* and end-systole *(2)* and of the interventricular septum *(3)* and posterior ventricular wall *(4)*.

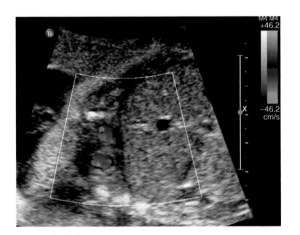

Figure 2–45   Color Doppler imaging to evaluate the ventricles in a short-axis view. No color is seen crossing the interventricular septum.

BOX 2–8

Uses for Aortic Arch View

Assess diameter of arch for areas of narrowing
Doppler imaging of aortic arch from aortic valve
   to descending aorta for coarctation
Confirm antigrade flow
Quantitate peak systolic velocity

(proximal to the valve) (Figs. 2–49 and 2–50) or stenosis (distal to the valve) (Figs. 2–51 and 2–52) because a reasonable Doppler interrogation angle is usually obtainable.

Simultaneous M-mode placement through the aorta and left atrium, which is located posterior to the aorta in this projection, is another useful method for evaluating fetal arrhythmias (Fig. 2–53). The atrial contraction will be depicted in atrial wall movement, whereas the ventricular response is reflected in the motion of the aortic valve or the wall of the right ventricle.

In the normal heart, this short-axis view confirms the perpendicular relationship of the aorta to the pulmonary artery, thereby excluding certain defects such as transposition of the great arteries and truncus arteriosus.

View of the Aortic Arch

The aortic arch view is obtained from a longitudinal plane of the fetal torso, with the transducer angled from the left shoulder to the right hemithorax (Fig. 2–54) (Box 2–8). The aortic arch can

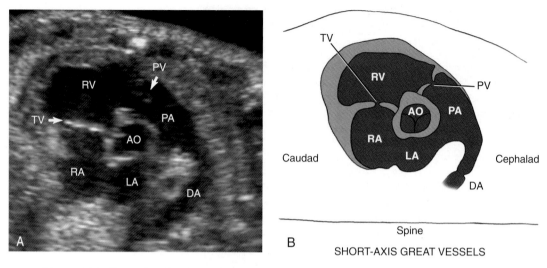

Figure 2–46   Sonogram of a short-axis view of the great vessels **(A)** and schematic of a short-axis view of the great vessels **(B)**. *AO,* Aorta; *DA,* ductus arteriosus; *LA,* left atrium; *PA,* pulmonary artery; *PV,* pulmonic valve; *RA,* right atrium; *RV,* right ventricle; *TV,* tricuspid valve.

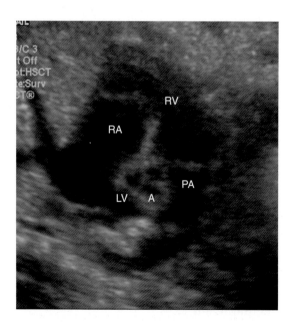

Figure 2–47   All three leaflets of the aortic valve *(A)* can often be identified in a short axis view of the great vessels. *LA,* Left atrium; *PA,* pulmonary artery; *RA,* right atrium; *RV,* right ventricle.

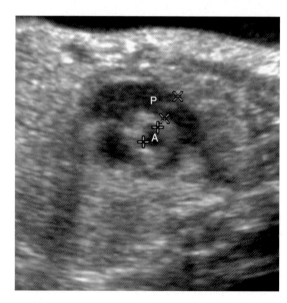

Figure 2–48   Measurement of the aortic *(A)* and pulmonary *(P)* arteries at the level of the valves in a short-axis view of the great vessels.

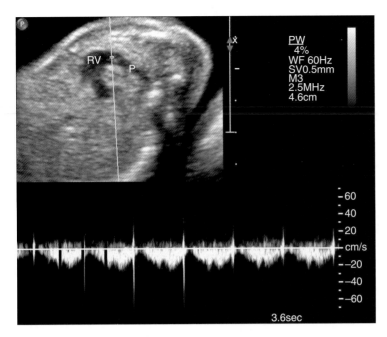

Figure 2–49 Pulsed Doppler imaging to evaluate the pulmonic valve for insufficiency from a short-axis view. Proper cursor placement is proximal to the valve, within the right ventricle *(RV)*. Normal inflow can be seen below the baseline. If valvular insufficiency was present, it would be displayed as retrograde flow (above the baseline) into the right ventricle during diastole. *P,* Pulmonary artery.

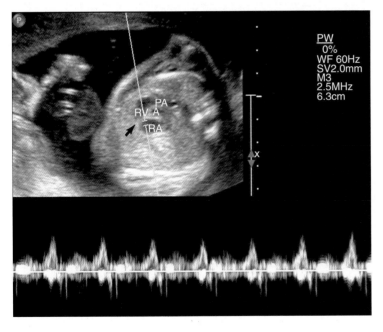

Figure 2–50 Pulsed Doppler imaging to evaluate the tricuspid valve for insufficiency from a short-axis view. The cursor is placed proximal to the tricuspid valve *(arrow)* in the right atrium *(RA)*. Normal tricuspid inflow is seen above the baseline. *A,* Aorta; *PA,* pulmonary artery; *RV,* right ventricle.

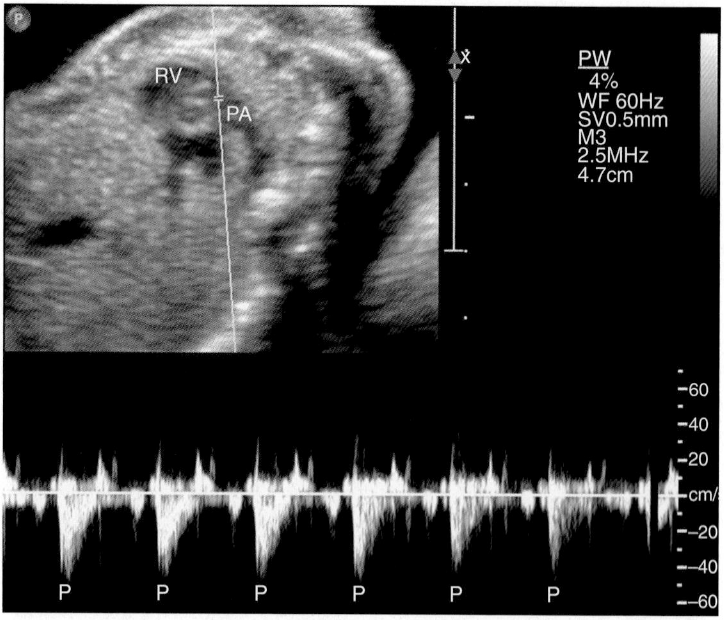

Figure 2–51 Pulsed Doppler imaging to evaluate the pulmonic valve for stenosis. Proper cursor placement is distal to the valve, in the pulmonary artery *(PA)*. Normal pulmonic outflow *(P)* is displayed below the baseline. *RV,* Right ventricle.

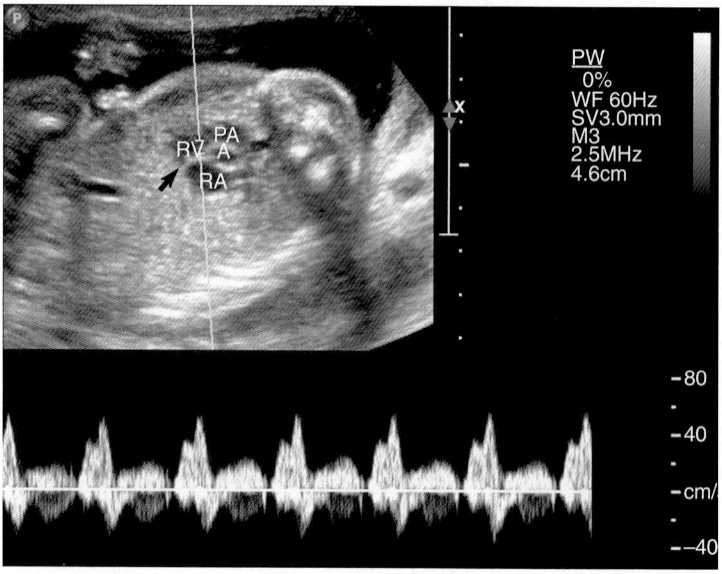

Figure 2–52 Pulsed Doppler imaging to evaluate the tricuspid valve for stenosis in a short axis view of the great vessels. Proper cursor placement is distal to the valve *(arrow),* in the right ventricle *(RV).* Normal tricuspid valve outflow is seen above the baseline. *A,* Aorta; *PA,* pulmonary artery; *RA,* right atrium.

be differentiated from the flatter, broader, more caudally located ductal arch by identifying the three head and neck vessels arising from its superior aspect (brachiocephalic artery, left common carotid artery, left subclavian artery) (Fig. 2–55).

The aortic arch has been described as having a rounded "candy cane" appearance.[61]

The diameter of the aortic arch can be measured at various levels in this view to aid in the diagnosis of coarctation or aortic atresia (see

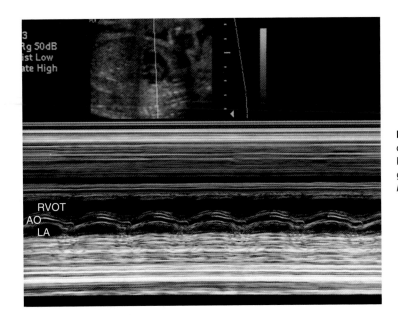

Figure 2–53 Directing an M-mode cursor through the aortic root *(AO)* and left atrium *(LA)* in a short-axis view of the great vessels to evaluate an arrhythmia. *RVOT,* Right ventricular outflow tract.

Chapter 11).[88] Color Doppler imaging may be useful for confirming patency and excluding areas of narrowing within the aorta (Fig. 2–56). Pulsed Doppler imaging should also be used to evaluate the arch from the aortic valve to the descending aorta, looking for areas of increased or decreased velocities (Fig. 2–57). Of particular importance is the section of the arch between the left subclavian artery takeoff and the insertion of the ductus arteriosus because this is where most in utero coarctations occur. Normal velocity through the aortic arch is usually defined as a peak systolic velocity of 120 cm/sec or less throughout gestation.[89] It should be borne in mind, however, that diagnosis of coarctation of the aorta is extremely difficult, and a coarctation may be present even in the setting of a normal-appearing aortic arch with normal velocities. Additionally, coarctations may not occur until after birth. When the aortic arch is being evaluated, it is also important to remember to confirm a left-sided location of the descending aorta. This is optimally done from the three-vessel view or by identifying the descending aorta to the left of the fetal spine in a transverse plane of the fetal chest.

View of the Ductal Arch

The ductal arch view is obtained by returning to a more anteroposterior axis of the thorax. It is

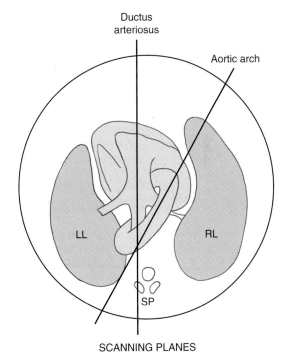

Figure 2–54 Diagram showing the appropriate transducer orientation for obtaining images of the ductus arteriosus and the aortic arch. *LL,* Left lung; *RL,* right lung; *SP,* spine. (Modified from Romero R, Pilu G, Jeanty P, et al: The heart. In: Romero R, Pilu G, Jeanty P, et al. [eds]: Prenatal Diagnosis of Congenital Anomalies. Norwalk, CT, Appleton & Lange, 1988, p 128.)

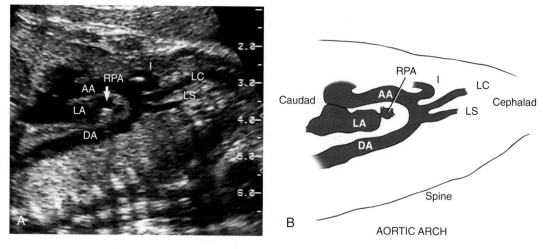

Figure 2–55 Sonogram of the aortic arch **(A)** and schematic of the aortic arch **(B)**. *AA,* Ascending aorta; *DA,* descending artery; *I,* innominate artery; *LA,* left atrium; *LC,* left carotid artery; *LS,* left subclavian artery; *RPA,* right pulmonary artery.

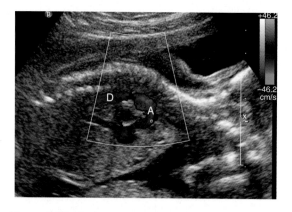

Figure 2–56 Evaluating the aortic arch with color Doppler imaging. Color shows blood flow moving from the ascending aorta, through the aortic arch *(A)* and down the descending aorta *(D).*

BOX 2–9

Uses for Ductal Arch View

Doppler imaging of ductal arch from pulmonary artery to descending aorta
Confirm antigrade flow
Quantitate peak systolic velocity

---

often helpful to image the short-axis view of the great vessels and then angle the transducer slightly until the pulmonary artery–ductus arteriosus confluence connects with the descending aorta (Fig. 2–58). The appearance of the ductal arch is flatter than that of the aortic arch. It is often referred to as a "hockey stick" appearance.[61] The ductal arch is composed of the pulmonary artery, ductus arteriosus, and descending aorta (Box 2–9).

The configuration of the ductus arteriosus is variable and has been reported to take on a greater curvature as pregnancy progresses.[87] By late in the third trimester, a majority of fetuses have a markedly curved ductus arteriosus with a configuration that appears as either a sharply angled C shape or an S shape. Such a configuration should not be misinterpreted as an anomaly in a fetus with an otherwise normal heart.

Brezinka et al[89] and Van der Mooren et al[90] have both published data showing that both peak systolic and diastolic velocities in the ductus arteriosus increase as gestational age increases. This linear increase has been confirmed by other studies.[91] No correlation between peak systolic velocity and fetal heart rate has been observed. [89-92]

Mielke and Benda[92] developed nomograms of normal ductal velocities based on a prospective study of 222 fetuses from 13 to 41 weeks of gestation (Fig. 2–59).

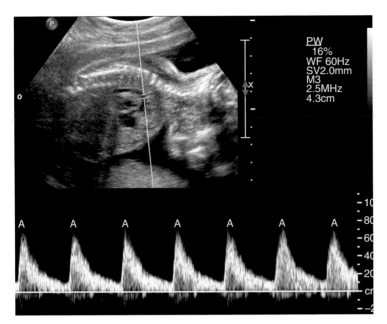

Figure 2–57 Pulsed Doppler evaluation of the aortic arch, showing normal aortic blood flow displayed above the baseline *(A)*.

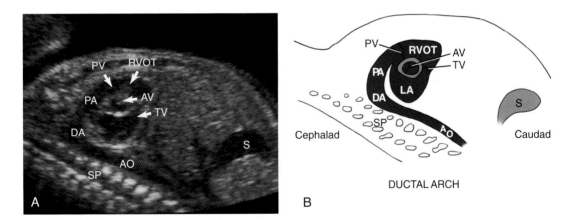

Figure 2–58 Sonogram of the ductal arch **(A)** and schematic of the ductal arch **(B)**. *AO,* Descending aorta; *AV,* aortic valve; *DA,* ductus arteriosus; *LA,* left atrium; *PA,* pulmonary artery; *PV,* pulmonary valve; *RVOT,* right ventricular outflow tract; *S,* stomach; *SP,* spine; *TV,* tricuspid valve.

An increase in peak systolic velocity in the ductus arteriosus of greater than 1.4 M/sec has been reported in cases of ductal constriction.[93] Ductal constriction in the fetus has been reported after maternal indomethacin, glucocorticoid, or nimesulide therapy. This is usually transient, with constriction regressing after medication is discontinued.[92-95] Increased peak velocity can also be observed in the presence of right ventricular outflow tract obstruction, anemia, and high cardiac output.[92] With severe right ventricular outflow tract obstruction, reversed blood flow across the

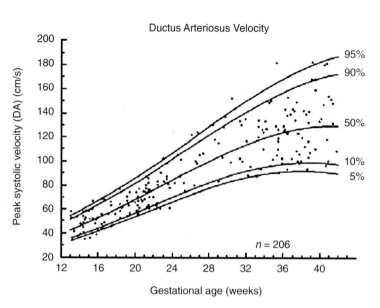

Figure 2–59 Peak systolic velocity (percentiles) plotted against gestational age in the ductus arteriosus. (From Mielek G, Benda N: Blood flow velocity waveforms of the fetal pulmonary artery and the ductus arteriosus: Reference ranges from 13 weeks to term. 2000; 15:213–218. © Ultrasound Obstet Gynecol. Reproduced with permission. Permission is granted by John Wiley & Sons Ltd on behalf of the ISUOG.)

ductus arteriosus may be present. Late in pregnancy, ductal velocities may increase as a result of increased tortuosity of the vessel.

Decreased peak velocities can be observed in the ductus arteriosus with intrauterine growth restriction.[96]

View of the Inferior Vena Cava and Superior Vena Cava

An inferior vena cava–superior vena cava or right atrial inflow view can be obtained by acquiring an aortic arch view and then sliding the transducer from the left parasagittal chest to the right parasagittal chest. In this view, the inferior vena cava and the superior vena cava should be identified entering the right atrium (Fig. 2–60)[72] (Box 2–10).

Three-Vessel View

The three-vessel view is very useful to access the great vessels (Box 2–11). It is obtained by acquiring an apical four-chamber view and then sliding the transducer cephalad. In this view the pulmonary artery at the level of the ductus arteriosus, the aortic arch, and the superior vena cava are seen in the same plane (Fig. 2–61).[97] This allows identification of the two great vessels and a side-by-side comparison of size. Color Doppler imaging in this view will confirm antegrade blood flow through both outflow tracts in a normal heart (Fig. 2–62). If reversed flow is visualized in one of the great vessels, severe outflow obstruction should be suspected. In a normal fetal heart, the pulmonary artery and the aorta lay in a "V" formation, in this plane, with the confluence of the V pointing to the posterior thorax (see Fig. 2–54). If this "V" formation is not present, anomalies of great vessel origination, such as transposition of the great arteries, should be investigated. By moving the transducer even more cephalad, the trachea can also be visualized and can be used to determine the situs of the aorta. In the normal fetal heart, both the aortic and ductal arches should be leftward of the trachea (Fig. 2–63). If a right-sided aortic arch is seen, an increased risk of other congenital heart abnormalities is present. The presence of a forth vessel at this level would be consistent with a persistent left superior vena cava (Fig. 2–64). The three-vessel view has also shown to be reliable for obtaining peak systolic velocities across the aortic arch, depending on the available Doppler angle.[98]

Surrounding Structures

In addition to evaluating the heart itself, attention should be paid to structures surrounding the heart that, if present may be indicative of congenital heart disease or associated abnormalities.

Interruption of the inferior vena cava with azygous continuation can be diagnosed in the fetus by identifying the "double-vessel" sign.[99] On a transverse image of the fetal chest, at the level of the

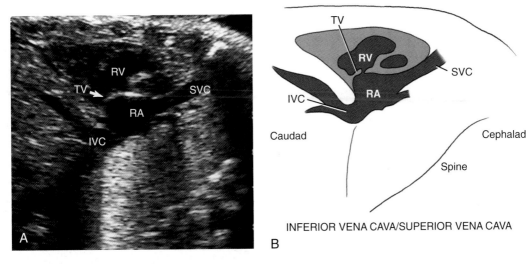

Figure 2–60 A, Sonogram of the inferior vena cava *(IVC)* and superior vena cava *(SVC).*
B, Schematic of the inferior and superior venae cavae. *RA,* Right atrium; *RV,* right ventricle;
TV, tricuspid valve.

BOX 2–10

Uses for Superior Vena Cava/Inferior Vena Cava View

Identify superior vena cava and inferior vena cava entering right atrium

Doppler imaging of superior vena cava and inferior vena cava to confirm presence, direction, and characteristics of waveforms

---

BOX 2–11

Uses for Three-Vessel View

Identify presence of pulmonary artery, aorta, and superior vena cava

Identify "V" configuration of pulmonary artery and aorta

Identify pulmonary artery and aorta to the left of the trachea

Subjective comparison of great vessel size

Apply color Doppler imaging to both great vessels to confirm same-direction blood flow

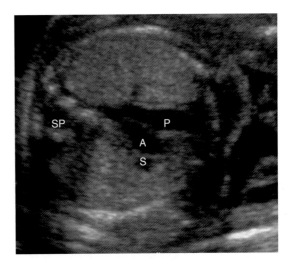

Figure 2–61 Three-vessel view used to evaluate the aorta *(A)* and pulmonary artery *(P)* at the level of the arches. The superior vena cava *(S)* can be seen to the right of the aorta. *SP,* Spine.

---

four-chamber view, the descending aorta should be seen as a circular structure just anterior to and leftward of the fetal spine. If two circular structures are identified at this level, the more rightward structure should be a dilated azygous vein, which acts as a collateral vessel when the inferior vena cava is interrupted (Fig. 2–65). Azygous continuation of the inferior vena cava has a very high association with the cardiosplenic syndromes, specifically polysplenia. Therefore, if a "double-vessel"

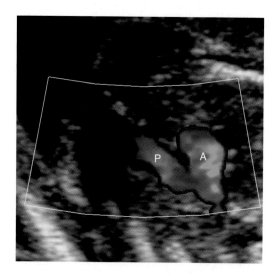

Figure 2–62 Color Doppler imaging in the three-vessel view to evaluate the direction of blood flow. *A,* Aorta; *P,* pulmonary artery.

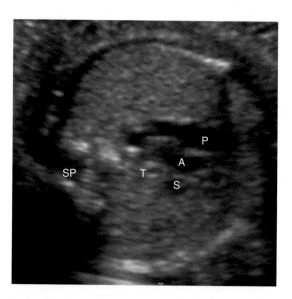

Figure 2–63 Three-vessel view showing the aorta *(A)* and pulmonary artery *(P)* normally positioned to the left of the trachea *(T). S,* Superior vena cava; *SP,* spine.

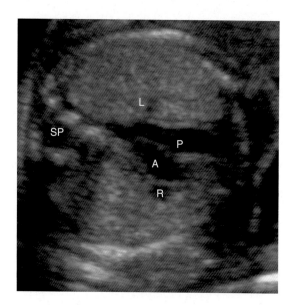

Figure 2–64 A persistent left superior vena cava *(L)* seen to the left of the pulmonary artery *(P)* in the three-vessel view. The right superior vena cava *(R)* is seen in its normal position to the right of the aorta *(A). SP,* Spine.

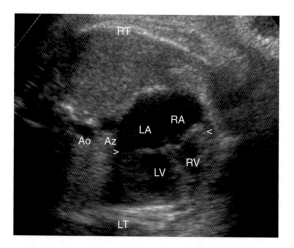

Figure 2–65 A dilated azygous vein *(Az)* anterior to the aorta *(Ao)* in a patient with an atrioventricular septal defect and polysplenia. The azygous vein is dilated as a result of interruption of the inferior vena cava. The *arrows* denote the single multileaflet atrioventricular valve. *LA,* Left atrium; *LT,* left side of fetal chest; *LV,* left ventricle; *RA,* right atrium; *RT,* right side of fetal chest; *RV,* right ventricle.

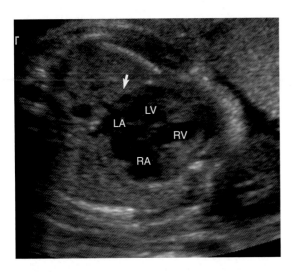

Figure 2–66 Persistent left superior vena cava *(arrow)* seen to the left of the fetal heart. *RA,* Right atrium; *RV,* right ventricle; *LA,* left atrium; *LV,* left ventricle.

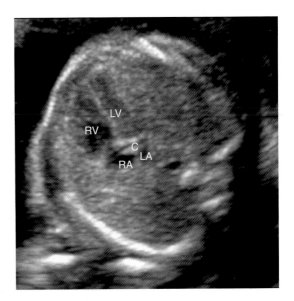

Figure 2–67 Normal coronary sinus *(C)* seen between the left atrium *(LA)* and the left ventricle *(LV),* draining into the right atrium *(RA)* in the four-chamber view. *RV,* Right ventricle.

sign is identified, the abdominal organs should be evaluated for abnormal situs, and the heart itself should be thoroughly evaluated for associated structural or rhythm abnormalities.

Another accessory vessel that is associated with an increased risk of congenital heart disease is a *persistent left superior vena cava.* On a transverse image of the fetal chest, at the level of the four-chamber view, a persistent left superior vena cava will appear as a circular structure to the left of the fetal heart, usually at the level of the AV groove (Fig. 2–66). A persistent left superior vena cava results from failure of degeneration of the left cardinal vein.[100] This anatomical variant is seen in approximately 0.3% of the general population. In neonates with known congenital heart disease, an increased prevalence is appreciated. Erdogan et al[100] reported an incidence of 3.3% in patients undergoing surgery for congenital heart disease. Therefore identification of this structure should also spur a thorough evaluation of the fetal heart. All persistent left superior vena cavae drain into the coronary sinus, usually causing it to enlarge.[101] The coronary sinus can be visualized in most fetal hearts as a tubular structure between the left atrium and left ventricle. It is easier to see in this setting because of its increase in size (Fig. 2–67). A right-sided superior vena cava is usually also

present with a persistent left superior vena cava. Absence of the normal right sided superior vena cava is reported in 20% of cases.[100]

The area surrounding the four-chamber heart should also be evaluated for extra structures arising from the heart itself, such as *cor triatriatum,* which is an additional chamber arising from the left atrium. Structures arising from the ventricles include *aneurysms* or *diverticula* (Fig. 2–68). A diverticulum is usually defined as a localized protrusion of the ventricular wall with a narrow connection to the ventricle.[102] Cardiac aneurysms, on the other hand, are defined as having large openings into the ventricle. All these anomalies can occur in isolation or in association with other congenital heart defects. Aneurysms or diverticula of the ventricles can also impede myocardial function, resulting is signs of congestive heart failure such as pericardial effusion.[102]

Pitfalls

Several potential pitfalls, such as the previously mentioned *pseudoventricular septal defect,* may be encountered during a fetal echocardiogram.[71] The following sections discuss the problems that may be encountered.

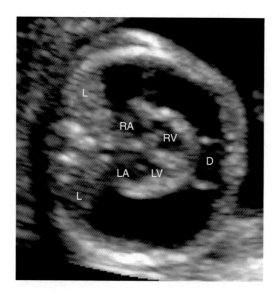

Figure 2–68 Diverticulum *(D)* arising from the right ventricle *(RV)*. A massive pericardial effusion that compresses the fetal lungs *(L)* is also visualized. *LA,* Left atrium; *LV,* left ventricle; *RA,* right atrium; *RV,* right ventricle.

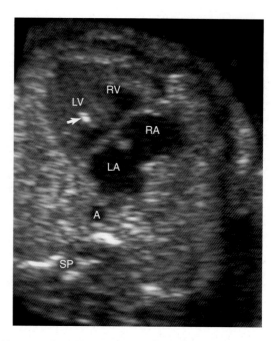

Figure 2–70 Echogenic focus *(arrow)* within the left ventricle *(LV)*. A, Aorta; *LA,* left atrium; *RA,* right atrium; *RV,* right ventricle; *SP,* spine.

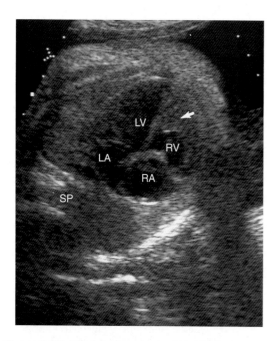

Figure 2–69 Thickened moderator band *(arrow)* mimicking an abnormality. *LA,* Left atrium; *LV,* left ventricle; *RA,* right atrium; *RV,* right ventricle; *SP,* spine.

Prominent Moderator Band

The moderator band located within the right ventricle may vary in prominence, occasionally mimicking a heart tumor or a thickened heart wall (Fig. 2–69). Evaluating this area in several projections should reassure the examiner that he or she is visualizing a normal variant.[71]

Echogenic Foci

Observing an echogenic focus within the ventricle in the region of the papillary muscle or chordae tendineae is not unusual (Fig. 2–70). As technology improves the resolution of ultrasound equipment, this finding has become commonplace. These foci are usually seen within the left ventricle (92.8%) but may be seen in the right ventricle (4.8%) or in both ventricles (2.4%).[103] This finding is thought to represent increased beam reflection on a normal papillary muscle or chordae tendineae and is commonly thought to be of no clinical significance.[71,104,105] Past literature reported an increased incidence of echogenic foci in the setting of a chromosome abnormality.[106-108] However, more recent literature indicates that echogenic foci found in isolation in an otherwise low-

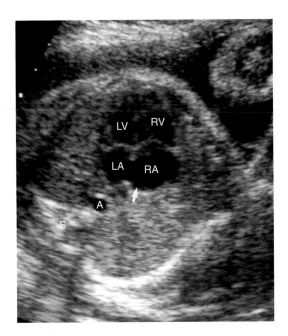

Figure 2–71 Normal eustachian valve *(arrow)* within the right atrium *(RA)*. *A,* Aorta; *LA,* left atrium; *LV,* left ventricle; *RV,* right ventricle; *S,* spine.

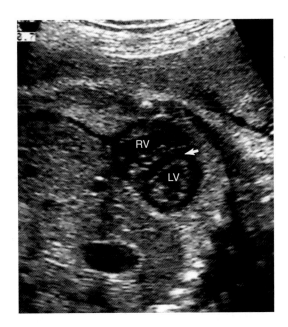

Figure 2–72 Short-axis view of the ventricles, showing the hypoechoic myocardium *(arrow)* transecting the interventricular septum. *LV,* Left ventricle; *RV,* right ventricle.

risk pregnancy carries no increase in the risk of trisomy and should be considered a normal variant.[109-111]

Linear Structure Within the Right Atrium

Several linear structures may be visualized within the right atrium. A fixed linear echo extending from the anterior junction of the inferior vena cava within the right atrium toward the foramen ovale represents the normal eustachian valve (Fig. 2–71).

Multiple linear echoes are unusual but can represent the Chiari network.[71] This network is visible when the resorptive process of the embryonic right valve of the sinus venosus leaves a fenestrated network of fibers. It is not believed to have any functional significance, although it has been reported in a fetus with premature atrial and ventricular contractions.[112]

Pseudopericardial Fluid

The peripheral rim of the myocardium usually appears hypoechoic and has been confused with a pericardial effusion.[113] This confusion is eliminated by obtaining a short-axis view of the ven-

tricles in which a pseudoeffusion will be seen coursing through the interventricular septum (Fig. 2–72). Obviously, a true effusion would not be within the septum; therefore normal myocardium can be confirmed. In a four-chamber view, a true pericardial effusion should extend above the AV groove, which is located at the level of the mitral and tricuspid valves. Hypoechoic myocardium will not extend above the AV groove (Fig. 2–73).

Pseudothickening of the Tricuspid Valve

An arch-shaped band of muscle, the parietal band or supraventricular crest, located between the tricuspid and pulmonary valves may be mistaken for a thickened tricuspid valve.[71] This misconception is usually created by angling too superiorly from the standard apical four-chamber view (Fig. 2–74). An inferior angulation correction will usually allow identification of the normal tricuspid valve leaflets.

Pseudo-Overriding of the Aorta

The appearance of a pseudo-overriding aorta is usually created in a long-axis view of the aorta or

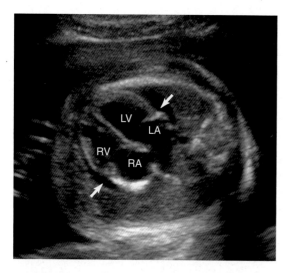

Figure 2–73 True pericardial effusion extending above the atrioventricular grooves *(arrow)* in the four-chamber view. *LA,* Left atrium; *LV,* left ventricle; *RA,* right atrium; *RV,* right ventricle.

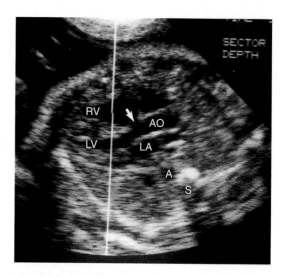

Figure 2–75 "Pseudo"-overriding of the aorta *(AO)*. A long-axis view with artifactual dropout of septal echos *(arrow)*, causing the appearance of an overriding aorta. *A,* Descending aorta; *LA,* left atrium; *LV,* left ventricle; *RV,* right ventricle; *S,* spine.

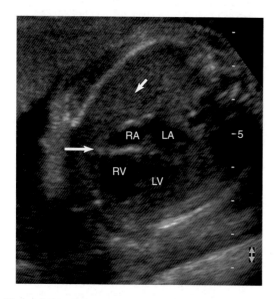

Figure 2–74 Parietal band *(arrow)* within the right side of the heart mimicking a thickened tricuspid valve. *LA,* Left atrium; *LV,* left ventricle; *RA,* right atrium; *RV,* right ventricle.

in an apical five-chamber view (Fig. 2–75). It is thought to be a result of the artifactual dropout that can be created in the thin membranous portion of the septum. To prevent mistaking this artifact for an abnormality, different views should

be obtained. True overriding would be apparent in several planes.[71]

Parallel Great Vessels

Parallel courses of the aorta and pulmonary artery can be indicative of several heart abnormalities, such as transposition of the great arteries or double-outlet right ventricle. However, this orientation can be created in the normal heart if these vessels are imaged distal to the valves at the level of the aortic arch (three-vessel view) (Fig. 2–76). At this level, the aorta and pulmonary artery–ductus arteriosus continuum normally run in a parallel fashion for a short segment. Imaging the normal orientation of the great vessels in a short-axis view should obviate mistaking this for an abnormal orientation.[71]

Whenever a questionable area is identified during a fetal echocardiogram, several different imaging planes should be attempted. In most cases, this should help distinguish normal variants from true abnormalities.

Pulsed Doppler Echocardiography

Pulsed Doppler imaging substantially enhances the ability to detect cardiac malformations in utero. It is an effective means of quantitating flow velocity in the heart vessels and across the heart valves and of determining flow direction. Additionally, it is a useful adjunct in differentiating arrhythmias.[114]

In a standard fetal echocardiogram, Doppler imaging should be used to evaluate all four cardiac valves, both proximal and distal to the valve. Doppler interrogation of the foramen ovale should be performed to document the presence of flow into the left atrium. The ductus arteriosus and aortic arch should also be interrogated to document the presence, direction, and velocity of flow. It should be borne in mind that measurement of absolute flow on the basis of flow velocity determinations is prone to error in the fetus. These inaccuracies occur because of the inability to obtain reasonable angles of insonation routinely in the fetus. This angle dependence, however, does not affect relative changes in flow velocity, such as during an ectopic beat, when the fetus acts as its own control.[115]

Technical factors to consider include attempting to place the Doppler cursor in the area of interest at an angle as close to 0 degrees as possible with use of the angle correction capabilities of the equipment. The sample gate should be set small enough so that interference from wall noise and transmitted flow from adjoining vessels or valves can be minimized.[116] The wall filter should be set to eliminate unnecessary noise without losing essential low-flow information, and the velocity scale (pulse repetition frequency) should be set to record maximum velocities accurately.[115–121]

Pulsed Doppler Imaging of the Aortic and Pulmonic Valves

Peak systolic velocities are measured across the aortic and pulmonic valves by placing the Doppler sample volume just distal to the valve. These peak velocities are predominantly determined by ventricular contractility and afterload. Normal peak systolic velocities of the aortic and pulmonic valves are usually reported to be around 120 cm/sec throughout gestation. However, these velocities may normally exceed the reported values late in gestation. In the setting of valvular stenosis, the peak systolic velocity will be markedly increased because of narrowing of the valve. In some instances, the valve may appear normal by two-dimensional imaging, with the stenosis only being diagnosed by pulsed Doppler evaluation. To access the aortic and pulmonic valves for insufficiency,

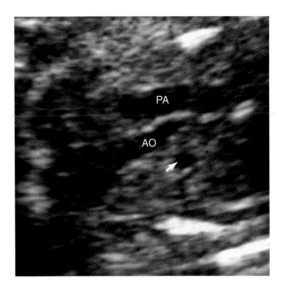

Figure 2–76 Normal parallel course of the aorta *(AO)* and pulmonary artery *(PA)* occurring distal to the semilunar valves at approximately the level of the aortic arch. The *arrow* shows the superior vena cava.

the pulsed Doppler cursor is placed proximal to the valve in the respective ventricle. Retrograde flow in the respective ventricular chamber during diastole is diagnostic for valvular insufficiency or regurgitation. When valvular insufficiency is appreciated, a downstream stenosis or atresia should be investigated.

Pulsed Doppler Imaging of the Mitral and Tricuspid Valves

Normal blood flow through the mitral and tricuspid valves occurs in diastole. The characteristic waveform of these valves has two peaks, representing early diastolic ventricular filling (E-point) and ventricular filling during atrial systole (A-point). In the normal fetal heart, a greater proportion of diastolic filling occurs during atrial systole, resulting in the A-point being higher than the E-point (see Fig. 2–13). Throughout gestation, this E/A ratio increases, but it never exceeds 1. After birth, as the myocardium matures, the relationship between the E-point and A-point reverses, with the E-point velocity exceeding that of the A-point. That relationship holds constant until the later decades of life, when an A-point dominance may reappear. Although peak velocity nomograms for the fetal mitral or tricuspid valves do exist, they are not usually used to access valve normalcy. It is the E-point–A-point relationship that is of greater importance. If an inverted E-point–A-point relationship (ratio >1) is observed in utero, two scenarios should be considered. The first is a technical "pseudo" reversal that can occur if the mitral or tricuspid valves are interrogated at an inappropriate Doppler angle. If this occurs, a more appropriate angle of insonation should be acquired, such as that found with an apical four-chamber view, and the valves should be reinterrogated. A true in utero reversal of the E and A points may result from abnormalities that affect the myocardium, such as intrauterine growth restriction (IUGR) (Fig. 2–77). In IUGR, hypoxemia and polycythemia are known to occur and to impair cardiac function.[122] Hypoxemia has been associated with impaired myocardial contractility, whereas polycythemia can alter blood viscosity and therefore preload.[123] Congenital cardiac anomalies that affect the myocardium, such as hypoplasia of the ventricle, may also result in a reversal of the E-point–A-point relationship in the ipsilateral AV valve.

Although absolute peak velocities are not usually used in accessing the mitral and tricuspid valves, a markedly increased velocity would be indicative of valvular stenosis. Valvular insufficiency or regurgitation of the AV valves would be detected by placing the pulsed Doppler sample volume proximal to the valve in the atrium. Retrograde flow visualized during systole would be indicative of valvular insufficiency. Some degree of mitral or tricuspid valve insufficiency in the fetus is a normal finding.[124] This would be seen on a spectral tracing as retrograde flow occurring only briefly at the beginning of the systolic phase of the cardiac cycle (see Fig. 2–9). Retrograde flow that lasts longer than just the beginning of systole should be considered abnormal (see Fig. 2–11). If an abnormal amount of mitral or tricuspid valve insufficiency is appreciated, the ipsilateral great vessel should be evaluated for stenosis or atresia. Abnormalities of valve placement, such as Ebstein anomaly, that result in the valve leaflets not coapting correctly can also cause insufficiency.

Pulsed Doppler Imaging of the Pulmonary Veins

Pulsed Doppler waveforms of at least the two superior pulmonary veins should be documented. The normal direction of flow is into the left atrium. A normal waveform pattern for the pulmonary veins consists of a first peak during ventricular systole (S), which represents atrial relaxation, a second peak during early diastolic filling of the ventricle

Figure 2–77 Reversal of the E and A points of the mitral valve waveform in a fetus with IUGR.

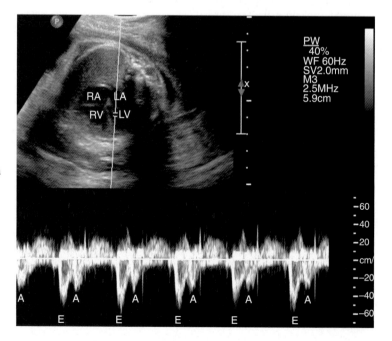

(D), and a forward end-diastolic velocity that represents atrial contraction (A). Specific systolic and diastolic velocities are not normally used; however, velocities have been shown to increase significantly during the second half of pregnancy.[125] Reversal of the A wave has been associated with cardiac defects that cause increased left atrial pressure, such as hypoplastic left heart syndrome with a restricted foramen ovale.

Ductus Venosus

The ductus venosus is an additional fetal shunt connecting the umbilical vein with the inferior vena cava. Abnormalities in the ductus venosus waveform have been suggested to be useful in the detection of early cardiac dysfunction.[126] The normal waveform consists of an S-wave representing peak systolic velocity, a D-wave reflecting ventricular diastole, and an A-wave representing atrial contraction (Fig. 2–78). In the setting of myocardial dysfunction or severe right heart obstruction caused by congenital heart disease, absent or reversed flow during atrial contraction may be present. This finding may predict a poorer outcome in fetuses with heart disease.[126] Reversal of the A-

wave may also be seen in fetuses with severe IUGR or severely affected twin-twin transfusion syndrome. Therefore, if this finding is present without an apparent cardiac cause, overall fetal well-being should be considered.

Color Doppler Echocardiography

Color Doppler imaging plays an essential role in fetal echocardiography. It provides a more efficient and expedient means of assessing normal and abnormal flow patterns in the fetal heart. Color Doppler imaging supplies information on the presence or absence of flow, flow direction, and flow patterns. Several authors have expressed the importance of using color Doppler imaging as an adjunct to all fetal echocardiograms.[77,127–132]

By superimposing color over the gray-scale image, morphological and hemodynamic information can be assessed simultaneously. Color allows visualization of flow in entire structures, such as the aortic arch, thus making it much more time efficient than pulsed Doppler imaging. This efficiency is also prudent when imaging a fetus because color Doppler imaging produces lower peak intensities than does pulsed Doppler imaging.[132]

Color Doppler imaging can simplify the investigation of valvular stenosis or insufficiency, again by sampling a large area and identifying areas of turbulence or flow reversal (see Fig. 2–10) In some cases, color may aid in visualizing heart structures, such as the outflow tracts, which may be difficult to see with gray-scale imaging alone. Also, it may occasionally lead to detection of an abnormality not obvious on the gray-scale image, such as valvular stenosis, small ventricular septal defects (Fig. 2–79), and flow reversal within the aortic or ductal arches.[127,128,130,132]

Color Doppler imaging is not without technical limitations. As with pulsed Doppler imaging, color Doppler imaging is angle dependent. Therefore insonation angles approaching 90 degrees result in no flow information (color) being displayed. Frame rate also influences the usefulness of color. The equipment used for fetal echocardiography should have specific fetal cardiac imaging capabilities with higher pulse repetition frequencies, which allow color imaging at a frame rate fast enough to evaluate the rapid fetal heart rate. Using a narrow color field or reducing the image depth, when possible, may be necessary to maintain an adequate frame rate.

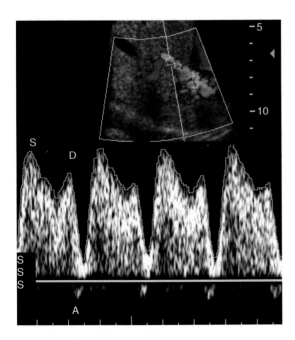

Figure 2–78 Normal Doppler waveform of the ductus venosus. *A,* Atrial contraction; *D,* diastolic peak; *S,* systolic peak.

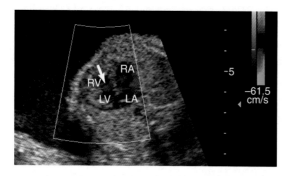

Figure 2–79 Color Doppler imaging to identify a ventricular septal defect *(arrow)* in a subcostal four-chamber view. *LA,* Left atrium; *LV,* left ventricle; *RA,* right atrium; *RV,* right ventricle.

Several artifacts specific to color Doppler imaging may be encountered. Moving tissue (i.e., myocardium) may be encoded with color because of transmitted pulsations from flow within the heart chambers and vessels. Increasing the wall filter, color priority, or velocity scale may decrease or eliminate this appearance. Additionally, slightly increasing gray-scale gain may decrease the presence of color noise over solid tissue.[132]

As with gray-scale imaging, color Doppler penetration decreases with higher frequencies. Thus, deeper flow may be difficult to detect with high-frequency transducers. Changing to a lower-frequency transducer may overcome this color limitation but will result in some sacrifice in gray-scale resolution.

It should be borne in mind that color Doppler imaging will provide mean velocity information only. This is due to the means by which color information is acquired. Usually a method of rapid sampling termed "autocorrelation" is incorporated. This requires several Doppler pulses to be transmitted over several lines of information at the same time. The acquisition of this large area of data is so time intensive that current equipment can provide only an average of this information efficiently.[132] It is for this reason that pulsed Doppler imaging is often a necessary adjunct to color Doppler imaging to provide quantitative information regarding peak velocities.

Power Doppler imaging in general may hold several advantages over color Doppler imaging. However, many of these advantages are not applicable in the fetal heart. Power Doppler imaging assesses the amplitude of the signal, as opposed to

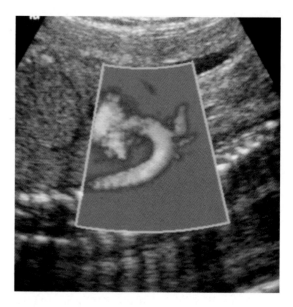

Figure 2–80 Color power image of the fetal aortic arch showing the presence of flow but no directional information. (Courtesy Advanced Technology Laboratories, Bothell, Wash.)

color Doppler imaging, which relies on signal frequency. For this reason, power Doppler imaging is not dependent on insonation angle, making it more sensitive than color Doppler imaging in detecting flow. However, the same acquisition parameters result in power Doppler imaging being able to display only the presence of flow, not direction or velocity information.

In the fetal heart, power Doppler imaging may be useful in identifying flow in structures such as the aortic arch (Fig. 2–80), but artifactual noise is often encountered when this modality is used, making it less desirable in other structures.

M-Mode Echocardiography

Although M-mode echocardiography may not be necessary routinely in fetal echocardiographic examinations, it is essential in differentiating some arrhythmias.[133] M-mode imaging is useful in acquiring measurements of chamber size and wall thickness, although not absolutely necessary. Cartier et al[86] measured the aorta and pulmonary artery with both two-dimensional and M-mode imaging in a prospective study of 403 fetuses. Their results showed a high correlation among two-dimensional and M-mode measurements for each vessel ($r = 0.992$ for the aorta, $r = 0.973$ for the pulmonary artery). They concluded that technically adequate measurements could be obtained in the fetal heart by either modality.

M-mode imaging is helpful in evaluating contractility in abnormalities that may affect wall motion, such as cardiomyopathies. Particularly important information derived from M-mode measurements when heart disease is suspected is fractional shortening. This equation gives an index of ventricular contractility and is calculated from the following formula by using M-mode ventricular dimensions:

$$\frac{\text{Diastolic ventricular dimension} - \text{Systolic ventricular dimension}}{\text{Diastolic ventricular dimension}} \times 100\%$$

Normal fractional shortening of the fetal heart is greater than 25%.[135]

More recently, nomograms of area fractional shortening, derived from tracing the endocardium on two-dimensional sonography, have been published.[135]

M-mode echocardiography can also be useful in evaluating valve motion, although the fetal heart valves are often difficult to visualize on M-mode echocardiography because of their small size. Even in the normal fetal heart, M-mode imaging is useful as a quick and accurate method of measuring fetal heart rate. Also, as mentioned previously, placing the M-mode cursor through an atrial and ventricular wall simultaneously is very useful in determining the type of arrhythmia present.

In summary, all cardiac structures should be evaluated as thoroughly as possible when a fetal echocardiogram is performed. An understanding of the importance of different scanning planes and modalities available will increase the ability to identify congenital heart disease.

References

1. Hoffman JIE: Incidence of congenital heart disease. II. Prenatal incidence. Pediatr Cardiol 1995; 16:155–165.
2. Hoffman JIE, Christianson R: Congenital heart disease in a cohort of 19,502 births with long-term follow-up. Am J Cardiol 1978; 42:640–647.
3. Hoffman JIE: Incidence of congenital heart disease. 1: Postnatal incidence. Pediatr Cardiol 1995; 16:103–113.
4. Mitchell SC, Korones SB, Berendes HW: Congenital heart disease in 56,109 births. Circulation 1971; 43:323–332.
5. Ianniruberto A: Management of fetal cardiac structural abnormalities. Fetal Ther 1986; 1:89–91.
6. McCurdy CM, Reed KL: Basic technique of fetal echocardiography. Semin US CT MRI 1993; 14:267–276.
7. Smrcek JM, Berg C, Geipel A, et al: Detection rate of early fetal echocardiography and in-utero development of congenital heart defects. J Ultrasound Med 2006; 25:187–196.
8. Hamar BD, Dziura J, Friedman A, et al: Trends in fetal echocardiography and implications for clinical practice, 1985–2003. J Ultrasound Med 2006; 25:197–202.
9. Allan LD, Crawford DC, Anderson RH, et al: Spectrum of congenital heart disease detected echocardiographically in prenatal life. Br Heart J 1985; 54:523–526.
10. Oberhaensli I, Extermann P, Friedli B, et al: Ultrasound screening for congenital cardiac malformations in the fetus: Its importance for peri- and postnatal care. Pediatr Radiol 1989; 19:94–99.
11. Allan LD, Crawford DC, Anderson RH, et al: Echocardiographic and anatomic correlates in fetal congenital heart disease. Br Heart J 1984; 52:542–548.
12. Benacerraf BR, Pober BR, Sanders SP: Accuracy of fetal echocardiography. Radiology 1987; 165:847–849.
13. Crawford DC, Chita SK, Allan LD: Prenatal detection of congenital heart disease: Factors affecting obstetric management and survival. Am J Obstet Gynecol 1988; 159:352–356.
14. Nyberg DA, Emerson DS: Cardiac malformations. In: Nyberg DA, Mahony BS, Pretorius DH (eds): Diagnostic Ultrasound of Fetal Anomalies: Text and Atlas. Chicago, Yearbook Medical, 1990, pp. 300–341.
15. Brown DL, Emerson DS, Carrier MS, et al: Congenital cardiac anomalies: Prenatal sonographic diagnosis. AJR Am J Roentgenol 1989; 153:109–114.
16. Wheller JJ, Reiss R, Allen HD: Clinical experience with fetal echocardiography. Arch Pediatr Adolesc Med 1990; 144:49–53.
17. Allan LD: Diagnosis of fetal cardiac abnormalities. Arch Dis Child 1989; 64:864-968.
18. Allan LD: Fetal cardiology. Ultrasound Obstet Gynecol 1994; 4:441–444.
19. AIUM Technical Bulletin: Performance of the Fetal Cardiac Ultrasound Examination.

American Institute of Ultrasound in Medicine, J Ultrasound Med 1998; 17:796.

20. Allan LD: Fetal echocardiography: Confidence limits and accuracy. Pediatr Cardiol 1985; 6:145–146.

21. DeVore GR, Medearis AL, Bear MB: Fetal echocardiography: Factors that influence imaging of the fetal heart during the second trimester of pregnancy. J Ultrasound Med 1993; 12:659–663.

22. Allan LD: Diagnosis of fetal cardiac abnormality: Br J Hosp Med 1988; 40:290–293.

23. Allan LD: Cardiac anatomy screening: what is the best time for screening in pregnancy? Curr Opin Obstet Gynecol 2003; 15:143–146.

24. Fyfe DA, Kline CH: Fetal echocardiographic diagnosis of congenital heart disease. Pediatr Clin North Am 1990; 37:45–67.

25. Nora JJ, Fraser FC: Cardiovascular disease. In: Nora JJ, Fraser FC (eds): Medical Genetics: Principles and Practice, 3rd ed. Philadelphia, Lea & Febiger, 1989, pp 321–337.

26. Nora JJ, Nora AH: Maternal transmission of congenital heart diseases: New recurrence risk figures and the question of cytoplasmic inheritance and vulnerability to teratogens. Am J Cardiol 1987; 59:459–463.

27. Stamm ER, Drose JA, Thickman D: The fetal heart. In: Rumack CM, Wilson SR, Charboneau JW (eds): Diagnostic Ultrasound, vol II. St Louis, Mosby–Year Book, 1991, pp 800–827.

28. McGahan JP: Sonography of the fetal heart: Findings of the four-chamber view. AJR Am J Roentgenol 1991; 156:547–553.

29. Copel JA, Kleinman CS: The impact of fetal echocardiography on perinatal outcome. Ultrasound Med Biol 1986; 4:327–335.

30. Bromley B, Estroff JA, Sanders SP, et al: Fetal echocardiography: Accuracy and limitations in a population at high and low risk for heart defects. Am J Obstet Gynecol 1992; 166:1472–1481.

31. Benacerraf BR, Sanders SP: Fetal echocardiography. Radiol Clin North Am 1990; 28:131–147.

32. Reed KL: Introduction to fetal echocardiography. Obstet Gynecol Clin North Am 1991; 18:811–822.

33. Berg KA, Boughman JA, Astemborski JA, et al: Implications for prenatal cytogenetic analysis from Baltimore-Washington study of liveborn infants with confirmed congenital heart defects (CHD). Am J Hum Genet 1986; 39:A50.

34. Berg KA, Clark EB, Astemborski JA, et al: Prenatal detection of cardiovascular malformations by echocardiography: An indication for cytogenetic evaluation. Am J Obstet Gynecol 1988; 159:477–481.

35. Wladimiroff JW, Stuart PA, Sachs ES, et al: Prenatal diagnosis and management of congenital heart defects: Significance of associated fetal anomalies and prenatal chromosome studies. Am J Med Genet 1985; 21:285–290.

36. Ferencz C, Neill CA: Cardiovascular malformations: Prevalence at livebirth. In: Freedom RM, Benson LN, Smallhorn JF (eds): Neonatal Heart Disease. London, Springer-Verlag, 1992, pp 19–29.

37. Stewart PA, Wladimiroff JW, Reuss A, et al: Fetal echocardiography: A review of six years experience. Fetal Ther 1987; 2:222–231.

38. Nicolaides K, Shawwa L, Brizot M, et al: Ultrasonographically detectable markers of fetal chromosomal defects. Ultrasound Obstet Gynecol 1993; 3:56–59.

39. Cleves MA, Hobbs CA, Cleves PA, et al: Congenital defects among liveborn infants with Down syndrome. Birth Defects Research (Part A) 2007; 79:657–663.

40. Pont SJ, Robbins JM, Bird TM, et al: Congenital malformations among liveborn infants with trisomies 18 and 13. Am J Med Genet 2006; 140A:1749–1756.

41. Rowland TW, Hubbel JP, Nadas AS: Congenital heart disease in infants of diabetic mothers. J Pediatr 1973; 83:815–820.

42. Becerra JE, Khoury MJ, Cordero JF, et al: Diabetes mellitus during pregnancy and the risks for specific birth defects: a population-based case-control study. Pediatrics 1990; 85:1–9.

43. Friedberg MK, Silverman NH: Changing indications for fetal echocardiography in a university center population. Prenat Diagn 2004; 24:781–786.

44. Wren C, Birrell G, Hawthorne G: Cardiovascular malformations in infants of diabetic mothers. Heart 2003; 89:1217–1220.

45. Levy HL, Waisbren SE: Effects of untreated maternal phenylketonuria and hyperphenylalaninemia on the fetus. N Engl J Med 1983; 309:1269–1274.

46. Lenke RR, Levy HL: Maternal phenylketonuria and hyperphenylalaninemia: An international survey of the outcomes of untreated and treated pregnancies. N Engl J Med 1980; 303:1202–1208.

47. Drose JA, Dennis MA, Thickman D: Infection in utero: Ultrasound findings in 19 cases. Radiology 1991; 178:369–374.

48. Confino E: Infectious causes of congenital cardiac anomalies. In: Elkayam U, Gleicher N (eds): Cardiac Problems and Pregnancy, 2nd ed. New York, Alan R. Liss, 1990, p 569.

49. Fogel M, Copel JA, Cullen MT, et al: Congenital heart disease and fetal thoracoabdominal anomalies: Associations in utero and the importance of cytogenetic analysis. Am J Perinatol 1991; 8:411–416.

50. Copel JA, Pilu G, Kleinman CS: Congenital heart disease and extracardiac anomalies: Associations and indications for fetal echocardiography. Am J Obstet Gynecol 1986; 154:1121–1132.

51. Abrams ME, Meredith KS, Kinnard R, et al: Hydrops fetalis: A retrospective review of cases reported to a large national database and identification of risk factors associated with death. Pediatrics 2007; 120:84–89.

52. Callan NA, Maggio M, Steger S, et al: Fetal echocardiography: Indications for referral, prenatal diagnoses, and outcomes. Am J Perinatol 1991; 8:390–394.

53. Reed KL, Sahn DJ: A proposal for referral patterns for fetal cardiac studies. Semin Ultrasound CT MRI 1984; 5:249–252.

54. McAuliffe FM, Hornberger LK, Winsor S, et al: Fetal cardiac defects and increased nuchal translucency thickness: A prospective study. Am J Obstet Gynecol 2004; 191:1486–1490.

55. Westin M, Saltvedt S, Bergman G, et al: Is measurement of nuchal translucency thickness a useful screening tool for heart defects? A study of 16,383 fetuses. Ultrasound Obstet Gynecol 2006; 27:632–639.

56. Müller MA, Clur SA, Timmerman E, et al: Nuchal translucency measurement and congenital heart defects: Modest association in low-risk pregnancies. Prenat Diagn 2007; 27:164–169.

57. Atzei A, Gajewska K, Huggon IC, et al: Relationship between nuchal translucency thickness and prevalence of major cardiac defects in fetuses with normal karyotype. Ultrasound Obstet Gynecol 2005; 26:154–157.

58. Comstock CH: Normal fetal heart axis and position. Obstet Gynecol 1987; 70:255–257.

59. Shipp TD, Bromley B, Hornberger LK: Levorotation of the fetal cardiac axis: A clue for the presence of congenital heart disease. Obstet Gynecol 1995; 85:97–102.

60. Smith RS, Comstock CH, Kirk JS, et al: Ultrasonographic left cardiac axis deviation: A marker for fetal anomalies. Obstet Gynecol 1995; 85:187–191.

61. DeVore GR: The prenatal diagnosis of congenital heart disease-a practical approach for the fetal sonographer. J Clin Ultrasound 1985; 13:229–245.

62. Hess LW, Hess DB, McCaul JF, et al: Fetal echocardiography. Obstet Gynecol Clin North Am 1990; 17:41–79.

63. McCurdy CM, Reed KL: Basic technique of fetal echocardiography. Semin Ultrasound CT MRI 1993; 14:267–276.

64. Cooke SG, Wilde P: Fetal echocardiography-four years experience in Bristol. Clin Radiol 1989; 40:568–572.

65. Allan LD: Fetal echocardiography. Clin Obstet Gynecol 1988; 31:61–79.

66. Axel L: Real-time sonography of fetal cardiac anatomy. AJR Am J Roentgenol 1983; 141:283–288.

67. Devore GR, Donnerstein RL, Kleinman CS, et al: Fetal echocardiography. I: Normal anatomy as determined by realtime-directed M-mode ultrasound. Am J Obstet Gynecol 1982; 144:249–260.

68. Huhta JC, Hagler DJ, Hill LM: Two-dimensional echocardiographic assessment of normal fetal cardiac anatomy. J Reprod Med 1984; 29:162–167.

69. Nimrod C, Nicholson S, Machin G, et al: In utero evaluation of fetal cardiac structure: A preliminary report. Am J Obstet Gynecol 1984; 148:516–518.

70. Shime J, Bertrand M, Hagan-Ansert S, et al: Two dimensional and M-mode echocardiography in the human fetus. Am J Obstet Gynecol 1984; 148:629–685.

71. Brown DL, DiSalvo DN, Frates MC, et al: Sonography of the fetal heart: Normal variants and pitfalls. AJR Am J Roentgenol 1993; 160:1251–1255.

72. Cyr DR, Guntheroth WG, Mack LA, et al: A systematic approach to fetal echocardiography using real-time/two-dimensional sonography. J Ultrasound Med 1986; 5:343–350.

73. AIUM Guidelines for Performance of the Antepartum Obstetrical Ultrasound Examination. Laurel, MD, American Institute of Ultrasound in Medicine, 1986.

74. Tegnander E, Williams W, Johansen OJ, et al: Prenatal detection of heart defects in a non-selected population of 30,149 fetuses-detection rates and outcome. Ultrasound Obstet Gynecol 2006; 27:252–265.

75. Wong SF, Chan FY, Cincotta RB, et al: Factors influencing the prenatal detection of structural congenital heart diseases. Ultrasound Obstet Gynecol 2003; 21:19–25.

76. Copel JA, Pilu G, Geen J, et al: Fetal echocardiographic screening for congenital heart disease: The importance of the four-

chamber view. Am J Obstet Gynecol 1987; 157:648–655.

77. DeVore GR: Color Doppler examination of the outflow tracts of the fetal heart: A technique for identification of cardiovascular malformations. Ultrasound Obstet Gynecol 1994; 4:463–471.

78. Leslie KK, Persutte WH, Drose JA, et al: Prenatal detection of congenital heart disease by basic ultrasonography at a tertiary care center: What should our expectations be? J Matern Fetal Invest 1996; 6:132–135.

79. DeVore GR, Siassi B, Platt LD: Fetal echocardiography. VIII: Aortic root dilatation—a marker for tetralogy of Fallot. Am J Obstet Gynecol 1988; 159:129–136.

80. DeVore GR: The aortic and pulmonary outflow tract screening examination in the human fetus. J Ultrasound Med 1992; 11:345–348.

81. Jaeffi ET, Sholler GF, Jones ODH, et al: Comparative analysis of pattern, management and outcome of pre- versus postnatally diagnosed major congenital heart disease: a population-based study. Ultrasound Obstet Gynecol 2001; 17:380–385.

82. Weil SR, Huhta JC: Sonographic differential diagnosis of fetal cardiac abnormalities. Semin US CT MRI 1993; 14:298–317.

83. Kleinman CS, Donnerstein RL: Ultrasonic assessment of cardiac function in the intact human fetus. J Am Coll Cardiol 1985; 5:84S–94S.

84. Anteby EY, Shimonovitz S, Yagal S: Fetal echocardiography: The identification of two of the pulmonary veins from the four chamber view during the second trimester of pregnancy. Ultrasound Obstet Gynecol 1994; 4:208–210.

85. Allan LD, Joseph MC, Boyd EG, et al: M-mode echocardiography in the developing human fetus. Br Heart J 1982; 47:573–583.

86. Cartier MS, Davidoff A, Warneke LA, et al: The normal diameter of the fetal aorta and pulmonary artery: Echocardiographic evaluation in utero. AJR Am J Roentgenol 1987; 149:1003–1007.

87. Benson CB, Brown PM, Doubilet DN, et al: Increasing curvature of the normal fetal ductus arteriosus with advancing gestational age. Ultrasound Obstet Gynecol 1994; 5:95–97.

88. Del Rio M, Martinez JM, Figueras F, et al: Reference ranges for Doppler parameters of the fetal aortic isthmus during the second half of pregnancy. Ultrasound Obstet Gynecol 2006; 28:71–76.

89. Brezinka C, Stifnen T, Wladimiroff JW: Doppler flow velocity wave forms in the fetal ductus arteriosus during the first half of pregnancy: A reproducibility study. Ultrasound Obstet Gynecol 1994; 4:121–123.

90. Van Der Mooren K, Barendregt LG, Wladimiroff JW: Flow velocity wave forms in the human fetal ductus arteriosus during the normal second half of pregnancy. Pediatr Res 1991; 30:487–490.

91. Tulzer G, Gudmundsson S, Sharkey AM, et al: Doppler echocardiography of fetal ductus arteriosus constriction versus increased right ventricular output. J Am Coll Cardiol 1991; 18:532–536.

92. Mielke G, Benda N: Blood flow velocity waveforms of the fetal pulmonary artery and the ductus arteriosus: reference ranges from 13 weeks to term. Ultrasound Obstet Gynecol 2000; 15:213–218.

93. Mielke G, Peukert U, Krapp M, et al: Fetal and transient neonatal right heart dilatation with severe tricuspid valve insufficiency in association with abnormally S-shaped kinking of the ductus arteriosus. Ultrasound Obstet Gynecol 1995; 5:338–341.

94. Respondek M, Weil SR, Huhta JC: Fetal echocardiography during indomethacin treatment. Ultrasound Obstet Gynecol 1995; 5:86–89.

95. Paladini D, Marasini M, Volpe P: Severe ductal constriction in the third-trimester fetus following maternal self-medication and nimesulide. Ultrasound Obstet Gynecol 2005; 25:357–361.

96. Rizzo G, Arduini D: Fetal cardiac function in intrauterine growth retardation. Am J Obstet Gynecol 1991; 165:876–882.

97. Viñals F, Heredia F, Giuliano A: The role of the three vessels and trachea view (3VT) in the diagnosis of congenital heart defects. Ultrasound Obstet Gynecol 2003; 22:358–367.

98. Del Rio M, Martinez JM, Figueras F, et al: Doppler assessment of fetal aortic isthmus blood flow in two different sonographic planes during the second half of gestation. Ultrasound Obstet Gynecol 2005; 26:170–174.

99. Sheley RC, Nyberg DA, Kapur R: Azygous continuation of the interrupted inferior vena cava: a clue to prenatal diagnosis of the cardiosplenic syndromes. J Ultrasound Med 1995; 14:381–387.

100. Erdogan M, Karakas P, Uygur F, et al: Persistent left superior vena cava: the anatomical and surgical importance. West Indian Med J 2007; 56:72–76.

101. Rein AJJT, Nir A, Nadjari M: The coronary sinus in the fetus. Ultrasound Obstet Gynecol 2000; 15:468–472.

102. McAuliffe FM, Hornberger LK, Johnson J, et al: Cardiac diverticulum with pericardial effusion: report of two new cases treated by in-utero pericardiocentesis and a review of the literature. Ultrasound Obstet Gynecol 2005; 25:401–404.

103. Petrikovsky BM, Challenger M, Wyse LJ: Natural history of echogenic foci within ventricles of the fetal heart. Ultrasound Obstet Gynecol 1995; 5:92–94.

104. Levy DW, Mintx MC: The left ventricle echogenic focus: A normal finding. AJR Am J Roentgenol 1988; 150:85–86.

105. Arda S, Cenk Sayin NC, Varol FG, et al: Isolated fetal intracardiac hyperechogenic focus associated with neonatal outcome and triple test results. Arch Gynecol Obstet 2007; 276:481–485.

106. Benacerraf BR: The second-trimester fetus with Down syndrome: Detection using sonographic features. Ultrasound Obstet Gynecol 1996; 7:147–155.

107. Lehman CD, Nyberg DA, Winter TC, et al: Trisomy 13 syndrome: Prenatal US findings in a review of 33 cases. Radiology 1995; 194:217–222.

108. Roberts DJ, Genest D: Cardiac histologic pathology characteristics of trisomies 13 and 21. Hum Pathol 1992; 23:1130–1140.

109. Wax JR, Cartin A, Pinette MG, et al: Are intracardiac echogenic foci markers of congenital heart disease in the fetus with chromosomal abnormalities: J Ultrasound Med 2004; 23:895–898.

110. Arda S, Cenk Saym N, Varol FG, et al: Isolated fetal intracardiac hyperechogenic focus associated with neonatal outcome and triple test results. Arch Gynecol Obstet 2007; 276:481–485.

111. Bethune M: Management options for echogenic intracardiac focus and choroid plexus cysts: a review including Australian Association of Obstetrical and Gynaecological Ultrasonologists consensus statement. Australas Radiol 2007; 51:324–329.

112. Clements J, Sobotka-Plojhar M, Exalto N, et al: A connective tissue membrane in the right atrium (Chiari's network) as a cause of fetal cardiac arrhythmia. Am J Obstet Gynecol 1982; 142:709–712.

113. Brown DL, Cartier MS, Emerson DS, et al: The peripheral hypoechoic rim of the fetal heart. J Ultrasound Med 1989; 81:603–608.

114. Reed LK, Sahn DJ, Marx GR, et al: Cardiac Doppler flows during fetal arrhythmias: Physiologic consequences. Obstet Gynecol 1987; 70:1–6.

115. Maulik D, Nanda NC, Moodley S, et al: Application of Doppler echocardiography in the assessment of fetal cardiac disease. Am J Obstet Gynecol 1985; 151:951–957.

116. Maulik D, Nanda N, Saini VD: Fetal Doppler echocardiography: Methods and characterization of normal and abnormal hemodynamics. Am J Cardiol 1984; 53:572–578.

117. Huhta JC, Strasburger JF, Carpenter RJ, et al: Pulsed Doppler fetal echocardiography. J Clin Ultrasound 1985; 13:247–254.

118. Shenker L, Reed KL, Marx GR, et al: Fetal cardiac Doppler flow studies in prenatal diagnosis of heart disease. Am J Obstet Gynecol 1988; 158:1267–1273.

119. Reed KL, Anderson CF, Shenker L: Fetal pulmonary artery and aorta: Two-dimensional Doppler echocardiography. Obstet Gynecol 1987; 69:175–178.

120. Reed KL, Meijboom EJ, Sahn DJ, et al: Cardiac Doppler flow velocities in human fetuses. Circulation 1986; 73:41–46.

121. Choi JY, Noh CI, Yun YS: Study on Doppler wave forms from the fetal cardiovascular system. Fetal Diagn Ther 1991; 6:74–83.

122. Severi FM, Rizzo G, Bocchi C, et al: Intrauterine growth retardation and fetal cardiac function. Fetal Diagn Ther 2000; 15:8–19.

123. Rizzo G, Arduini D, Romanini C: Doppler echocardiographic assessment of fetal cardiac function. Ultrasound Obstet Gynecol 1992; 2:434–445

124. Messing B, Porat S, Imbar T, et al: Mild tricuspid regurgitation: a benign feta finding at various stages of pregnancy. Ultrasound Obstet Gynecol 2005; 26:606–610.

125. Lenz F, Chaoui R: Reference ranges for Doppler-assessed pulmonary venous blood flow velocities and pulsatility indices in normal human fetuses. Prenatal Diagn 2002; 22:786–791.

126. Bianco K, Small M, Julien S, et al: Second-trimester ductus venosus measurement and adverse perinatal outcome in fetuses with congenital heart disease. J Ultrasound Med 2006; 25:979–982.

127. Rice MJ, McDonald RW, Sahn DJ: Contribution of color Doppler to the evaluation of cardiovascular abnormalities in the fetus. Semin US CT MRI 1993; 14:277–285.

128. Sharland GK, Chita SK, Allan LD: The use of colour Doppler in fetal echocardiography. Int J Cardiol 1990; 28:229–236.

129. Chiba Y, Kanzaki T, Kobayashi H, et al: Evaluation of fetal structural heart disease using

color flow mapping. Ultrasound Med Biol 1990; 16:221–229.

130. Copel JA, Hobbins JC, Kleinman CS: Doppler echocardiography and color flow mapping. Obstet Gynecol Clin North Am 1991; 18:845–851.

131. Stewart PA, Wladimiroff JW: Fetal echocardiography and color Doppler flow imaging: The Rotterdam experience. Ultrasound Obstet Gynecol 1993; 2:168–175.

132. Mitchell DG: Color Doppler imaging: Principles, limitations and artifacts. Radiology 1990; 177:1–10.

133. DeVore GR, Siassi B, Platt LD: M-mode assessment of ventricular size and contractility during the second and third trimesters of pregnancy in the normal fetus. Am J Obstet Gynecol 1984; 150:981–988.

134. Cyr DR, Guntheroth WG, Mack LA: Fetal Echocardiography. In: Berman MC (ed): Diagnostic Medical Sonography, vol I: Obstetrics and Gynecology. Philadelphia, JB Lippincott, 1991, pp 249–271.

135. Goldinfeld M, Weiner E, Peleg D, et al: Evaluation of fetal cardiac contractility by two-dimensional ultrasonography. Prenat Diagn 2004; 24:799–803.

CHAPTER 3

Cardiac Malposition

Paul D. Russ
Julia A. Drose

Axis and position are two basic morphological features of the fetal heart.[1-4] Axis describes the rotational orientation of the heart in the thorax.[1-3] It refers to the degree that the cardiac apex points to the left or right. Position describes the translational relationship or overall location of the heart in the chest.[1,3,4] It indicates the hemithorax that the heart predominantly occupies. Many anomalies alter either the cardiac axis or the cardiac position. In general, abnormal axis is a manifestation of intrinsic congenital heart disease (CHD), whereas altered position results from an extracardiac defect.

Both axis and position can be readily evaluated with the four-chamber view during either routine obstetrical ultrasonography or formal fetal echocardiography.[1-4] Cardiac axis can be considered in two ways. Axis can be measured as the angle between a line along the interventricular septum and an anteroposterior line that bisects the thorax (Fig. 3–1).[1] This defines the rotational orientation of the heart with respect to the chest wall. In normal fetuses, this angle is about 45 degrees, plus or minus 20 degrees, leftward of midline.[1-4] This does not change significantly during gestation.[2] Another aspect of axis is the comparison of the heart's orientation to the location of other organs, particularly those of the upper abdomen. For example, the cardiac apex normally points toward the stomach on the left side of the fetus.[4]

Cardiac position can be described by a line extending along the interatrial septum (Fig. 3–2). A point is defined at its intersection with the posterior margin of the heart.[1] This point is relatively independent of axis and normally is just to the right of midline, close to the center of the thorax. Expressed more simply, most of the fetal heart, especially the ventricles, is positioned in the left anterior quadrant of the chest.[1] The right ventricle is normally near the left anterior chest wall, and the left atrium is anterior to the descending aorta and spine.[5]

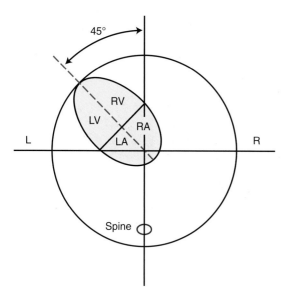

Figure 3–1 Diagram showing measurement of the cardiac axis from the four-chamber view of the heart. Axis can be measured as the angle between a line along the interventricular septum and an anteroposterior line that bisects the thorax. *L,* Left; *LA,* left atrium; *LV,* left ventricle; *R,* right; *RA,* right atrium; *RV,* right ventricle. Normal axis is defined as 45 degrees between these two points, ±20 degrees.

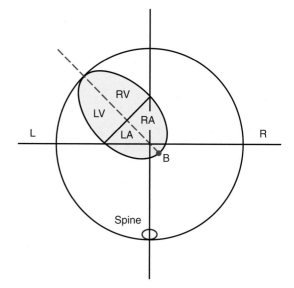

Figure 3–2 Diagram showing assessment of the position of the fetal heart from the four-chamber view. A line through the interventricular septum is extended to the base of the heart to produce point *(B)*. If point B lies within the shaded area, cardiac position is considered normal. *L,* Left; *LA,* left atrium; *LV,* left ventricle; *R,* right; *RA,* right atrium; *RV,* right ventricle.

Abnormal Cardiac Axis

Abnormal axis is often associated with complex intracardiac defects and sometimes with intractable arrhythmias. Because the structural abnormalities can be complicated, a systematic or segmental evaluation of the heart is recommended.[4–6] Such an evaluation includes determining venoatrial, atrioventricular (AV), and ventriculoarterial (VA) connections.[4,6] The segmental approach also establishes the relationship of the heart chambers and cardiac axis to the arrangement of other intrathoracic and abdominal organs. This description of body configuration is defined in terms of situs.[4–11]

Although the terminology is variable and sometimes confusing, abnormalities of cardiac axis can be generally categorized as dextrocardia, mesocardia, and severe levocardia.[6–12] With dextrocardia, the cardiac apex points to the right. If mesocardia is present, the apex is in a midline position. With severe levocardia, it is directed further leftward than the angle previously described.[1,6,11]

Abdominal Situs

There are three types of situs: situs solitus, situs inversus, and situs ambiguous.[4,8,11] Situs solitus is the normal organ arrangement, which includes the liver on the right side and the stomach on the left side. With situs inversus, there is a mirror-image configuration so that the liver is on the left and the stomach is on the right. If there is neither situs solitus nor situs inversus, there is situs ambiguous, also referred to as indeterminate situs or heterotaxy.[7,8,10,11]

The terms atrial or visceroatrial situs are often used in discussions of situs solitus, situs inversus, and situs ambiguous.[4,6,8,10–12] These modifiers emphasize the anatomical interrelationship of atrial and upper abdominal organ arrangement. Although there are exceptions, atrial and visceral situs are usually concordant in situs solitus or situs inversus[4,6,8,10,11]; that is, the morphological right atrium is located on the same side as the liver. This reflects the fact that the systemic venous connections to the right atrium tend to be the most anatomically constant.[7]

In bilateral right-sidedness and bilateral left-sidedness, the two major subtypes of situs ambiguous, visceroatrial situs has a different but consistent pattern. With bilateral right-sidedness (asplenia syndrome), both atria have the morphological features of right atria. When there is bilateral left-sidedness (polysplenia syndrome), both atria have the morphological characteristics of left atria.[4-6,8,10,11]

The likelihood and type of CHD can be predicted by evaluating the cardiac axis as a function of situs.[6-11] For each situs-axis pair, several permutations are possible if AV and VA connections are considered.[6-10] Anomalous AV anatomy is usually manifested as ventricular inversion; the ventricles are switched so that the right atrium drains into the morphological left ventricle and the left atrium drains into the morphological right ventricle.[6,7,9] Abnormal or discordant VA connections correspond to transposition of the great vessels; the aorta arises from the anatomical right ventricle and the pulmonary artery arises from the left ventricle.[4,6-8,10] In corrected transposition, there is ventricular inversion with transposition of the great vessels.[6-9] Fetal echocardiography is facilitated by considering the more common combinations of axis, situs, and AV and VA connections.

Situs Solitus

Situs solitus with levocardia is the normal body configuration (Fig. 3–3). It is associated with CHD in fewer than 1% of cases.[11] However, an extreme leftward axis deviation or levorotation (severe levocardia) of greater than 57 to 75 degrees correlates with a significantly increased risk of a heart defect (Fig. 3–4).[2,3] Abnormalities that can have pronounced levorotation include truncus arteriosus, Ebstein anomaly, pulmonary stenosis, coarctation of the aorta, tetralogy of Fallot (TOF), transposition of the great arteries, and double-outlet right ventricle (DORV). Because of the frequent conotruncal and great vessel defects, the

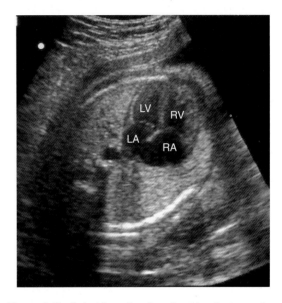

Figure 3–3 Apical four-chamber view showing normal cardiac axis, or levocardia. *LA*, Left atrium; *LV*, left ventricle; *RA*, right atrium; *RV*, right ventricle. The apex of the heart is approximately 45 degrees leftward of midline.

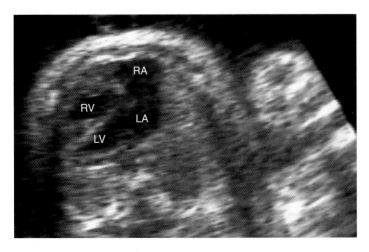

Figure 3–4 Subcostal four-chamber view in a fetus with tetralogy of Fallot showing abnormal left axis deviation or severe levocardia, or levorotation of the heart. *LA*, Left atrium; *LV*, left ventricle; *RA*, right atrium; *RV*, right ventricle.

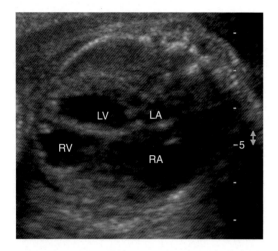

Figure 3–5 Subcostal four-chamber view in a fetus with Ebstein anomaly, showing abnormal levorotation as a result of the enlarged right atrium *(RA)*. *LA,* Left atrium; *LV,* left ventricle; *RV,* right ventricle.

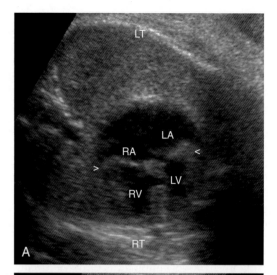

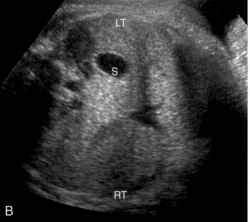

Figure 3–6 Isolated dextrocardia in a fetus with an atrioventricular septal defect (arrowheads showing a single atrioventricular valve). The apex of the heart is directed toward the right side of the fetal chest **(A),** but the fetal stomach *(S)* is positioned normally in the left upper quadrant of the abdomen **(B).** *LA,* Left atrium; *LT,* left; *LV,* left ventricle; *RA,* right atrium; *RT,* right; *RV,* right ventricle.

echocardiographic examination should be more extensive than the four-chamber view alone.[2,3]

The reason that CHD occurs with extreme levorotation in situs solitus is not known. Abnormal chamber size, for example, the enlarged right atrium in Ebstein anomaly, could cause the leftward axis deviation (Fig. 3–5).[2] It is also postulated that defective hearts overrotate from right to left during embryogenesis.[2,3] Extracardiac anomalies such as omphalocele, hydrocephalus, Dandy-Walker malformation, diaphragmatic hernia, and renal agenesis can be present. Abnormal karyotypes are not infrequent and include trisomy 21, trisomy 18, and trisomy 13.[2,3]

Situs solitus with dextrocardia is also referred to as dextroversion or isolated dextrocardia (Fig. 3–6, *A* and *B*).[6-8] This condition is found in 1 in 29,000 individuals in the general population. It is associated with CHD in 95% of cases.[11]

Situs solitus with dextrocardia can be divided into two subgroups. In one type, the AV and VA relationships are usually normal.[6,8-10] Sometimes there is complete transposition of the great arteries.[8] There are often other abnormalities such as atrial septal defect (ASD), ventricular septal defect (VSD), atrioventricular septal defect (AVSD), coarctation of the aorta, and anomalous pulmonary venous connections.[6] This dextroversion can be complicated by an ectopia cordis variant,

namely, herniation of a left ventricular diverticulum through the anterior diaphragm into the epigastrium.[8]

The other type of situs solitus with dextrocardia is associated with both AV and VA discordance or corrected transposition. Corrected transposition is common in dextroversion, occurring in up to 90%

of cases.[6,7,10] This type of situs solitus is often also complicated by VSD and pulmonary stenosis.[6,8] Other abnormalities that can be present include AVSD, TOF, pulmonary atresia, Ebstein anomaly, and anomalous systemic and pulmonary venous connections.[6,7]

Situs Inversus

Situs inversus is rare. It occurs in about 0.00005% of patients.[11] In most cases of situs inversus, the atrial and visceral situs are concordant; that is, there is dextrocardia.[8,11] Occasionally, the cardiac apex points leftward in situs inversus, a condition termed levoversion or isolated levocardia.[6-9,11]

Situs inversus with dextrocardia is referred to as mirror-image dextrocardia (Fig. 3–7, *A* and *B*).[6-11] Although the right atrium and right ventricle are on the left side and the left atrium and left ventricle are on the right side, there are usually physiological AV and VA connections.[6,7,9] Consequently, CHD is not common. Associated cardiac defects are found in 0.3% to 5% of patients.[7,11] Abnormalities that occur include ASD, VSD, AVSD, pulmonary atresia, TOF, and DORV.[6,10] If there is VA or AV plus VA discordance, the mirror-image equivalent of complete transposition or corrected transposition, respectively, is found.[6,10]

Situs inversus with levoversion or isolated levocardia is extremely rare.[11] It is the mirror-image of situs solitus with dextroversion.[8] CHD occurs in almost 100% of cases.[11] The inverted equivalent of corrected transposition is common.[6,8,10] There is also an association with DORV.[6,10] Systemic venous anomalies such as the lack of an inferior vena cava can be present.[9]

Mesocardia is uncommon (Fig. 3–8).[6] In one study, only 17 cases were noted among 3150 patients with CHD.[12] In another series that was based on a registry of about 3000 specimens, only seven of 65 malpositioned hearts manifested mesocardia.[10] The low frequency of mesocardia could be artificial because cases tend to be grouped according to either dextroversion or levoversion.[6] For example, in situs solitus, mesocardia reflects incomplete dextroversion.[6-9,12] In situs inversus, a heart in the midline corresponds to partial levoversion.[6,12]

Mesocardia occurs with situs solitus, situs inversus, and situs ambiguous.[6,10,12] As expected, the cardiac defects in mesocardia resemble those found in dextroversion and levoversion.[6] Many cases are associated with corrected transposition and complete transposition.[6,7,10,12] Other abnormalities that can be found include DORV, a single

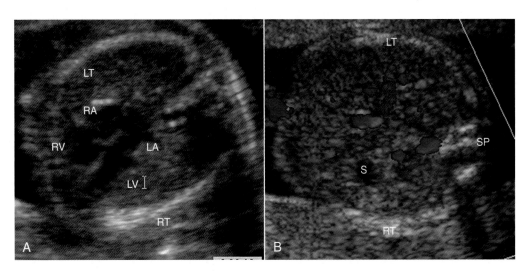

Figure 3–7 Apical four-chamber view in a fetus with dextrocardia and situs inversus totalis.
A, The heart is normal, although the apex is directed toward the right side of the fetal chest.
B, The fetal stomach *(S)* is located in the right abdomen, whereas the liver (color shows portal sinus) is in the left abdomen. *LA,* Left atrium; *LT,* left; *LV,* left ventricle; *RA,* right atrium; *RT,* right; *RV,* right ventricle; *SP,* spine.

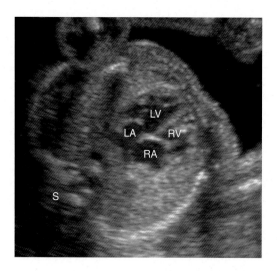

Figure 3–8 Mesocardia. The apex is directed midline. *LA*, Left atrium; *LV*, left ventricle; *RA*, right atrium; *RV*, right ventricle; *S*, spine.

ventricle, AVSD, and pulmonary stenosis or pulmonary atresia.[10,12]

Situs Ambiguous

Situs ambiguous is associated with two distinct syndromes: asplenia and polysplenia.[11] The visceroatrial situs in both is unusual. In asplenia or Ivemark syndrome, there is right atrial isomerism and bilateral right-sidedness.* Both atria have symmetrical right atrial morphological features.[11] Each lung is trilobed with an epiarterial bronchus.[8] The liver is often in a midline position, and the spleen is absent.[11,14] The stomach can be in the midepigastrium or located to either side of the abdomen.[11]

In polysplenia syndrome, there is left atrial isomerism and bilateral left-sidedness.[6,8,11,14] Both atria have features of the left atrium.[8] The lungs are bilobed with hyparterial bronchi.[11] In polysplenia, the abdominal organs tend to be less symmetrical than is the case in asplenia.[10] The liver is in a midline position in about one half of patients.[8] Multiple clumped splenules are usually unilateral and are located along the greater curvature of the stomach.[6,8,11] In up to 60% of patients, the position of the stomach is either in the midline or to the left.[14]

*References 6, 8, 9, 11, 13, 14.

Asplenia syndrome is associated with CHD in 99% to 100% of patients.[11] Dextrocardia, mesocardia, and levocardia can occur.[6,11] The cardiac anomalies in asplenia syndrome tend to be more severe than those in polysplenia syndrome.[11] There is often corrected or complete transposition of the great arteries.[6,8,10] ASD and AVSD are common.[6,8,10,11] There is a single ventricle in 50% of individuals and pulmonary stenosis or atresia in 75%.[8] Total anomalous pulmonary venous connection, particularly with return to the portal vein, often occurs.[8] Systemic venous abnormalities include bilateral superior venae cavae.[6,8,10]

There is a lower incidence of CHD in polysplenia syndrome. About 5% to 10% of patients have no heart disease. Associated cardiac defects tend to be milder compared with those of asplenia syndrome.[11] In polysplenia syndrome, the cardiac apex is rotated rightward in about 50% of cases and otherwise points to the left.[8,10] Mesocardia is uncommon.[10,15] Transposition of the great arteries is less frequent than in asplenia syndrome.[10] Although complete or corrected transposition can occur, the aorta–pulmonary arterial interrelationship is normal in 70% of patients. ASD, VSD, and AVSD are common.[8,10] A single ventricle is present in only 5% of hearts, but DORV is found in about 30%.[10] In contrast to asplenia syndrome, pulmonary stenosis or atresia is absent in two thirds of patients.[6–8,10] However, 40% to 50% of patients have left-sided obstructive lesions such as coarctation of the aorta, aortic stenosis, left ventricular hypoplasia, and mitral stenosis.[8,11] An anomalous pulmonary venous connection is common, but it is usually partial rather than total.[10] A characteristic feature of polysplenia is interruption of the hepatic portion of the inferior vena cava with azygous or hemiazygous continuation.[8,10,11,14] This condition occurs in about two thirds of patients.[8,14]

Complete heart block with bradycardia is common in polysplenia syndrome (Fig. 3–9).[4,5,11,14–16] It is often associated with an AVSD (Fig. 3–10).[4,5,14–16] AV block is apparently related to malformation and degeneration of the conduction system in these hearts.[15–17]

Polysplenia syndrome has been detected and diagnosed prenatally with ultrasound.[4,5,14,16,18] Nonimmune hydrops fetalis, the stomach on the right side, an interrupted inferior vena cava with azygous continuation, AVSD, and complete heart block have been demonstrated (see Figs. 3–9 and

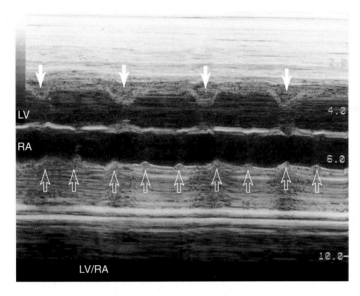

Figure 3–9 M-mode tracing of a fetal heart in a patient with polysplenia syndrome and an AVSD. Complete heart block was seen with an atrial rate *(open arrows)* of 142 beats per minute and a ventricular rate *(arrows)* of 60 beats per minute. *LV,* Left ventricle; *RA,* right atrium.

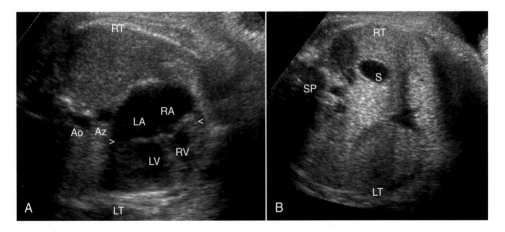

Figure 3–10 Four-chamber view in a fetus with a complete AVSD and polysplenia. **A,** The single AV valve *(arrows)* can be seen in addition to an ASD between the right atrium *(RA)* and the left atrium *(LA)*. A VSD is also present between the right ventricle *(RV)* and the left ventricle *(LV)*. Additionally, a dilated azygous vein *(Az)* resulting from an interrupted inferior vena cava is seen anterior to the fetal descending aorta *(Ao)*. The apex of the heart is correctly oriented toward the left chest. **B,** The fetal stomach *(S)* is seen on the right side of the fetal abdomen. *LT,* Left; *RT,* right; *SP,* spine.

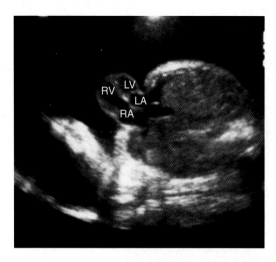

Figure 3-11 Thoracoabdominal ectopia cordis in a fetus with pentalogy of Cantrell. The heart lies outside the chest wall in this anomaly because of a sternal defect. *LA*, Left atrium; *LV*, left ventricle; *RA*, right atrium; *RV*, right ventricle.

3-10, *A* and *B*). The prognosis for fetuses with left atrial isomerism, complete AV block, and AVSD is poor. In utero and neonatal mortality rates are high.[5,14-16]

Abnormal Cardiac Position

As previously noted, fetal heart position can be defined separately from cardiac axis.[1] An abnormal position often indicates the presence of congenital defects that are different from those associated with an axis deviation. This distinction is emphasized by using the terms "dextroposition" and "levoposition" to describe the pathological displacement of the heart into the right or left thorax, respectively.[1,3,8,10,11] Extracardiac malformations are common and are often responsible for the abnormal location of the heart. In essence, the extracardiac defect pushes the heart out of its more midline location. These malformations include thoracoabdominal wall and diaphragmatic defects, a variety of pulmonary lesions, pleural disease, and miscellaneous intrathoracic tumors.

Ectopia Cordis

Ectopia cordis represents partial or complete displacement of the heart from the thoracic cavity.[6] It can be classified into five types according to heart location: cervical, thoracocervical, thoracic,

thoracoabdominal, and abdominal.[6,19,20] In the cervical form, the heart is in the neck and the sternum is intact. In the thoracocervical type, the heart protrudes through a defect in the superior sternum.[6,20] In thoracic ectopia cordis, there is a sternal defect and the heart lies outside the chest wall.[20,21] The thoracoabdominal type is associated with a common defect of the ventral lower thorax and midepigastrium (Fig. 3-11). In the abdominal form of ectopia cordis, a diaphragmatic gap allows the heart to enter the upper abdomen (Fig. 3-12).[6,20,21]

The thoracoabdominal type accounts for 7% of cases.[19,21] This malformation complex is known as the pentalogy of Cantrell (see Fig. 3-11).[19] In its complete form, ectopia cordis is associated with a deficient anterior pericardium, an inferior sternal defect, a ventral diaphragmatic opening, a supraumbilical abdominal wall defect (usually omphalocele), and congenital heart anomalies.[19,22-28] Pentalogy of Cantrell variants have been reported.[19,27] Some patients manifest three major features, including diaphragmatic, abdominal wall, and intracardiac defects.[19] In others, all the syndrome abnormalities are expressed except for either the cardiac or diaphragmatic defects.[27]

The cause of ectopia cordis is not known.[29] The cervical type may represent failure of the heart to descend from its embryonic location in the neck.[6,20] Other forms of ectopia cordis are thought to reflect abnormal mesodermal development at 14 to 18 days of gestation.[19,25,26,30] The chest and abdominal wall defects likely result from failure of ventromedial migration and fusion of the paired anterior body folds.[19,25,29] Thoracoabdominal ectopia cordis also involves defective formation of the transverse septum, a structure that later becomes the anterior diaphragm and associated pericardium.[19,20,25]

In some cases, ectopia cordis is part of the amniotic band syndrome.[21,27,29-31] Strands of amnion can be found attached to the ectopic heart and to the margins of thoracic and abdominal wall defects.[21,30,31] It is suggested that these adherent bands interfere with subsequent fetal development.[30]

Ectopia cordis can also be a feature of the limb-body wall complex.[19,27,32,33] This syndrome is postulated to result from amniotic rupture during the third to fifth weeks of embryogenesis, potentially as a result of an early vascular insult.[32,33] Along with neural tube defects, facial clefts, and limb reduction anomalies, the limb-body wall complex

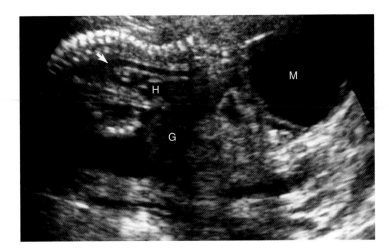

Figure 3–12 Sagittal image of a fetus with abdominal ectopia cordis. The aortic arch *(arrow)* and the fetal heart *(H)* can be seen in the fetal abdomen. Also noted were a gastroschisis *(G)* and a sacral meningomyelocele *(M).*

is associated with thoracoabdominoschisis. These large lateral body wall defects allow the gross evisceration of internal organs, including the heart, into the extraembryonic coelom.

Ectopia cordis is diagnosed prenatally with ultrasound by determining that the fetal heart is outside the thoracic cavity (see Figs. 3–11 and 3–12).[19,21,23–27,29–31,34] Because it is present from embryogenesis, ectopia cordis is detectable early in the second trimester of pregnancy.[19,21,29,31] Its diagnosis can be facilitated by endovaginal scanning.[21] Ectopia cordis can be missed in utero.[19,30] A partial ectopic position of the heart in association with a small omphalocele can be difficult to recognize during ultrasonography.[19]

Structural intracardiac defects are often present with ectopia cordis.[6,19,22–27,29–30,34] TOF complicates both the thoracic and thoracoabdominal forms.[6,19–22,34] ASD and VSD are not uncommon.[6,19,25,26,29–31] Many other congenital heart lesions can occur with ectopia cordis, including coarctation of the aorta, transposition of the great arteries, truncus arteriosus, aortic stenosis, pulmonary stenosis or pulmonary atresia, a single or hypoplastic ventricle, DORV, AVSD, mitral stenosis, tricuspid atresia, Ebstein anomaly, and anomalous pulmonary venous connections.* In some patients, the heart is intrinsically normal.[20,27,30]

Extracardiac defects can also be associated with ectopia cordis (see Fig. 3–12).[6] As noted, omphalocele is common and gastroschisis is sometimes present.[6,19] Neural tube anomalies include anencephaly, exencephaly, encephalocele, microcephaly, hydrocephalus, meningocele, and kyphoscoliosis.[6,19,25–27,29–31] Cleft lip, cleft palate, and a variety of skeletal deformities can occur.* The midline craniofacial and skeletal defects potentially reflect the association of ectopia cordis with amniotic band syndrome and limb–body wall complex.[21,27,30]

Chromosomal analysis is usually normal in cases of ectopia cordis.[19,25,26,29] Trisomy 18 has been reported.[19–27,29] Trisomy 13 and Turner syndrome have also been described.[19]

Ectopia cordis has a poor prognosis.[19,25,29,34] Postnatal survival is uncommon, particularly with the thoracic and thoracoabdominal types.[25,29] Although occasionally successful, the hazards of cardiac compression and kinking of the great vessels while reducing the heart into a small thorax makes surgical correction difficult at best.† In addition, complex intracardiac lesions can threaten survival despite the presence of repairable thoracic and abdominal wall defects.‡

Congenital Diaphragmatic Hernia

Congenital diaphragmatic defects occur in about 1 in 2000 to 3000 births.[35] Abnormalities include hernia, eventration, and agenesis. Congenital diaphragmatic hernia (CDH) is most common.[36]

---

*References 6, 19, 23, 26, 29, 31.

---

*References 6, 19, 21, 25, 26, 29–31.
†References 6, 20, 22, 24, 25, 29, 30, 34.
‡References 19, 20, 23, 24, 29, 30.

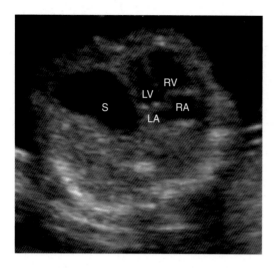

Figure 3–13 Transverse image through the chest of a fetus with a diaphragmatic hernia. The fetal heart is located in the right hemithorax. The cardiac apex points toward the left side. The fetal stomach *(S)* can be seen in the left hemithorax, causing the heart to be pushed to the right. *LA,* Left atrium; *LV,* left ventricle; *RA,* right atrium; *RV,* right ventricle.

CDH results from incomplete embryological development of the diaphragm. Posterolateral anomalies or Bochdalek defect occurs at 8 to 10 weeks of gestation because of incomplete closure of the pleuroperitoneal canals.[35–41] Anteromedial or Morgagni hernias result from maldevelopment of the retrosternal transverse septum.[35,37,39]

More than 90% of fetal diaphragmatic anomalies are Bochdalek hernias.[35] Most of these hernias are unilateral.[36,37] Although either hemidiaphragm can be affected, 75% to 90% of defects are left sided.[35,36,41]

Morgagni hernia is much rarer.[36,37] These hernias often lack an investing peritoneal sac.[35] Associated defects in the diaphragmatic pericardium can result in herniation of abdominal contents into the pericardial space.[35,37,42]

Left-sided CDHs usually contain stomach and bowel. The spleen and liver, particularly the left lobe, can be involved.[35,37–39,43–45] Intrathoracic liver, gallbladder, and bowel can be present with right-sided defects.*

The prenatal ultrasonographic diagnosis of CDH is often indirect. Actual visualization of the diaphragm is uncommon. Identifying some of the diaphragm is not necessarily helpful because CDH usually involves only a portion of this structure.[38,40]

CDH is suggested by cardiac dextroposition or levoposition (Fig. 3–13). A mediastinal shift is often caused by the mass effect of the hernia. Finding peristalsing bowel or a fluid-filled stomach or gallbladder in the chest helps confirm the presence of CDH.[35–38,40,41,43,46–48] In the absence of fetal swallowing of amniotic fluid, a nondistended stomach can be inconspicuous despite its intrathoracic location.[37] Because the liver is relatively isoechoic to fetal lung, detecting it in either right- or left-sided CDH can be difficult.[36–39,40,41]

Polyhydramnios occurs frequently with CDH.* It develops later in pregnancy, commonly after 24 weeks' gestation.[46,48] Although the etiology is uncertain, polyhydramnios is thought to be related to obstruction of the upper gastrointestinal tract from bowel herniation and mediastinal shift.[32,43,48]

CDH is associated with other anomalies in about 50% of cases.[35–37,39,43] Cardiac defects are found in association with 9% to 23% of CDHs.[35,36] Almost every kind of congenital heart lesion can develop; no single abnormality is more likely to occur than is another.[42] Structural cardiac anomalies that have been noted include coarctation of the aorta, transposition of the great arteries, truncus arteriosus, pulmonary stenosis, TOF, DORV, ASD, VSD, AVSD, tricuspid atresia, mitral atresia, and ectopia cordis.[35,42,43,49]

Reduced size and underdevelopment of the ipsilateral cardiac ventricle can complicate CDH.[36,49,50] This is postulated to result from the mass effect of the hernia. Alternatively, distortion of intrathoracic vessels or fetal lung compression could alter intracardiac hemodynamics, causing a potentially reversible type of chamber hypoplasia. Normal ventricular development can occur after surgical correction of the CDH.[50]

Noncardiac anomalies associated with CDH are not uncommon. Neural tube, gastrointestinal, genitourinary, and musculoskeletal defects occur.[35–37,39,40,42,48] Central nervous system abnormalities include anencephaly, holoprosencephaly, encephalocele, hydrocephalus, and spina bifida.[35,37,39] Gastrointestinal lesions include omphalocele, annular pancreas, bowel malrotation, and imperforate anus.[34,42,48] Genitourinary tract

---

*References 36–38, 39, 40, 41, 43, 46.

*References 35, 36, 39, 43, 47, 48.

anomalies include renal agenesis, cystic renal dysplasia, ureteropelvic junction obstruction, hydronephrosis, and uterine defects.[35,37,43] CDH and pulmonary sequestration can occur together.[45] Asplenia and polysplenia are among a variety of syndromes associated with CDH.[35,37,42]

Chromosomal analysis reveals an abnormal karyotype in up to 21% of patients with CDH.[40,48,51] Trisomy 13, trisomy 18, and trisomy 21 can occur.[35-37,39,42,43,48] Turner syndrome can also be found.[35]

Although the prognosis for fetuses with CDH remains poor, with an overall survival rate of around 50%, survival has improved over time.[51-54] This reflects the continuing improvement in conventional management. Factors that correlate with a poor outcome include the prenatal detection of a large hernia before 24 weeks' gestation, a marked mediastinal shift, ventricular underdevelopment, the presence of other anomalies, nonimmune hydrops fetalis, and intrauterine growth restriction.[35,36,47,49] Polyhydramnios may or may not be a poor prognostic indicator.[36,47,49]

The cause of perinatal morbidity and death in cases of CDH is pulmonary hypoplasia, pulmonary hypertension, and persistent fetal circulation associated with in utero lung compression.[36,37,43,47,48] Because of impaired fetal lung development, postnatal surgical reduction and repair of a CDH does not guarantee survival.[43,46-48] Prenatal intervention could improve pulmonary development, resulting in a better outcome at birth.[43,47]

Cystic Adenomatoid Malformation

Cystic adenomatoid malformation (CAM) is a hamartomatous lesion of the lung that accounts for about 25% of congenital pulmonary malformations.[35,55-58] It is thought to result from arrested bronchiolar development and overgrowth of mesenchymal tissues.[35] CAM can be divided into three subtypes in part on the basis of differing histological and macroscopic pathological features.[35,55-61] Type I CAM has one or more 2- to 10-cm cysts of variable size with adjacent smaller cysts.[35,36,55] The insult that causes this lesion probably occurs before 10 weeks of gestation.[35] Type II CAM consists of multiple, smaller (<1 to 2 cm), more uniform, and evenly spaced cysts.[35,36,58,59] It likely results from a developmental defect occurring before 31 days of gestation.[35] Type III CAM is made up of large, bulky masses with microscopic cysts that are usually no larger than 0.3 to 0.5 cm.[35,55,59]

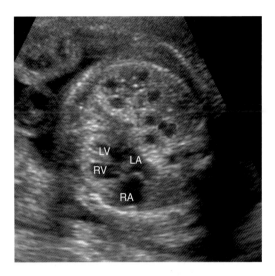

Figure 3–14 Transverse image through the thorax in a fetus with a type I CAM containing multiple macroscopic cysts. The CAM is pushing the fetal heart to the right hemithorax, but the cardiac apex is still directed leftward. *LA,* Left atrium; *LV,* left ventricle; *RA,* right atrium; *RV,* right ventricle.

These lesions are thought to be caused by an insult at 26 to 28 days of embryogenesis.[35]

CAM can be detected and diagnosed with antenatal ultrasonography as early as 12 weeks of gestation.[60] However, the average gestational age at diagnosis has been reported to be between 19 to 22 weeks' gestation.[56,58-68] Among the cases evaluated by prenatal ultrasonography, 57% are type 1, 6% are type II, and 37% are type III.[35] In utero, type I CAM looks like macroscopic cystic intrathoracic masses (Fig. 3–14).[55,58,65,69] With type II CAM, smaller cysts in a heterogeneous, more solid-appearing lesion are seen (Fig. 3–15).[69] Because its microscopic cysts result in innumerable acoustic interfaces, a type III CAM appears as a homogeneous echogenic solid mass (Fig. 3–16).[55,56,59,62]

CAM often displaces the fetal heart and mediastinum toward the contralateral hemithorax.* A CAM is usually unilateral and can occur in either the right or left lung. These lesions are occasionally bilateral.[56] The mass effect of a CAM can flatten or invert the diaphragm.[35,36,56,66] The positions of intra-abdominal organs remain normal.

CAM has also been reported to regress in utero, usually after 29 weeks' gestation.[70-72] However, it

---

*References 55, 56, 58, 59, 62, 64, 70.

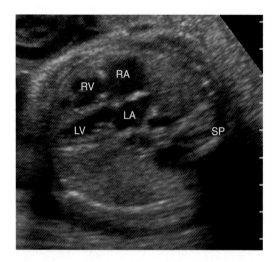

Figure 3–15 Transverse image through the thorax in a fetus with type II CAM. A discrete cyst is noted to the left of the descending aorta within a more solid-appearing mass. The heart is displaced to the right hemithorax, but the cardiac apex is still directed leftward. *LA*, Left atrium; *LV*, left ventricle; *RA*, right atrium; *RV*, right ventricle; *SP*, spine.

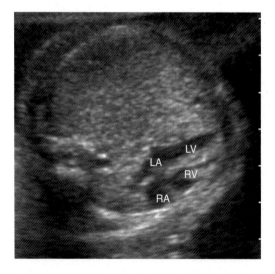

Figure 3–16 Transverse image of the chest in a fetus with type III CAM. The solid lesion can be seen displacing the fetal heart into the right hemithorax, but the cardiac apex is still directed leftward. *LA*, Left atrium; *LV*, left ventricle; *RA*, right atrium; *RV*, right ventricle.

is not entirely clear if the mass is actually decreasing in size or if it is becoming more isoechoic to the surrounding lung tissue.[72]

Polyhydramnios occurs in 68% of prenatally detected cases of CAM, and hydrops fetalis occurs in 62% of such cases.[35] Possible mechanisms for polyhydramnios include esophageal obstruction from the thoracic mass effect, overproduction of fluid by abnormal lung parenchyma, and decreased absorption of fluid by hypoplastic, malformed tissue. Hydrops fetalis could be caused by compression of the heart and vena cava or by antidiuretic hormone secretion or protein loss from the lesion.[56,61–64,66,73]

CAM can be associated with other anomalies. Although the reported frequency varies, additional congenital malformations complicate up to 26% of cases.[74] Concomitant lesions predominate in the type II subgroup. Cardiac, gastrointestinal, and genitourinary abnormalities can occur.[56,74–76] Congenital heart defects found include truncus arteriosus, tetralogy of Fallot, coarctation of the aorta, complete transposition of the great arteries, hypoplastic left heart syndrome, and VSD.[75] Gastrointestinal anomalies that can be present include gastric duplication cyst, jejunal and ileal atresia, imperforate anus, and omphalocele. Possible genitourinary lesions include renal agenesis and uterine duplication. CDH and pulmonary sequestration can also be found with CAM. Among a variety of miscellaneous defects are hydrocephalus, tracheoesophageal fistula, and tracheal atresia. Additionally, karyotyping is recommended in cases of CAM to detect any associated chromosomal abnormalities.[36]

The prognosis for fetuses with CAM is variable. Although overall survival is 50%, the outcome is related to the histopathological characteristics of the lesion.[58,59,66,69] The survival rate for macrocystic CAM (type I and type II) is 71% compared with 20% for microcystic CAM (type III).[66] Excess mortality is attributed to lethal anomalies associated with type II lesions.[53] The mass effect of large, bulky type III CAM increases the likelihood of pulmonary hypoplasia, hydrops fetalis, and polyhydramnios.[59,66,69] In general, polyhydramnios and hydrops fetalis are poor prognostic indicators.* Ultimate survival depends on the degree of pulmonary hypoplasia.[64]

In some cases, CAM is noted to decrease in size spontaneously.[69,73,77] Improvement or resolution of the mediastinal shift and fetal ascites and polyhydramnios can be seen.[56,58,69,73,77] Mechanisms

---

*References 56, 58, 61, 63, 64, 66.

that could explain this phenomenon include (1) decompression of the CAM into the tracheobronchial tree, (2) involution of the mass as it outgrows its blood supply, and (3) greater growth of normal surrounding structures relative to the lesion.[69,73,77] Irrespective of cause, the prognosis in these cases is excellent, and neonates do well with appropriate postnatal care.[56,58,69,73,77]

Several therapeutic options are available in the management of CAM.[66–68,78] Prenatal intervention is intended to reduce mass effect and optimize pulmonary development. If fetal surgery is not performed, the CAM is excised shortly after birth. Prompt resection is necessary to obviate respiratory embarrassment and cardiovascular compromise from air trapping and mass effect, to allow for full development of adjacent compressed lung, and to avoid superinfection.[63,64,70,72] In addition, all CAMs should be removed because malignancy can eventually arise in these lesions.[56,63,77]

Bronchopulmonary Sequestration

Bronchopulmonary sequestration is uncommon, representing 0.15% to 6.4% of congenital lung malformations.[35] It is a mass of nonfunctioning pulmonary parenchyma without connection to the normal bronchial tree.[35,45] It has an anomalous systemic arterial blood supply arising from either the descending thoracic or abdominal aorta.[35,36,45,79] Bronchopulmonary sequestration probably represents a bronchopulmonary foregut abnormality.[36] This could be potentiated by the aberrant systemic artery during embryogenesis.[35,79]

There are two kinds of bronchopulmonary sequestration: intralobar and extralobar. Both have a systemic arterial supply and do not communicate with the airway. Both occur most often in the posterior basal segment of a lower lobe.[35]

Seventy-five percent of bronchopulmonary sequestrations are intralobar[36,80] and occur with equal frequency in the right and left lungs.[35] They are contained within the visceral pleura along with the adjacent normal lung and display pulmonary venous drainage to the left atrium.[79,80]

Twenty-five percent of sequestrations are extralobar.[36,80] About 80% of extralobar bronchopulmonary sequestrations are left sided,[35] and approximately 5% are infradiaphragmatic.[80] An extralobar sequestration is enclosed within its own separate pleura.[35,36,79,81] Venous drainage is to the inferior vena cava, portal or other abdominal vein,

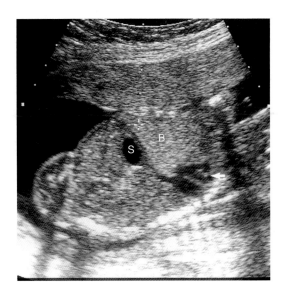

Figure 3–17 Coronal image of a fetus with a bronchopulmonary sequestration *(B)* displacing the fetal heart *(arrow)* to the right. *S*, Stomach.

azygous vein, hemiazygous vein, intercostal vein, or pulmonary vein.[82]

Bronchopulmonary sequestrations appear as relatively well-defined, rounded to triangular echogenic masses on prenatal ultrasonography (Fig. 3–17)[45,77,79–85] Demonstrating the anomalous feeding artery with color Doppler imaging can confirm the diagnosis.[45,77,86] As with other intrathoracic space–occupying lesions, bronchopulmonary sequestrations can have a mass effect, causing mediastinal shift, cardiac displacement, hydrops fetalis, and polyhydramnios.[77,79,82,83] This can be compounded by an associated pleural effusion.[82] Superimposed high output cardiac failure can occur from arteriovenous shunting through the sequestration.[77]

Bronchopulmonary sequestration is associated with other abnormalities. About 14% of intralobar sequestrations are associated with concomitant cerebral, cardiac, diaphragmatic, foregut, renal, and skeletal defects.[35] Approximately 50% to 60% of extralobar sequestrations have accompanying congenital anomalies,[36,84,85] which include cardiac, pericardial, other pulmonary, foregut, and vertebral abnormalities.[35,79,82–84] There is a strong association of bronchopulmonary sequestration with

CDH.[35,45,79,82–85] Patients with bronchopulmonary sequestration do not appear to have an increased frequency of chromosomal anomalies.[36]

The prognosis for fetal bronchopulmonary sequestration is related to the type of sequestration and its mass effect; to associated pulmonary hypoplasia, hydrops fetalis, and polyhydramnios; and to the presence or absence of other congenital anomalies.[35,77,81–83,85] In general, survival is better with intralobar sequestration than with extralobar sequestration.[36] This is because both hydrops fetalis and concomitant malformations are less likely with intralobar bronchopulmonary sequestration.[35] As with CAM, spontaneous regression of bronchopulmonary sequestration can occur in utero.[77]

Pleural Fluid Collections

Fetal pleural fluid collections can accumulate for many reasons.[35] Pleural effusion can be one of several features of generalized hydrops fetalis (Fig. 3–18),[35] which has both immune and nonimmune causes.[36] Nonimmune hydrops fetalis is associated with many conditions, including anatomical cardiac defects and arrhythmias, CDH, CAM, and bronchopulmonary sequestration.[35,36,87,88]

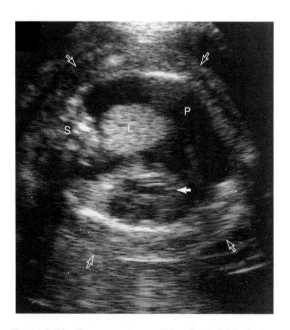

Figure 3–18 Transverse image through the fetal chest showing the heart *(solid arrow)* being displaced to the right side by a large pleural effusion *(P)*. Marked skin edema *(open arrows)* is also noted. *L*, Lung; *S*, spine.

Chylothorax is the most common cause of primary pleural effusion.[36] It can be an isolated abnormality.[35] Chylothorax can also be associated with congenital pulmonary lymphangiectasia, trisomy 21, and Turner syndrome.[35,79,89]

Isolated or congenital chylothorax potentially results from disruption or maldevelopment of the thoracic duct.[35,79,90] In most cases, the pleural fluid is unilateral and in the right hemithorax. Sometimes there is bilateral involvement. Males are affected more often than are females.[79,90]

Ultrasonographically, congenital chylothorax appears as uncomplicated, anechoic fluid within the fetal chest.[35,36,90] Although it can conform to the contours of the hemithorax,[36] a large chylothorax can cause mediastinal shift, cardiac displacement, and diaphragmatic inversion.[90–92] Hydrops fetalis, polyhydramnios, and pulmonary hypoplasia can result from the increased intrathoracic pressure.[79,90–94] Congenital chylothorax can be suspected at prenatal ultrasonography when unilateral pleural fluid is the only finding, when it is much larger than other identified effusions, and when it precedes other features of hydrops fetalis.[36]

The perinatal mortality rate is about 50% for fetuses with congenital chylothorax.[36] Chylothorax and hydrothorax can be managed aggressively with in utero thoracentesis and pleuroamniotic shunting.[92,94–98] Objectives of prenatal intervention include (1) diagnostic sampling for fluid analysis, (2) unmasking underlying structural pathological conditions, (3) preventing pulmonary hypoplasia, (4) alleviating hydrops fetalis and polyhydramnios, and (5) facilitating postnatal resuscitation and care.[35,36,79,92,94–98] A newly described treatment involves intrapleural injections of OK-432 in fetuses with pleural effusions.[99] A study published by Nygaad et al[99] reported total remission of pleural effusions in seven fetuses treated in utero. Other studies have also shown promising results; however, long-term postnatal follow-up is continuing.[99–102]

Miscellaneous Thoracic Lesions

Many other thoracic lesions can cause cardiac displacement, either directly or indirectly. Mediastinal tumors with mass effect include teratoma and neuroblastoma.[35,103–105] Foregut malformations such as bronchogenic, duplication, and neurenteric cysts can sometimes produce a mediastinal shift.[35,106–108] Bronchial atresia can cause an intrathoracic mass effect from postobstructive fluid accumulation and resultant expansion of the ipsilateral lung.[35,36,109] With unilateral pulmonary agenesis, the fetal heart can shift toward the affected hemithorax.[1,35] Chest wall lesions that can displace the heart include hamartoma and hemangioma.[35,110,111]

Axis and position are two important features of the fetal heart. Both can be assessed easily with the four-chamber view during either routine obstetrical ultrasonography or fetal echocardiography. An abnormal axis is often associated with structural cardiac defects. It requires the segmental evaluation of visceroatrial situs and cardiac anatomy. An abnormal position is often caused by an extracardiac congenital malformation. When detected, a careful examination of the fetus for a thoracic or infradiaphragmatic anomaly is warranted.

References

1. Comstock CH: Normal fetal heart axis and position. Obstet Gynecol 1987; 70:255–259.
2. Shipp TD, Bromley B, Hornberger LK, et al: Levorotation of the fetal cardiac axis: A clue for the presence of congenital heart disease. Obstet Gynecol 1995; 85:97–102.
3. Smith RS, Comstock CH, Kirk JS, et al: Ultrasonographic left cardiac axis deviation: A marker for fetal anomalies. Obstet Gynecol 1995; 85:187–191.
4. Nyberg DA, Emerson DS: Cardiac malformations. In: Nyberg DA, Mahony BS, Pretorius DH (eds): Diagnostic Ultrasound of Fetal Anomalies: Text and Atlas. St Louis, Mosby–Year Book, 1990, pp 300–341.
5. Silverman NH, Schmidt KG: Ultrasound evaluation of the fetal heart. In: Callen PW (ed): Ultrasonography in Obstetrics and Gynecology. Philadelphia, WB Saunders, 1994, pp 291–332.
6. Hagler DJ, O'Leary PW: Cardiac malpositions and abnormalities of atrial and visceral situs. In: Emmanouilides GC, Riemenschneider TA, Allen HD, et al (eds): Heart Disease in Infants, Children, and Adolescents Including the Fetus and Young Adult, 5th ed. Baltimore, Williams & Wilkins, 1995, pp 1307–1336.
7. Daves ML: Cardiac Roentgenology: Shadows of the Heart. Chicago, Year Book Medical, 1981.
8. Amplatz K, Moller JH: Radiology of Congenital Heart Disease. St Louis, Mosby–Year Book, 1993, pp 945–976.
9. Swischuk LE, Sapire DW: Basic Imaging in Congenital Heart Disease, 3rd ed. Baltimore, Williams & Wilkins, 1986.
10. Stanger P, Rudolph AM, Edwards JE: Cardiac malpositions: An overview based on study of sixty-five necropsy specimens. Circulation 1977; 56:159–172.
11. Winer-Muram HT, Tonkin ILD: The spectrum of heterotaxic syndromes. Radiol Clin North Am 1989; 27:1147–1170.
12. Lev M, Liberthson RR, Golden JG, et al: The pathologic anatomy of mesocardia. Am J Cardiol 1971; 28:428–435.
13. De Vore GR, Sarti DA, Siassi B, et al: Prenatal diagnosis of cardiovascular malformations in the fetus with situs inversus viscerum during the second trimester of pregnancy. J Clin Ultrasound 1986; 14:454–457.
14. Sheley RC, Nyberg DA, Kapur R: Azygous continuation of the interrupted inferior vena cava: A clue to prenatal diagnosis of the cardiosplenic syndromes. J Ultrasound Med 1995; 14:381–387.
15. Garcia OL, Mehta AV, Pickoff AS, et al: Left isomerism and complete atrioventricular block: A report of six cases. Am J Cardiol 1981; 48:1103–1107.
16. de Araujo LML, Silverman NH, Filly RA, et al: Prenatal detection of left atrial isomerism by ultrasound. J Ultrasound Med 1987; 6:667–670.
17. Dickinson DF, Wilkinson JL, Anderson KR, et al: The cardiac conduction system in situs ambiguous. Circulation 1979; 59:879–885.
18. Stoker AF, Tonnes SV, Spence J: Ultrasound diagnosis of situs inversus in utero. S Afr Med J 1983; 64:832–834.
19. Ghidini A, Sirtori M, Romero R, et al: Prenatal diagnosis of pentalogy of Cantrell. J Ultrasound Med 1988; 7:567–572.
20. Dobell ARC, Williams HB, Long RW: Staged repair of ectopia cordis. J Pediatr Surg 1982; 17:353–358.
21. Fleming AD, Vintzileos AM, Rodis JF, et al: Diagnosis of fetal ectopia cordis by transvaginal ultrasound. J Ultrasound Med 1991; 10:413–415.
22. Finberg HJ: Case of the day. Pentalogy of Cantrell. J Ultrasound Med 1993; 4:247.
23. Harrison MR, Filly RA, Stanger P, et al: Prenatal diagnosis and management of omphalocele and ectopia cordis. J Pediatr Surg 1982; 17:64–66.
24. Mercer LJ, Petres RE, Smeltzer JS: Ultrasonic diagnosis of ectopia cordis. Obstet Gynecol 1983; 61:523–525.
25. Abu-Yousef MM, Wray AB, Williamson RA, et al: Antenatal ultrasound diagnosis of variant of pentalogy of Cantrell. J Ultrasound Med 1987; 6:535–538.

26. Wicks JD, Levine MD, Mettler FA Jr: Intrauterine sonography of thoracic ectopia cordis. AJR Am J Roentgenol 1981; 137:619–621.

27. Denath FM, Romano W, Solcz M, et al: Ultrasonographic findings of exencephaly in pentalogy of Cantrell: Case report and review of the literature. J Clin Ultrasound 1994; 22:351–354.

28. Desselle C, Herve P, Toutain A, et al: Pentalogy of Cantrell: Sonographic assessment. J Clin Ultrasound 2007; 35:216–220

29. Klingensmith WC III, Cioffi-Ragan DT, Harvey DE: Diagnosis of ectopic cordis in the second trimester. J Clin Ultrasound 1988; 16:204–206.

30. Haynor DR, Shuman WP, Brewer DK, et al: Imaging of fetal ectopia cordis: Roles of sonography and computed tomography. J Ultrasound Med 1984; 3:25–27.

31. Bieber FR, Mostoufi-Zadeh M, Birnholz JC, et al: Amniotic band sequence associated with ectopia cordis in one twin. J Pediatr 1984; 105:817–819.

32. Patten RM, Van Allen M, Mack LA, et al: Limb-body wall complex: In utero sonographic diagnosis of a complicated fetal malformation. AJR Am J Roentgenol 1986; 146:1019–1024.

33. Goncalves LF, Jeanty P: Ultrasound evaluation of fetal abdominal wall defects. In: Callen PW (ed): Ultrasonography in Obstetrics and Gynecology, 3rd ed. Philadelphia, WB Saunders, 1994, pp 370–388.

34. Todros T, Presbitero P, Montemurro D, et al: Prenatal diagnosis of ectopia cordis. J Ultrasound Med 1984; 3:429–431.

35. Hilpert PL, Pretorius DH: The thorax. In: Nyberg DA, Mahony BS, Pretorius DH (eds): Diagnostic Ultrasound of Fetal Anomalies: Text and Atlas. St Louis, Mosby–Year Book, 1990, pp 262–299.

36. Goldstein RB: Ultrasound evaluation of the fetal thorax. In: Callen PW (ed): Ultrasonography in Obstetrics and Gynecology. Philadelphia, WB Saunders, 1994, pp 333–346.

37. Comstock CH: The antenatal diagnosis of diaphragmatic anomalies. J Ultrasound Med 1986; 5:391–396.

38. Chinn DH, Filly RA, Callen PW, et al: Congenital diaphragmatic hernia diagnosed prenatally by ultrasound. Radiology 1983; 148:119–123.

39. Stiller RJ, Roberts NS, Weiner S, et al: Congenital diaphragmatic hernia: Antenatal diagnosis and obstetrical management. J Clin Ultrasound 1985; 13:212–215.

40. Botash RJ, Spirt BA: Color Doppler imaging aids in the prenatal diagnosis of congenital diaphragmatic hernia. J Ultrasound Med 1993; 12:359–361.

41. Whittle MJ, Gilmore DH, McNay MB, et al: Diaphragmatic hernia presenting in utero as a unilateral hydrothorax. Prenat Diagn 1989; 9:115–118.

42. Greenwood RD, Rosenthal A, Nadas AS: Cardiovascular abnormalities associated with congenital diaphragmatic hernia. Pediatrics 1976; 57:92–97.

43. Nakayama DK, Harrison MR, Chinn DH, et al: Prenatal diagnosis and natural history of the fetus with a congenital diaphragmatic hernia: Initial clinical experience. J Pediatr Surg 1985; 20:118–124.

44. Bootstaylor BS, Filly RA, Harrison MR, et al: Prenatal sonographic predictors of liver herniation in congenital diaphragmatic hernia. J Ultrasound Med 1995; 14:515–520.

45. Luet'ic T, Crombleholme TM, Semple JP, et al: Early prenatal diagnosis of bronchopulmonary sequestration with associated diaphragmatic hernia. J Ultrasound Med 1995; 14:533–535.

46. Benacerraf BR, Greene MF: Congenital diaphragmatic hernia: US diagnosis prior to 22 weeks' gestation. Radiology 1986; 158:809–810.

47. Adzick NS, Harrison MR, Glick PL, et al: Diaphragmatic hernia in the fetus: Prenatal diagnosis and outcome in 94 cases. J Pediatr Surg 1985; 20:357–361.

48. Benacerraf BR, Adzick NS: Fetal diaphragmatic hernia: Ultrasound diagnosis and clinical outcome in 19 cases. Am J Obstet Gynecol 1987; 156:573–576.

49. Crawford DC, Wright VM, Drake DP, et al: Fetal diaphragmatic hernia: The value of fetal echocardiography in the prediction of postnatal outcome. Br J Obstet Gynaecol 1989; 96:705–710.

50. Crawford DC, Drake DP, Kwaitkowski D, et al: Prenatal diagnosis of reversible cardiac hypoplasia associated with congenital diaphragmatic hernia: Implications for postnatal management. J Clin Ultrasound 1986; 14:718–721.

51. Beck C, Alkasi O, Nikischin W, et al: Congenital diaphragmatic hernia, etiology and management, a 10-year analysis of a single center. Arch Gynecol Obstet. Published on-line, Aug 7, 2007.

52. Kalache KD, Mkhitaryan M, Bamberg C, et al: Isolated left-sided congenital diaphragmatic hernia: cardiac axis and displacement before fetal viability has no role in predicting postnatal outcome. Prenat Diagn 2007; 27:322–326.

53. Downard CD, Jaksic T, Garza JJ, et al: Analysis of an improved survival rate for congenital diaphragmatic hernia. J Pediatr Surg 2003; 38:729–732.

54. Harrison MR, Keller RI, Hawgood SB, et al. A randomized trial of fetal endoscopic tracheal occlusion for severe fetal congenital

diaphragmatic hernia. N Engl J Med 2003; 349:1916–1924.

55. Rosado-de-Christenson ML, Stocker JT: From the archives of the AFIP: Congenital cystic adenomatoid malformation. Radiographics 1991; 11:865–886.

56. Rempen A, Feige A, Wunsch P: Prenatal diagnosis of bilateral cystic adenomatoid malformation of the lung. J Clin Ultrasound 1987; 15:3–8.

57. Husler MR, Wilson D, Rychik J, et al: Prenatally diagnosed fetal lung lesions with associated conotruncal heart defects: Is there a genetic association? Prenat Diagn. Published on-line, Sept 5, 2007.

58. Graham D, Winn K, Dex W, et al: Prenatal diagnosis of cystic adenomatoid malformation of the lung. J Ultrasound Med 1982; 1:9–12.

59. Diwan RV, Brennan JN, Philipson EH, et al: Ultrasonic prenatal diagnosis of type III congenital cystic adenomatoid malformation of lung. J Clin Ultrasound 1983; 11:218–221.

60. Illanes S, Hunter A, Evans M, et al: Prenatal diagnosis of echogenic lung: Evolution and outcome. Ultrasound Obstet Gynecol 2005; 26:145–149.

61. Pezzuti RT, Isler PJ: Antenatal ultrasound detection of cystic adenomatoid malformation of lung: Report of a case and review of the recent literature. J Clin Ultrasound 1983; 11:342–346.

62. Johnson JA, Rumack CM, Johnson ML: Cystic adenomatoid malformation: Antenatal demonstration. AJR Am J Roentgenol 1984; 142:483–484.

63. Cohen RA, Moskowitz PS, McCallum WD: Sonographic diagnosis of cystic adenomatoid malformation in utero. Prenat Diagn 1983; 3:139–143.

64. Donn SM, Martin JN Jr, White SJ: Antenatal ultrasound findings in cystic adenomatoid malformation. Pediatr Radiol 1981; 10:180–182.

65. Stauffer UG, Savoldelli G, Mieth D: Antenatal ultrasound diagnosis in cystic adenomatoid malformation of the lung: Case report. J Pediatr Surg 1984; 19:141–142.

66. Adzick NS, Harrison MR, Glick PL, et al: Fetal cystic adenomatoid malformation: Prenatal diagnosis and natural history. J Pediatr Surg 1985; 20:483–488.

67. Blott M, Nicolaides KH, Greenough A: Postnatal respiratory function after chronic drainage of fetal pulmonary cyst. Am J Obstet Gynecol 1988; 159:858–859.

68. Adzick NS, Harrison MR, Flake AW, et al: Fetal surgery for cystic adenomatoid malformation of the lung. J Pediatr Surg 1993; 28:806–812.

69. Saltzman DH, Adzick NS, Benacerraf BR: Fetal cystic adenomatoid malformation of the lung: Apparent improvement in utero. Obstet Gynecol 1988; 71:1000–1002.

70. Harmath A, Csaba A, Hauzman E, et al: Congenital lung malformations in the second trimester: Prenatal ultrasound diagnosis and pathologic findings. J Clin Ultrasound 2007; 35:250–255.

71. Wilson RD, Hedrick HL, Liechty KW, et al: Cystic adenomatoid malformation of the lung: Review of genetics, prenatal diagnosis, and in utero treatment. Am J Med Gen 2006; 140A:151–155.

72. Gornall AS, Budd JLS, Draper ES, et al: Congenital cystic adenomatoid malformation: accuracy of prenatal diagnosis, prevalence and outcome in a general population. Prenat Diagn 2003; 23:997–1002.

73. Fine C, Adzick NS, Doubilet PM: Decreasing size of a congenital cystic adenomatoid malformation in utero. J Ultrasound Med 1988; 7:405–408.

74. Stocker JT, Madewell JE, Drake RM: Congenital cystic adenomatoid malformation of the lung: Classification and morphologic spectrum. Hum Pathol 1977; 8:155–171.

75. Miller RK, Sieber WK, Yunis EJ: Congenital adenomatoid malformation of the lung: A report of 17 cases and review of the literature. Pathol Annu 1980; 15:387–407.

76. Bale PM: Congenital cystic malformation of the lung: A form of congenital bronchiolar ("adenomatoid") malformation. Am J Clin Pathol 1979; 71:411–420.

77. MacGillivray TE, Harrison MR, Goldstein RB, et al: Disappearing fetal lung lesions. J Pediatr Surg 1993; 28:1321–1325.

78. Harrison MR, Adzick NS, Jennings RW, et al: Antenatal intervention for congenital cystic adenomatoid malformation. Lancet 1990; 336:965–967.

79. Reece EA, Lockwood CJ, Rizzo N, et al: Intrinsic intrathoracic malformations of the fetus: Sonographic detection and clinical presentation. Obstet Gynecol 1987; 70:627–632.

80. Mariona F, McAlpin G, Zador I, et al: Sonographic detection of fetal extrathoracic pulmonary sequestration. J Ultrasound Med 1986; 5:283–285.

81. Maulik D, Robinson L, Daily DK, et al: Prenatal sonographic depiction of intralobar pulmonary sequestration. J Ultrasound Med 1987; 6:703–706.

82. Thomas CS, Leopold GR, Hilton S, et al: Fetal hydrops associated with extralobar pulmonary sequestration. J Ultrasound Med 1986; 5:668–671.

83. Romero R, Chervenak FA, Kotzen J, et al: Antenatal sonographic findings of extralobar pulmonary sequestration. J Ultrasound Med 1982; 1:131–132.

84. Davies RP, Ford WDA, Lequesne GW, et al: Ultrasonic detection of subdiaphragmatic pulmonary sequestration in utero and postnatal diagnosis by fine-needle aspiration biopsy. J Ultrasound Med 1989; 8:47–49.

85. Baumann H, Kirkinen P, Huch A: Prenatal ultrasonographic findings in extralobar subdiaphragmatic lung sequestration: A case report. J Perinat Med 1988; 16:67–69.

86. Ruano R, Benachi A, Aubry MC, et al: Prenatal diagnosis of pulmonary sequestration using three-dimensional power Doppler ultrasound. Ultrasound Obstet Gynecol 2005; 25:128–133.

87. Chinn DH: Ultrasound evaluation of hydrops fetalis. In: Callen PW (ed): Ultrasonography in Obstetrics and Gynecology, 3rd ed. Philadelphia, WB Saunders, 1994, pp 420–439.

88. Rustico MA, Lanna M, Coviello D, et al: Fetal pleural effusion. Prenat Diagn 2007; 27:793–799.

89. Kerr Wilson RHJ, Duncan A, Hume R, et al: Prenatal pleural effusion associated with congenital pulmonary lymphangiectasia. Prenat Diagn 1985; 5:73–76.

90. Meizner I, Carmi R, Bar-Ziv J: Congenital chylothorax-prenatal ultrasonic diagnosis and successful post partum management. Prenat Diagn 1986; 6:217–221.

91. Defoort P, Thiery M: Antenatal diagnosis of congenital chylothorax by gray scale sonography. J Clin Ultrasound 1978; 6:47–48.

92. Schmidt W, Harms E, Wolf D: Successful prenatal treatment of non-immune hydrops fetalis due to congenital chylothorax: Case report. Br J Obstet Gynaecol 1985; 92:685–687.

93. Lange IR, Manning FA: Antenatal diagnosis of congenital pleural effusions. Am J Obstet Gynecol 1981; 140:839–840.

94. Petres RE, Redwine FO, Cruikshank DP: Congenital bilateral chylothorax: Antepartum diagnosis and successful intrauterine surgical management. JAMA 1982; 248:1360–1361.

95. Benacerraf BR, Frigoletto FD Jr, Wilson M: Successful midtrimester thoracentesis with analysis of the lymphocyte population in the pleural effusion. Am J Obstet Gynecol 1986; 155:398–399.

96. Blott M, Nicolaides KH, Greenough A: Pleuroamniotic shunting for decompression of fetal pleural effusions. Obstet Gynecol 1988; 71:798–800.

97. Rodeck CH, Fisk NM, Fraser DI, et al: Long-term in utero drainage of fetal hydrothorax. N Engl J Med 1988; 319:1135–1138.

98. Seeds JW, Bowes WA Jr: Results of treatment of severe fetal hydrothorax with bilateral pleuroamniotic catheters. Obstet Gynecol 1986; 68:577–579.

99. Nygaard U, Sundberg K, Nielsen HS, et al: New treatment of early fetal chylothorax. Obstet Gynecol 2007; 109:1088–1092.

100. Okawa T, Takano Y, Fujimori K, et al: A new fetal therapy for chylothorax: Pleurodesis with OK-432. Ultrasound Obstet Gynecol 2001; 18:376–377.

101. Jorgensen C, Brocks V, Bang J, et al: Treatment of severe fetal chylothorax associated with pronounced hydrops with intrapleural injection of OK-432. Ultrasound Obstet Gynecol 2003; 21:66–69.

102. Chen M, Shih JC, Wang BT, et al: Fetal OK-432 pleurodesis: Complete or incomplete? Ultrasound Obstet Gynecol 2005; 26:791–793.

103. Cyr DR, Guntheroth WG, Nyberg DA, et al: Prenatal diagnosis of an intrapericardial teratoma: A cause for nonimmune hydrops. J Ultrasound Med 1988; 7:87–90.

104. Farooki ZQ, Arciniegas E, Hakimi M, et al: Real-time echocardiographic features of intrapericardial teratoma. J Clin Ultrasound 1982; 10:125–128.

105. deFilippi G, Canestri G, Bosio U, et al: Thoracic neuroblastoma: Antenatal demonstration in a case with unusual postnatal radiographic findings. Br J Radiol 1986; 59:704–706.

106. Albright EB, Crane JP, Shackelford GD: Prenatal diagnosis of a bronchogenic cyst. J Ultrasound Med 1988; 7:91–95.

107. Young G, L'Heureux PR, Krueckeberg ST, et al: Mediastinal bronchogenic cyst: Prenatal sonographic diagnosis. AJR Am J Roentgenol 1989; 152:125–127.

108. Newnham JP, Crues JV III, Vinstein AL, et al: Sonographic diagnosis of thoracic gastroenteric cyst in utero. Prenat Diagn 1984; 4:467–471.

109. McAlister WH, Wright JR Jr, Crane JP: Mainstem bronchial atresia: Intrauterine sonographic diagnosis. AJR Am J Roentgenol 1987; 148:364–366.

110. Brar MK, Cubberley DA, Baty BJ, et al: Chest wall hamartoma in a fetus. J Ultrasound Med 1988; 7:217–220.

111. Lewis BD, Doubilet PM, Heller VL, et al: Cutaneous and visceral hemangiomata in the Klippel-Trenaunay-Weber syndrome: Antenatal sonographic detection. AJR Am J Roentgenol 1986; 147:598–600.

CHAPTER 4

Atrial Septal Defects

Elizabeth R. Stamm

OUTLINE

Definition

Embryology

Occurrence Rate

Sonographic Criteria

Treatment

Prognosis

Associated Anomalies

Definition

Any defect in the atrial septum other than a normal patent foramen ovale represents an atrial septal defect (ASD).

ASDs are classified according to their embryogenesis, their location relative to the fossa ovalis, and their size. There are four types of ASDs, listed here in order of frequency, with ostium secundum ASDs making up approximately 80% of cases (Fig. 4–1):

1. Ostium secundum
2. Ostium primum
3. Sinus venosus
4. Coronary sinus

The most common type of ASD, the ostium secundum ASD, generally occurs in isolation. It is located centrally in the atrial septum, superimposed on the fossa ovalis. The ostium primum ASD is the second most common type. Although ostium primum defects may occur alone, they usually occur as part of a more complex congenital cardiac anomaly, the atrioventricular septal defect. The ostium primum ASD is located low in the atrial septum immediately adjacent to the atrioventricular valves. Sinus venosus ASDs are rare and can be divided into two types:

1. Sinus venosus ASDs of the superior vena cava (SVC) type are located just inferior to the orifice of the SVC in the right atrium so that the SVC overrides the ASD, providing blood to both atria. Sinus venosus ASDs of the SVC type closely approximate the site where the right pulmonary veins enter the left atrium, allowing anomalous pulmonary venous drainage through the ASD. This type of ASD is present in partial anomalous pulmonary venous return to the right atrium.[1]

2. Sinus venosus ASDs of the inferior vena cava type are located in the atrial septum, adjacent to the orifice of the inferior vena cava in the right atrium.

The rare coronary sinus ASD is located at the expected site of the ostium of the coronary sinus in the right atrium. In this anomaly, the deficient or "unroofed" coronary sinus opens, through a defect in its distal wall, directly into the left atrium. The coronary sinus may enlarge greatly, resulting from increased flow. Usually, a persistent left SVC enters the upper left aspect of the left atrium. Rarely, the coronary sinus is absent rather than simply "unroofed." This variation is associated with cyanosis after birth because a large volume of desaturated (anomalous) left SVC blood pours into the left atrium where it mixes with and dilutes the oxygen-rich blood returning from the lungs.

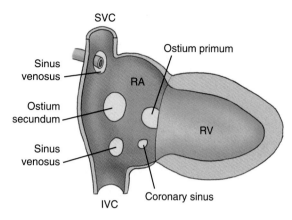

Figure 4–1   Location of the four types of ASD as viewed from the right atrium. *IVC,* Inferior vena cava; *RA,* right atrium; *RV,* right ventricle; *SVC,* superior vena cava.

The common atrium, the most severe form of ASD, is defined as an ASD involving >50% of the interatrial septum. Common atrium is rarely an isolated anomaly.[1]

Embryology

Between the fourth and sixth weeks of gestation, the primitive atrium is divided into right and left halves by a complex series of events. Throughout this process, some degree of interatrial blood flow is maintained. The septum primum, a thin, mobile, crescent-shaped membrane, develops along the cephalad portion of the atrium and grows caudally toward the endocardial cushions (Fig. 4–2, *A*). The space between the septum primum and the endocardial cushions, termed the ostium primum, is eventually obliterated when the septum primum fuses with the endocardial cushion (Fig. 4–2, *B* to *D*). Before complete fusion, however, multiple small fenestrations develop in the septum primum, coalescing to form the ostium secundum (Fig. 4–2, *B* to *D*), maintaining free blood flow from the right to the left primitive atrium.

A second crescent-shaped membrane, the septum secundum, subsequently develops just to the right of the septum primum (Fig. 4–2, *D* to *F*). The thick muscular septum secundum is formed from invagination of the roof of the primitive common atrium. As this membrane grows toward the endocardial cushions, it covers the ostium secundum (Fig. 4–2, *E* and *F*). Its crescent-shaped lower border never fuses entirely with the endo-

cardial cushion, leaving an opening that represents the foramen ovale (Fig. 4–2, *E* and *F*). The upper portion of the septum primum is gradually resorbed, and the remaining lower portion becomes the valve of the foramen ovale or foraminal flap (Fig. 4–2, *G* and *H*).

The most common type of ASD, the ostium secundum defect, is caused by a shortened valve of the foramen ovale (foraminal flap) resulting from excessive resorption of the septum primum or to deficient growth of the septum secundum (Fig. 4–3).

The ostium primum ASD occurs when the lower portion of the atrial septum, which is partially formed from the endocardial cushions, is deficient and fuses incompletely with the endocardial cushions (Fig. 4–4). This defect can occur in isolation but is usually part of the more complex atrioventricular septal defect, also referred to as an endocardial cushion defect or an atrioventricular canal defect, in which a single large abnormal atrioventricular valve separates the atria and ventricles in the presence of a large ASD and ventricular septal defect (VSD) (Fig. 4–5).

The sinus venosus ASD occurs during embryogenesis when the right horn of the sinus venosus, which normally encompasses the orifice of the SVC and the inferior vena cava, develops abnormally, leaving an opening in the atrial septum near one of these orifices (see Fig. 4–1).

The coronary sinus ASD occurs when improper development of the coronary sinus allows it to communicate directly with the left atrium through a defect in the wall of its distal extremity, leaving an open channel from the right atrium through the coronary sinus and into the left atrium (see Fig. 4–1). Even in the absence of structural defects, the anatomy of the normal neonatal atrial septum is complex (Fig. 4–6).

Occurrence Rate

ASDs occur in 1 in 1500 live births,[2,3] and they comprise approximately 6.7% of congenital heart disease in live-born infants.[4] Overall, ASDs are twice as common in female infants than in male infants.[5,6]

ASD is the fifth most common form of congenital heart disease, and it is the most common form in adult patients. A patient's life span without surgery can easily reach 50 years, and frequently ASDs are discovered incidentally at autopsy in asymptomatic individuals.

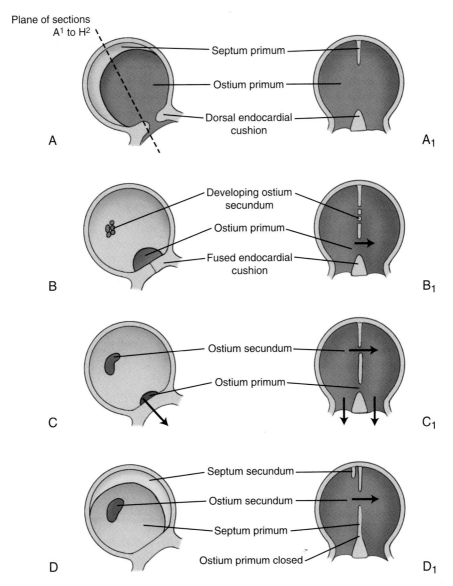

Plane of sections
A¹ to H²

Figure 4–2 Differentiation of the atrial septum as viewed from the right side (lateral) and the anteroposterior direction (subscript letters). **A,** The beginning of the septum primum. **B,** Growth of the septum primum toward the fused endocardial cushions; perforations are developing as the early ostium secundum. **C,** The septum primum is nearly fused to the endocardial cushions. The coalesced perforations form the ostium secundum. **D,** The ostium primum is closed—the beginning of the septum secundum.

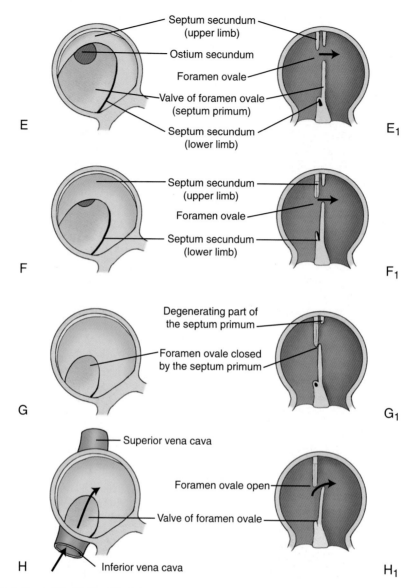

Figure 4–2, cont'd   E, Growth of the septum secundum. **F,** The septum secundum is covering the ostium secundum; the foramen ovale. **G,** The continued growth of the septum secundum; closure of the foramen ovale. **H,** Relationship between the inferior vena cava and the valve of the foramen ovale.

Ostium secundum defects account for more than 80% of all ASDs[5] and occur twice as often in female patients.[7] Sinus venosus defects account for 5% to 10% of all ASDs and occur with equal frequency in male and female patients.[8] Coronary sinus defects are rare. Various combinations of these types of ASD can occur together.

Rarely, ostium secundum ASDs are familial and may occur through multiple generations.[9–12] Perhaps the best known example of familial inheritance of ASD is the Holt-Oram syndrome.[13] This disorder is characterized by an autosomal dominant pattern of inheritance with a penetrance of nearly 100%. In addition to a septum secundum

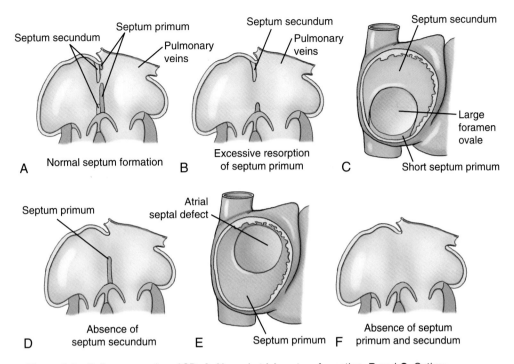

Figure 4–3 Ostium secundum ASD. **A,** Normal atrial septum formation. **B** and **C,** Ostium secundum defect caused by excessive resorption of the septum primum. **D** and **E,** Similar defect caused by failure of development of the septum secundum. **F,** Common atrium or cor triloculare biventriculare—complete failure of the septum primum and septum secundum to form.

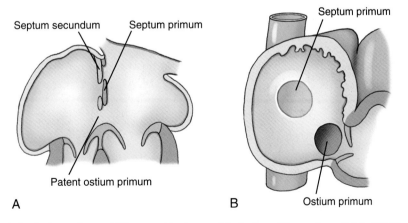

Figure 4–4 Ostium primum ASD caused by incomplete fusion of the endocardial cushions. **A,** View of the heart parallel with the interatrial septum. **B,** View from the right atrium, perpendicular to the interatrial septum.

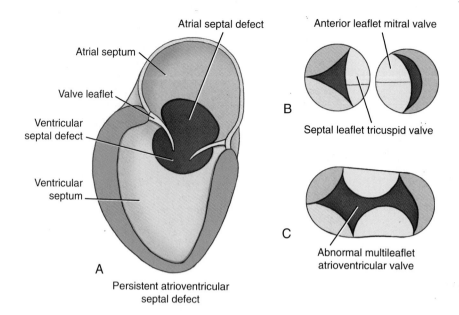

Figure 4–5 AVSD. **A,** Persistent atrioventricular septal defect. This abnormality is always accompanied by a septal defect in the atrial and ventricular septae. **B,** Normal valves in the atrioventricular orifices. **C,** Abnormal multileaflet valve in an atrioventricular canal defect.

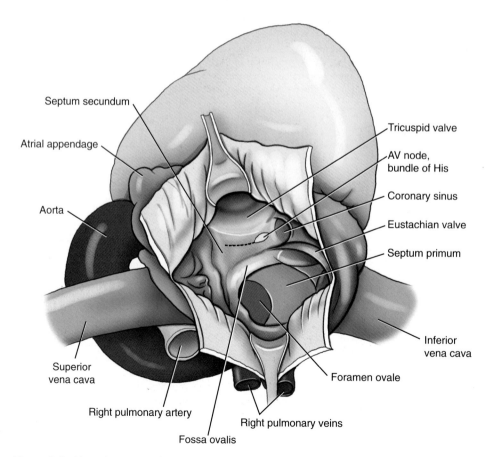

Figure 4–6 Normal anatomy of the neonatal atrial septum as viewed from the right atrium.

ASD, patients have congenital deformities of the upper limbs (most commonly with absent or hypoplastic radii) and cardiac rhythm abnormalities such as a right bundle branch block or first-degree atrioventricular block. Approximately 40% of these cases represent new mutations. The remainder are inherited from a parent.

A second example of familial inheritance of ASD (also ostium secundum type) is the syndrome of familial ASD with prolonged atrioventricular conduction.[14] Like Holt-Oram syndrome, this defect is inherited in an autosomal dominant manner. It is important to identify these syndromes before counseling patients whose fetuses have ASDs because if one of these syndromes is present, 50% of first-degree relatives will be affected with the syndrome and thus with ASDs. With the more common sporadically occurring ASD, only 3% of first-degree relatives are affected.

Sonographic Criteria

It is difficult to make the diagnosis of ASD with fetal echocardiography because the examination is complicated by the normal patent foramen ovale, which allows blood flow from the right atrium to the left atrium. With the currently available high-resolution equipment, the atrial septum can be evaluated in detail. The septum primum (the foraminal flap) is routinely visualized on the apical or subcostal four-chamber view as it opens into the left atrium at two times the fetal heart rate (Fig. 4–7). The septum primum has a configuration that resembles a "loose pocket" and thus, depending on the plane of section, it can appear circular or linear (Figs. 4–8 and 4–9).[15,16] The foraminal flap is easily demonstrated and has a characteristic appearance on M-mode echocardiography (Fig. 4–10). The thicker, relatively immobile septum secundum that makes up the bulk of the interatrial septum is perforated by the foramen ovale. It is visualized optimally on the subcostal four-chamber view (Fig. 4–11) because in this view the ultrasound beam is perpendicular to the interatrial septum.

Most in utero ASDs are best visualized in the subcostal four-chamber view (Fig. 4–12). The ostium secundum ASD appears as a larger-than-expected area of dropout in the central portion of the septum secundum in the vicinity of the foramen ovale or as a deficient foraminal flap (septum primum) that fails to cover the foramen ovale entirely (Fig. 4–13).

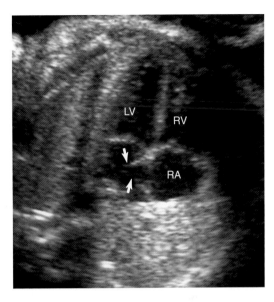

Figure 4–7 Apical four-chamber view with the septum primum (the foraminal flap) opening into the left atrium *(arrows)*. *LV*, Left ventricle; *RA*, right atrium; *RV*, right ventricle.

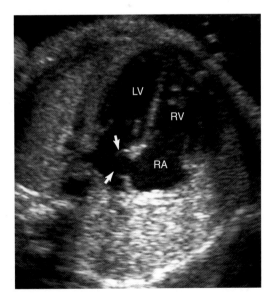

Figure 4–8 Apical four-chamber view showing the foraminal flap as a circular structure *(arrows)* within the left atrium. *LV*, Left ventricle; *RA*, right atrium; *RV*, right ventricle.

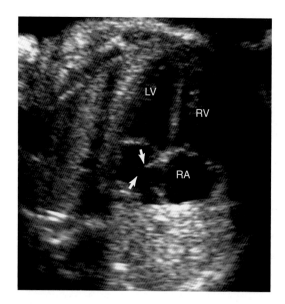

Figure 4–9 Apical four-chamber view showing the foraminal flap as a linear structure *(arrows)* within the left atrium. *LV,* Left ventricle; *RA,* right atrium; *RV,* right ventricle.

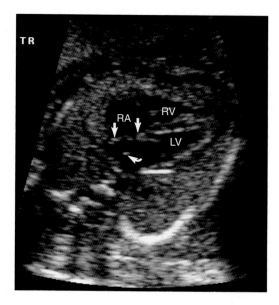

Figure 4–11 Subcostal four-chamber view showing the septum secundum *(arrows)* and the septum primum (foraminal flap) within the left atrium *(curved arrow).* *LV,* Left ventricle; *RA,* right atrium; *RV,* right ventricle.

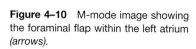

Figure 4–10 M-mode image showing the foraminal flap within the left atrium *(arrows).*

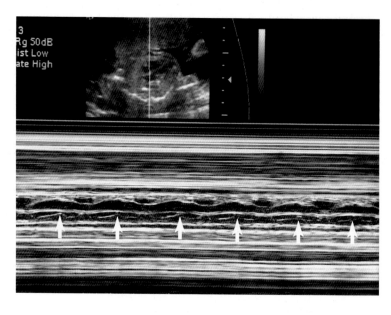

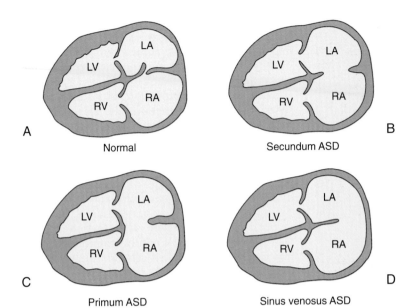

A — Normal
B — Secundum ASD
C — Primum ASD
D — Sinus venosus ASD

Figure 4–12 Diagram showing the appearance of the different types of ASDs as visualized in a subcostal four-chamber view of the fetal heart. **A,** Normal. **B,** Secundum ASD. **C,** Primum ASD. **D,** Sinus venosus ASD. *LA,* Left atrium; *LV,* left ventricle; *RA,* right atrium; *RV,* right ventricle.

The ostium primum ASD is characterized by the absence of the lower portion of the atrial septum (just above the atrioventricular valves). Frequently, the remaining portion of the atrial septum adjacent to the defect appears thickened and bulbous (Fig. 4–14).

Normally, the septal leaflet of the tricuspid valve inserts slightly more apically than does the anterior mitral valve leaflet, although this normal difference is subtle in the fetal population. The septal leaflet of the tricuspid valve and the anterior leaflet of the mitral valve insert at the same level in the presence of a septum primum ASD. This reflects the fact that the septum primum ASD represents part of the spectrum of the endocardial cushion defect. Although generally not evident in the fetus, the normal "fish mouth" appearance of the mitral valve in a short-axis view is absent because in most septum primum ASDs the anterior leaflet of the mitral valve contains a large cleft.

The antenatal diagnosis of sinus venosus ASD has not yet been reported.

Color flow imaging is helpful in the setting of large ASDs; however, the normal rapid flow through the foramen ovale may obscure smaller defects (Fig. 4–15).

Treatment

Because a right-to-left shunt at the atrial level is physiological in utero, the fetus is generally unaf-

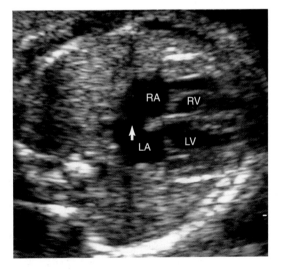

Figure 4–13 Subcostal four-chamber view showing an ostium secundum ASD *(arrow)* within the central portion of the septum secundum. *LA,* Left atrium; *LV,* left ventricle; *RA,* right atrium; *RV,* right ventricle.

fected by an isolated ASD, and in utero treatment is unnecessary. Indeed, the diagnosis of isolated ASD is rarely made prenatally. As with any fetal cardiac anomaly, the detection of a fetal ASD is an indication for a formal fetal echocardiogram along with careful obstetrical ultrasonography to exclude

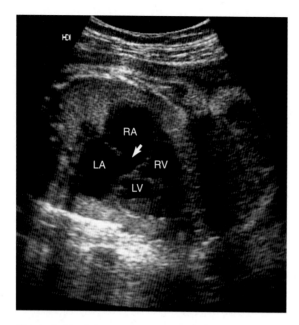

Figure 4–14   Subcostal four-chamber view demonstrating an ostium primum ASD *(arrow)* as characterized by the absence of the lower portion of the atrial septum. *LA,* Left atrium; *LV,* left ventricle; *RA,* right atrium; *RV,* right ventricle.

additional cardiac or extracardiac anomalies. Karyotyping should be considered because ASD may be associated with chromosomal anomalies.

Most ASDs remain asymptomatic in early life. Classically, diagnosis is first made when a murmur is heard in an asymptomatic child during a pre-school physical examination. The repair of ASDs in asymptomatic children is recommended to avoid worsening symptoms and complications such as supraventricular arrhythmias, congestive heart failure, or pulmonary vascular disease, which may develop later in life. Unrepaired ASDs are associated with a shortened life expectancy.[17] The timing of repair in the asymptomatic patient is flexible, with most surgeons recommending repair for the asymptomatic or mildly symptomatic child at 4 to 5 years of age. This general time frame was based on the fact that in the past the technical difficulty associated with repairing the child's small heart was considerable, and early repair generally offered no particular advantage. Because technical considerations are no longer a compelling reason to delay surgery, it is reasonable to perform elective closure of an ASD earlier. Elective repair generally is not performed before 1 year of age in asymptomatic patients because spontaneous closure of the ASD may occur in greater than

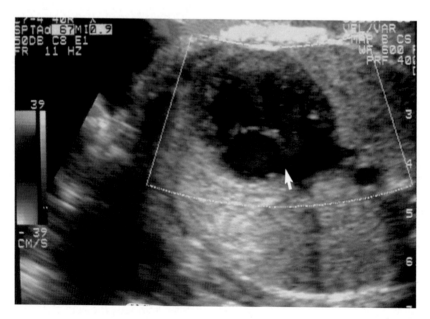

Figure 4–15   Apical four-chamber view showing color flow through the normal foramen ovale *(arrow).*

60% of these patients.[6,18-23] Few large ASDs close spontaneously after 1 year of life, so delaying surgery beyond the first year solely on the basis of possible spontaneous closure is unnecessary.

Rarely, symptoms may occur at birth[24] or in the first week of life.[25,26] Congestive heart failure or failure to thrive develops in infancy in approximately 5% of untreated isolated ASDs[27,28] with a mortality rate as high as 10% without surgical correction.[29] The initial management for the symptomatic infant includes the administration of digitalis and diuretics. Early surgical repair should be considered.

Percutaneous transcatheter repair of ASDs was first accomplished in 1976.[30] In general, the success rate has been high and the morbidity rate low. There is a growing interest in these minimally invasive surgical ASD repairs, which have become increasingly popular over the last 10 years.[31-34] Benefits include reduced postoperative pain and decreased recovery time. Totally endoscopic atrial septal repair (TEASR) is performed through an 8-mm incision and has proved both safe and effective and provides an excellent cosmetic result.[35]

Robotically assisted, totally endoscopic ASD repair is now widely performed with excellent success.[36-39]

Large ASDs may require a patch for complete closure. A wide variety of materials have been used to accomplish closure, including autologous or bovine pericardium and various synthetic products. Recently it has been demonstrated that autologous free right atrial wall can be safely used in ASD repair. This technique appears to offer important advantages over other materials. Research in this area is continuing.[40]

Prognosis

The prognosis for an isolated ASD in a fetus is excellent because shunting of blood from the right atrium to the left atrium through the foramen ovale occurs normally in utero so that the normal physiology is altered little. Most patients remain asymptomatic through early childhood. ASDs of all types can be safely and successfully repaired, even in small infants. The operative mortality rate in children is less than 1%—only slightly higher than it is in adults. With the advent of nonsurgical techniques, even the infant with severe symptoms can commonly undergo repair with relatively little risk.

Frequently, untreated patients survive well into their 50s, and there have been numerous reports of patients with ASDs remaining asymptomatic throughout life.

Associated Anomalies

ASDs often occur in conjunction with other congenital cardiac anomalies (Table 4–1), including VSD, patent ductus arteriosus, transposition of the great arteries, coarctation of the aorta, and others. Although usually the associated lesions are of primary importance, the ASD may play an important role in the physiology of the complex congenital heart disease. For example, in complete transposition of the great arteries, absence of an associated defect that allows continued mixing of the pulmonary and systemic circulations after closure of the foramen ovale would be fatal after birth. In total anomalous pulmonary venous connection, an ASD provides a route by which pulmonary venous blood can return to the systemic circulation. The absence of such a pathway would be incompatible with life. Partial anomalous pulmonary venous connection from the right lung is almost always associated with ASD.[41]

A total of 10% to 15% of ostium secundum ASDs are associated with partial anomalous pulmonary venous connection. Ostium primum ASDs are associated with an increased incidence of trisomy 21 and with cleft mitral valve and mitral regurgitation. A total of 80% to 90% of sinus venosus defects of the superior vena cava type are associated with an anomalous pulmonary connection of the right superior pulmonary vein to the right atrium or superior vena cava.[8,42,43] Coronary sinus ASD is usually associated with a persistent left superior vena cava that terminates on the roof of the left atrium. This anomaly may also be associated with atrioventricular septal defect and the asplenia syndrome.

A number of syndromes are associated with ASD. The best known of these is Holt-Oram syndrome. This autosomal dominant disorder with nearly 100% penetrance is characterized by an ASD (with or without other cardiac anomalies), upper limb deformities (most commonly hypoplastic or absent radii), and cardiac rhythm abnormalities, including first-degree atrioventricular block and right bundle-branch block. Fifty percent of first-degree relatives can be expected to be affected with this syndrome and thus to have an ASD.

TABLE 4–1   Conditions Associated with Atrial Septal Defect

| Maternal | | Fetal | | |
Condition	Drug Use	Associated Cardiac Abnormalities	Chromosome Abnormalities	Syndromes
Cytomegalovirus Diabetes	Alcohol Dilantin (phenytoin)	Coarctation Complete heart block Supravalvular aortic stenosis Atrioventricular septal defect Partial anomalous pulmonary venous connection Supraventricular tachycardia Wolfe-Parkinson-White syndrome Transposition of the great vessels Cleft mitral Valve Anomalous right pulmonary vein Persistent left superior vena cava	Monosomy medial 2q Monosomy 14q Trisomy 8 Trisomy 13 (Patau syndrome) Trisomy 16p Trisomy 16q Trisomy 21 Triploidy Golabi-Ito-Hall X-linked 45 X (Turner syndrome)	Acromicric dysplasia Alagille syndrome Arthrochalasis multiplex-congenita Cardiac-limb syndrome Cardiofacial syndrome Cardiomelic syndrome Cat-eye syndrome Cayler syndrome CHARGE (coloboma of the eye, heart anomaly, choanal atresia, retardation, and genital and ear anomalies) syndrome Chondroectodermal dysplasia Cryptophthalmos-syndactyly Cryptophthalmos syndrome Dermofaciocardioskeletal syndrome Duane syndrome Dysencephalia syndrome Eagle-Barrett syndrome Ehlers-Danlos syndrome Elfin facies syndrome Factor V deficiency Ferrell-Okihiro-Halal syndrome Fraser syndrome Geleophysic dwarfism Halarz syndrome Hand-heart syndrome Holt-Oram syndrome Hypogonadotropic syndrome Kallmann syndrome Kallmann-deMorsier syndrome Locking digits–growth defect Lutembacher syndrome Majewski syndrome malformations Marshall-Smith syndrome McDonough syndrome Meckel-Gruber syndrome Mutchinick syndrome Neurofibromatosis Noonan syndrome Okihiro syndrome Pentalogy of Cantrell Polysplenia Polystydactyly-cardiac syndrome Prune-belly syndrome Pulmonary venolobar syndrome Radial-renal-ocular syndrome Retardation Scimitar syndrome Short rib polydactyly syndrome, type II Situs inversus viscerum Sternal-cardiac malformation association TAR (thrombocytopenia with absent radius) syndrome Tracheal agenesis Venolobar syndrome Williams syndrome Williams-Beuren syndrome

References

1. Munoz-Castellanos L, Espinola-Zavaleta N, Kuri-Nivon M, et al: Atrial septal defect: Anatomoechocardiographic correlation. J Am Soc Echocardiogr 2006; 19:1182–1189.

2. Keith JD: Atrial septal defect: Ostium secundum, ostium primum and atrioventricularis communis (common AV canal). In: Keith JD, Rowe RD, Vlad P (eds): Heart Disease in Infancy and Childhood, 3rd ed. New York, MacMillan, 1978, pp 330–404.

3. Samanek M: Children with congenital heart disease: Probability of natural survival. Pediatr Cardiol 1992; 13:152–158.

4. Hoffman JIE, Christianson MA: Congenital heart disease in a cohort of 19,502 births with long term follow-up. Am J Cardiol 1978; 42:641–647.

5. Fyler DC: Atrial septal defect secundum. In: Fyler DC (ed): Nadas' Pediatric Cardiology. Philadelphia, Hanley and Belfus, 1992, pp 513–524.

6. Feldt RH, Avasthey P, Yoshim ASVF, et al: Incidence of congenital heart disease in children born to residents of Olmsted County, Minnesota 1950-1969. Mayo Clin Proc 1971; 46:794–799.

7. Fyler DC, Buckley LP, Hellenbrand WE, et al: Report of the New England Regional Infant Cardiac Program. Pediatrics 1980; 65(Suppl):375–461.

8. Davia JE, Cheiten MD, Bedynek JL: Sinus venosus atrial septal defect: analysis of fifty cases. Am Heart J 1973; 85:177–185.

9. Davidsen GH: Atrial septal defects in a mother and her children. Acta Med Scand 1958; 160:447–454.

10. Howitt G: Atrial septal defect in three generations. Br Heart J 1961; 23:494–496.

11. Johansson B, Sievers J: Inheritance of atrial septal defect. Lancet 1967; 1:1224–1225

12. Nora JJ, McNamara DG, Fraser FC: Hereditary factors in atrial septal defects. Circulation 1967; 35:448–456.

13. Holt M, Oram S: Familial heart disease with skeletal malformations. Br Heart J 1960; 22:236–242.

14. Bizarro RO, Callahan JA, Feldt RH, et al: Familial atrial septal defect with prolonged atrioventricular conduction: A syndrome showing the autosomal dominant pattern of inheritance. Circulation 1970; 41:677–683.

15. Crelin ES: Anatomy of the Newborn. An Atlas. Philadelphia, Lea & Febiger, 1969.

16. Kachalia P, Bowie JD, Adams DB, et al: In utero sonographic appearance of the atrial septum primum and septum secundum. J Ultrasound Med 1991; 10:423–426.

17. Campbell M: Natural history of atrial septal defect. Br Heart J 1970; 32:820–826.

18. Hanslik A, Pospisil U, Salzer-Muhar U, et al: Predictors of spontaneous closure of isolated secundum atrial septal defect in children: a longitudinal study. Pediatrics 2006; 118:1560–1565.

19. Garne E: Atrial and ventricular septal defects: Epidemiology and spontaneous closure. J Matern Fetal Neonat Med 2006; 19:271–276.

20. Ghisla RP, Hannon DW, Meyer RA, et al: Spontaneous closure of isolated secundum atrial septal defects in infants: An echocardiographic study. Am Heart J 1985; 109:1327–1333.

21. Cummings DR: Functional closure of atrial septal defects. Am J Cardiol 1968; 22:888–892.

22. Cayler GG: Spontaneous functional closure of symptomatic atrial septal defects. N Engl J Med 1967; 276:65–73.

23. Mody MR: Serial hemodynamic observations in secundum atrial septal defects with reference to spontaneous closure. Am J Cardiol 1973; 32:978–981.

24. Hastreiter AR, Wennemark JR, Miller RA, et al: Secundum atrial septal defects with congestive heart failure during infancy and early childhood. Am Heart J 1962; 64:467–472.

25. Phillips SJ, Okres JE, Henken D, et al: Complex secundum atrial septal defect and congestive heart failure in infants. J Thorac Cardiovasc Surg 1975; 70:696–700.

26. Toews WH, Nora JJ, Wolfe RR: Presentation of atrial septal defect in infancy. JAMA 1975; 234:1250–1251.

27. Navajas A, Pastor E, laFuente P, et al: Symptomatic atrial septal defect in infancy. An Esp Pediatr 1981; 14:25–32.

28. Gordovilla-Zurdo G, Cabo-Salvador J, Moreno-Granados F, et al: Surgery of symptomatic interauricular communication in the first year of life. An Esp Pediatr 1988; 29:94–98.

29. Hunt CE, Lucas RV Jr: Symptomatic atrial septa defects in infancy. Circulation 1973; 47:1042–1048.

30. King TD, Mills NL: Secundum atrial septal defects: nonoperative closure during cardiac catheterization. JAMA 1976; 235:2506–2509.

31. Kharouf R, Lusenberg DM, Khalid O, Abdulla R: Atrial septal defect: spectrum of care. Pediatr Cardiol 2008; 29:271–280.

32. Chang CH, Lin PJ, Chu JJ, et al: Surgical closure of atrial septal defect. Minimally invasive cardiac surgery or median sternotomy? Surg Endosc 1998; 12:820–824.

33. Formigar R, Donato RMD, Mazzere E, et al: Minimally invasive or interventional repair of

atrial septal defects in children: Experience in 171 cases and comparison with conventional strategies. J Am Coll Cardiol 2001; 37:1707–1712.

34. Cremer JT, Boning A, Anssar MB, et al: Different approaches for minimally invasive closure of atrial septal defects. Ann Thorac Surg 1999; 67:1648–1652.

35. Ak K, Aybek T, Wimmer-Greinecker G, et al: Evolution of surgical techniques for atrial septal defect repair in adults: A 10 year single-institution experience. J Thorac Cardiovasc Surg 2007; 134:757–764.

36. Baird CW, Stamou SC, Skipper E, et al: Total endoscopic repair of a pediatric atrial septal defect using the da Vinci robot and hypothermic fibrillation. Interact Cariovasc Thorac Surg 2007; 6:828–829.

37. Suematsu Y, Kiaii B, Bainbridge DT, et al: Robotic-assisted closure of atrial septal defect under real-time three-dimensional echo guide: in vitro study. Eur J Cardiothorac Surg 2007; 32:573–576.

38. Argenziano M, Oz MC, Kohmoto T, et al: Totally endoscopic atrial septal defect repair with robotic assistance. Circulation 2003; 108(1 Suppl):II101–II194.

39. Nikolaos B, Schachner T, Oehlinger A, et al: Robotically assisted totally endoscopic atrial septal defect repair: insights from operative times, learning curves, and clinical outcome. Ann Thorac Surg 2006; 82:687–693.

40. Talwar S, Choudhary SK, Mathur A, et al: Autolgous right atrial wall patch for closure of atrial septal defects. Ann Thorac Surg 2007; 84:913–916.

41. VanMeter C, LeBlanc JG, Culpepper WJ, et al: Partial anomalous pulmonary venous return. Circulation 1990; 82(5 Suppl):IV195–IV198.

42. Gotsman MS, Astley R, Parsons CG: Partial anomalous pulmonary venous drainage in association with atrial septal defect. Br Heart J 1965; 27:566–571.

43. Ettedgui JA, Siewers RD, Anderson RH, et al: Diagnostic echocardiographic features of the sinus venosus defect. Br Heart J 1990; 64:329–331.

CHAPTER 5

Ventricular Septal Defects

Amanda K. Auckland

Definition

The interventricular septum (IVS) is a musculo-membranous, complex, helical structure that separates the right ventricular chamber from the left ventricular chamber. This divider normally extends from the apex of the heart to unite with the atrial septum at the level of the atrioventricular valves (endocardial cushions). A ventricular septal defect (VSD) is a malformation that results in a hemodynamic communication between the right and the left ventricles.

Most VSDs occur in isolation; however, 40% occur as part of one or more other structural cardiac abnormalities.[1] Isolated VSDs are the most commonly recognized cardiac defect, accounting for 30% of cardiac defects in live-born infants and 9.7% in fetuses.[2] They may vary in size and may be single or multiple. VSDs have the highest recurrence rate and are the most teratogen-associated defect.[3]

Embryology

The partitioning of the primitive embryonic heart into the chambers of the atria and ventricles begins at approximately 28 days of gestation. Initially, the IVS forms as a median muscular ridge in the floor of the ventricle near the apex. The early primitive physiological septal defect that occurs as the septum closes is called the interventricular foramen. As a concave, thick, crescent-shaped fold, the IVS grows (primarily because of dilation of the ventricles on either side). Later, active proliferation of the myoblasts occurs and the thick muscular septum grows. The free edge of the primitive septum joins with the fused endocardial cushions at approximately 49 days of gestation. The interventricular foramen closes at about 56 days of gestation as a fusion of tissue from (1)

105

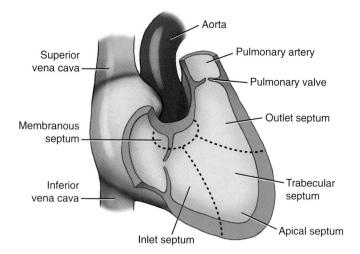

Figure 5–1 Diagram of the regions of the IVS as viewed from the right ventricle.

Labels: Aorta, Pulmonary artery, Pulmonary valve, Superior vena cava, Membranous septum, Outlet septum, Inferior vena cava, Trabecular septum, Inlet septum, Apical septum

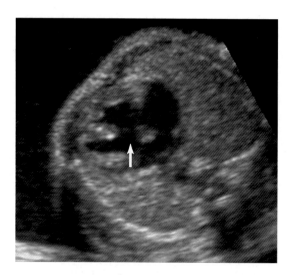

Figure 5–2 Subcostal four-chamber view showing a perimembranous VSD *(arrow)*. The defect involves both the membranous and upper portion of the muscular IVS.

the right bulbar ridge, (2) the left bulbar ridge, and (3) the endocardial cushions.[4,5] The IVS is thickest at the apex, and it narrows to become thinnest at the level of the atrioventricular valves.

A VSD results from either:

- A cessation of closure of the subaortic portion of the IVS because of maldevelopment of the following[4]:
  - The embryonic muscular septum
  - The endocardial cushions
  - Conal swellings

or
- From excess reabsorption of myocardial tissue in the formation of the trabeculae in the muscular septum.[4,6]

Classifications

The IVS can be divided into two distinct regions: (1) the membranous septal region and (2) the muscular septal region. The muscular septal region can be subdivided into (1) the inlet, (2) the outlet, and (3) the trabecular regions (Fig. 5–1).[6]

According to these criteria, VSDs can be classified as membranous defects or as muscular defects.

Membranous Defects

The membranous region of the septum is a small area close to the base of the heart that is bordered by the inlet and the outlet of the muscular septum and the commissure between the right and non-coronary cusps of the aortic valve. Because most defects in the membranous septum also involve a portion of the muscular septum, they are commonly described as perimembranous defects (Fig. 5–2).[7,8] Perimembranous defects constitute 75% of all VSDs.[8-11] Membranous VSDs are commonly associated with other structural cardiac abnormalities.[12]

Malalignment defects often involve the perimembranous septum. A malaligned perimembranous defect refers to a defect causing malalignment of the septum and great arteries (Fig. 5–3). When this occurs, both ventricles may empty into the

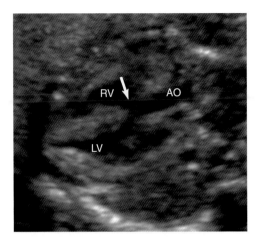

Figure 5–3 Long-axis view of the aorta *(AO)* showing malalignment of the IVS and aorta from a perimembranous VSD *(arrow)*. *LV,* Left ventricle; *RV,* right ventricle.

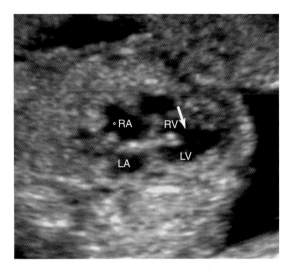

Figure 5–5 Subcostal four-chamber view of a fetal heart with a muscular VSD *(arrow)*. *LA,* Left atrium; *LV,* left ventricle; *RA,* right atrium; *RV,* right ventricle.

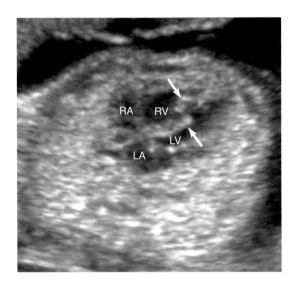

Figure 5–4 Subcostal four-chamber view showing a malalignment muscular VSD *(arrows)*. The septal defect resulted in separation of the septum. *LA,* Left atrium; *LV,* left ventricle; *RA,* right atrium; *RV,* right ventricle.

overriding great artery. Conversely, the malalignment defect may obstruct the ventricular outflow, depending on the size of the defect and the extent of malalignment. An anterior shift of the septum may cause a right ventricular outflow obstruction, whereas a posterior shift could result in a left ventricular outflow obstruction.[13] Malalignment defects can also occur in the muscular portion of the septum. In this setting the malalignment is between different portions of the septum (Fig. 5–4).

Muscular Defects

VSDs that are completely surrounded by muscular tissue make up 10% to 15% of VSDs (Fig. 5–5).[11] These defects vary in size and are frequently multiple.[13–15] Defects of the muscular septum are characterized by their location.[16]

Inlet Defects. Inlet defects are found in the predominantly smooth-walled muscular septum that extends from the muscular attachments of the tricuspid valve leaflets to the distal attachments of the tricuspid valve apparatus.[17] They are posterior and inferior to the membranous defects and account for 5% to 8% of VSDs.[18] VSDs that occur as part of an atrioventricular septal defect (AVSD) are inlet defects (Fig. 5–6).[13]

Outlet Defects. Outlet defects are anterior to the septal band of the right ventricle and occur in the most superior portion of the IVS, adjacent to the pulmonary and aortic valves. If the defect is found above the crista supraventricularis, it is described as a supracristal muscular VSD. Outlet defects are also referred to as subaortic, subpulmonary, or doubly committed subarterial defects.[11,13]

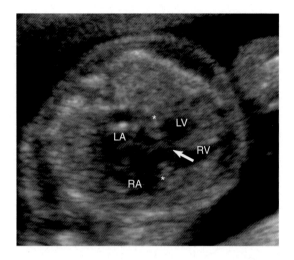

Figure 5–6   Subcostal four-chamber view in a fetus with an AVSD. An inlet VSD *(arrow)* is seen below the common atrioventricular valve *(asterisks)*. An atrial septal defect is also present. *LA,* Left atrium; *LV,* left ventricle; *RA,* right atrium; *RV,* right ventricle.

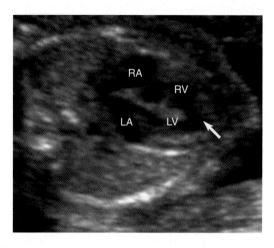

Figure 5–7   Subcostal four-chamber view of a fetal heart with a VSD in the apical portion of the muscular septum *(arrow). LA,* Left atrium; *LV,* left ventricle; *RA,* right atrium; *RV,* right ventricle.

Five percent to 7% of VSDs are the outlet type, except in the Asian population, where the incidence is much higher, approximating 30%.[8,19]

Trabecular Defects.   Trabecular defects are posterior to the trabecula septomarginalis (septal band of the crista) and the mid portion of the septum. Marginal or anterior defects are usually small, multiple, and tortuous, occurring near the septal free wall margins; they may be distributed all along the margin.[14] Trabecular defects are also termed midmuscular or central defects.

Apical Defects.   Apical defects are often included with trabecular defects. They occur close to the apex of the heart, distal to the insertion of the right moderator band. They are difficult to visualize with echocardiography even when large (Fig. 5–7).[14]

The term "Swiss cheese defect" has been used to describe the VSD that presents with multiple interventricular communications between the ventricles. These are typically apical in location. Nine percent of patients with VSDs have two or more defects.[17]

The frequency of occurrence of these types of muscular defects in the neonate is shown in Table 5–1.[17] Central trabecular defects are identified most frequently (44%), and apical defects are seen least often (5%). On the basis of these pub-

TABLE 5–1   Frequency of Muscular Ventricular Septal Defects in Neonates

Position	Frequency of All Muscular Ventricular Septal Defects (%)
Apical	25
Anterior	26
Midmuscular	44
Posterior	5

From Ramaciotti C, Vetter JV, Bornemeier RA, et al: Prevalence, relation to spontaneous closure and association of muscular ventricular septal defects with other cardiac defects. Am J Cardiol 1995; 75:61–65.

lished data, anterior and central defects tend to be identified in the immediate postpartum period, with a mean age of diagnosis of 1.3 and 2.2 weeks, respectively. Conversely, inlet and apical defects tend to be identified later (14 and 18 months, respectively).

Occurrence Rate

VSDs occur in 1% to 2% of live-born infants.[20-23] VSD is the most common congenital heart defect in children, accounting for 20% to 57% of cases.[21,24-29] The VSD has an incidence that is 20 times more common than the next most frequently encountered congenital heart defects.[21] VSDs are slightly more common in female patients than in male patients (56% versus 44%).[30]

The risk of congenital heart disease in a fetus with a VSD-affected sibling is approximately 3%. If two previous siblings are affected, this risk increases to 10%. If the mother of the fetus is the affected relative, the risk of congenital heart disease is 6% to 10%. If the affected relative is the father, the risk is approximately 2%.[22]

The occurrence rate of VSDs has been observed to decrease with prenatal and postnatal age. This is largely accounted for by spontaneous or elective termination of complicated pregnancies and spontaneous closure of VSDs with advancing gestational age.[23-26]

Spontaneous Closure of a Ventricular Septal Defect

In 74% of pregnancies in which an isolated fetal VSD was confirmed by two independent observers, the VSD resolved spontaneously before birth.[21,27] Of those that do not close prenatally, 75% to 90% will close within the first year of life.[25,26,28] The size and location of the defect influence the rate of spontaneous closure.[17] In general, large or malalignment defects tend to remain patent, whereas smaller perimembra-

nous defects have a greater tendency to close (Table 5-2).*

These data imply that very few isolated VSDs will require surgical repair.[29-31]

Sonographic Criteria

The ability to diagnose VSDs prenatally has been firmly established, although the efficacy of such diagnosis has not.[32] Although VSD is the most common congenital cardiac defect, it is only the fifth most common cardiac defect to be identified prenatally, accounting for only 5% of diagnoses (after AVSDs, 18%; hypoplastic left heart syndrome, 16%; coarctation, 11%; and Ebstein malformation, 7%).[33,34]

Color and pulsed Doppler imaging may increase the ability to identify in utero defects; however, the small size of many VSDs, and inherent limitations in fetal echocardiography, continue to make it a very difficult diagnosis.

The diagnosis of VSD is based on the ultrasonographic demonstration of a clear and distinct interruption in the usual contour of the septum. To interrogate the fetal heart, it is best to use the highest frequency transducer allowable (preferably 5 to 7.5 MHz). When the diagnosis of a VSD is made, a complete fetal echocardiogram is warranted to identify associated structural abnormalities.[11]

---

*References 3, 7, 17, 21, 25, 27, 28.

TABLE 5-2 Closure of VSD by Location of Defect			
Site of VSD	Closure in Utero (No. [%])	Closure after Birth (No. [%])	No Closure (No. [%])
Perimembranous	12 (52.2)	4 (17.4)	7 (30.4)
Muscular	1 (16.7)	2 (33.3)	3 (50)
Malalignment	—	—	8 (100)
Large VSD	—	—	3 (100)
TOTAL*	13 (32.5)	6 (15)	21 (52.5)
Perimembranous	11 (57.9)	4 (21.05)	4 (21.05)
Muscular	1 (10)	2 (40)	2 (40)
Malalignment	—	—	2 (100)
TOTAL†	12 (46.1)	6 (23.1)	8 (30.8)

From Paladini D, Palmieri S, Lamberti A, et al: Characterization and natural history of ventricular septal defects in the fetus. Ultrasound Obstet Gynecol 2000; 16:118–122.
*Included all continuing pregnancies (40 cases).
†Included only neonates who reached 1 year of age (26 cases).

The four-chamber view is commonly relied on for the prenatal diagnosis of a VSD.[35–37] Because axial resolution provides more detail than does lateral resolution, the best approach to the IVS is with the direction of the beam perpendicular to the septum (subcostal four-chamber view) (Fig. 5–8). When a VSD exists, it presents ultrasonographically as an anechoic area in the septum that is demonstrable from more than one tomographic plane (Figs. 5–9 and 5–10). If this anechoic area can be demonstrated from only one scanning plane or if the IVS is approaching a parallel orientation to the beam, such as in an apical four-chamber view, a false-positive or "pseudo" VSD should be suspected. (Fig. 5–11). The "T sign" has

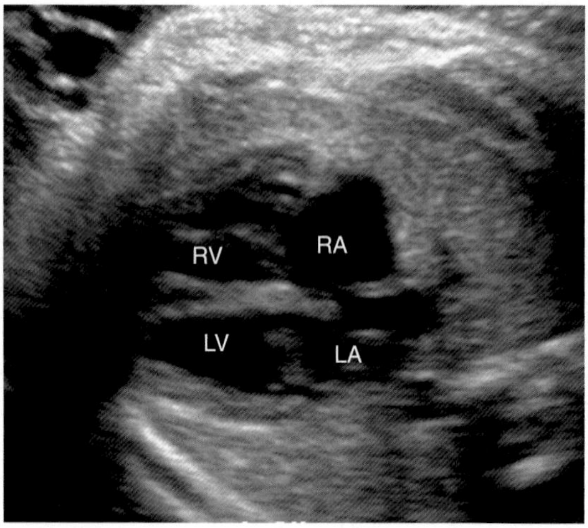

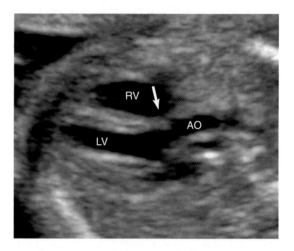

Figure 5–10　Long-axis view of the aorta *(AO)* showing the VSD *(arrow)* seen in Figure 5–9, in a different plane of view. *LV,* Left ventricle; *RV,* right ventricle.

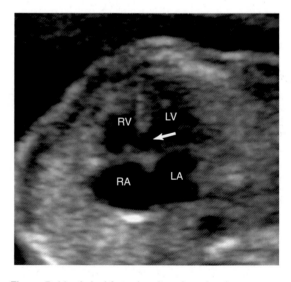

Figure 5–11　Apical four-chamber view showing artifactual dropout *(arrow)* resulting from the IVS being parallel to the angle of insonation, a "pseudo" VSD. *LA,* Left atrium; *LV,* left ventricle; *RA,* right atrium; *RV,* right ventricle.

(Figure 5–8 image)

Figure 5–8　Subcostal four-chamber view in a normal fetal heart showing the IVS in a perpendicular plane to the angle of insonation. *LA,* Left atrium; *LV,* left ventricle; *RA,* right atrium; *RV,* right ventricle.

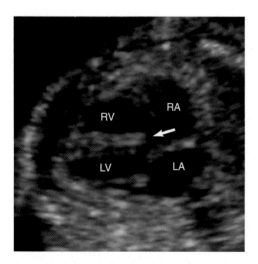

Figure 5–9　Subcostal four-chamber view showing a perimembranous VSD *(arrow)*. *LA,* Left atrium; *LV,* left ventricle; *RA,* right atrium; *RV,* right ventricle.

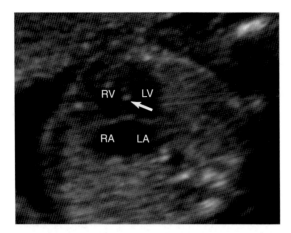

Figure 5–12 Apical four-chamber view showing the "T-sign" *(arrow)* often associated with a true VSD. The hyperechoic specular reflection is caused by the blunted end of the septal defect. *LA*, Left atrium; *LV*, left ventricle; *RA*, right atrium; *RV*, right ventricle.

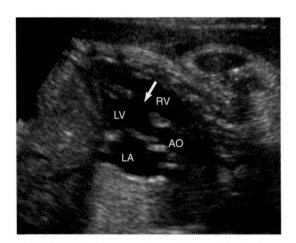

Figure 5–13 Long-axis view of the aorta *(AO)* showing a large VSD *(arrow)*. *LA*, Left atrium; *LV*, left ventricle; *RV*, right ventricle.

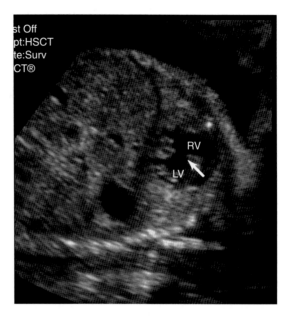

Figure 5–14 Short-axis view through the right *(RV)* and left *(LV)* ventricles, showing a VSD *(arrow)*.

been described as being helpful in distinguishing a real from a pseudo VSD in the apical projection. The "T sign" refers to an area of dropout that is bordered by a high-amplitude, hyperechoic, sharp, specular reflector (Fig. 5–12). This represents the blunted edge of the intact portion of the septum, and it is thought to not occur if the area of dropout is artifactual. Although this may be useful in some cases, it is not 100% reliable. False-positive and false-negative results, which are usually the consequence of image artifact, have plagued the identification of VSDs.[38,39]

Unfortunately, the four-chamber view allows the identification of only a small portion of inlet and trabecular defects[7] Other standard planes of orientation are helpful in assessing the IVS.[7] They include (1) the long-axis view of the left ventricular outflow tract (Fig. 5–13), (2) the long-axis view of the right ventricular outflow tract, and (3) the apex-to-base sweep of the ventricles in short-axis view (Fig. 5–14).

Perimembranous defects have the highest probability of detection, and apical defects are least likely to be detected.[7] VSDs as small as 3 mm have been identified.[32] Unfortunately, the resolution limitations of 1 to 2 mm do not allow the reliable visualization of very small defects.[7,37,38] Similarly, fetal echocardiography has been shown to be notoriously poor for quantifying the size of VSDs. This is intuitively reasonable because ultrasonography has been shown to have a 1- to 2-mm standard error of measure, for example, when measuring a 6-mm defect, a 30% error is simply too great to be reliable.

New techniques have been reported to allow better visualizaton of the IVS. Paladini et al[40]

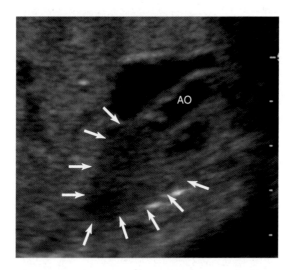

Figure 5–15   In-plane view of the IVS showing a surface view of the septum *(arrows)*. *AO*, Aorta.

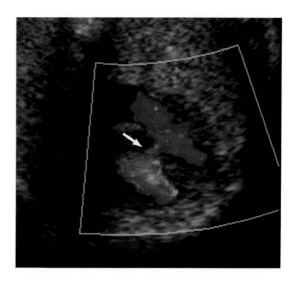

Figure 5–16   Subcostal four-chamber view with color Doppler imaging in the ventricles to confirm a VSD *(arrow)*.

describe the "in-plane" view of the IVS, which is acquired by turning the transducer perpendicular from a long-axis view of the left ventricle (Fig. 5–15). This plane allows a surface view through the anteroposterior diameter of the septum. The in-plane view may be useful in defining the extent of a VSD and confirming its presence. Three-dimensional ultrasonography and spatiotemporal imaging correlation techniques have also been reported as means to increase sensitivity.[41]

Color and pulsed Doppler imaging are valuable tools for assessing the fetal heart for a VSD (Figs. 5–16 and 5–17).[40,42–45] However, isolated or small VSDs may not result in hemodynamic disturbances in-utero.[4] This is due to the equalization of pressures of the ventricles that is present in the normal fetal heart as a result of the foramen ovale and ductus arteriosus. If there is shunting, it usually occurs in a low-velocity passive fashion, resulting in low-velocity flow. VSDs may demonstrate either bidirectional or unidirectional shunting (bidirectional is left-to-right shunting in systole and right-to-left shunting in diastole; unidirectional is left-to-right shunting).[44,46,47] Sharland et al[45] found bidirectional shunting identifiable with color Doppler imaging in the fetus to be an inconsistent finding, occurring in some patients but not in others. Chao et al[46] reported fluctuations of flow through the VSD throughout gesta-

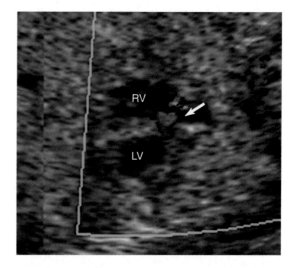

Figure 5–17   Short-axis view through the right *(RV)* and left *(LV)* ventricles with color Doppler imaging to confirm the presence of a VSD *(arrow)*.

tion. When color imaging is used, it is important to decrease the velocity scale to identify low flow and increase color-write priority settings. The angle of insonation is also very important with color Doppler imaging. In an apical four-chamber view, color has a tendency to artifactually override the thin membranous portion of the septum, giving the false impression of a defect.

Limitations of Sonographic Diagnosis of Ventricular Septal Defects

Early Diagnosis

The feasibility of first-trimester assessment of the fetal heart continues to be reported.[48] However, when cardiac defects are identified early in pregnancy, they are commonly complex defects. Most VSDs, particularly those that occur in isolation, will not be detected in the first trimester of pregnancy.

It is important to emphasize that a program of early assessment should not be implemented independent of mid second-trimester assessment. The fetal heart doubles in size between 14 and 18 weeks of gestation, and early assessment has been shown to be inaccurate and to yield incomplete results. Therefore, early assessment must be used in conjunction with later assessment.[48]

Reliability of Diagnosis

Because the accuracy of fetal echocardiography improves with the severity of the cardiac defect and given the benign nature of most isolated VSDs, it may reasonably be concluded that the VSD is least likely of all cardiac malformations to be detected. Although small isolated defects are exceeding difficult to detect prenatally, even moderate and larger defects can be difficult to see. In general, VSDs do not alter the structure of the heart. Therefore, they are very easily overlooked. Crawford et al[49] and Benacerraf et al[50] missed 35% and 70% of VSDs, respectively. In the study by Crawford et al,[49] 90% of the cases in which a VSD was seen were referred for evaluation because of a high index of suspicion on the basis of identification of a concomitant complex congenital heart defect or extracardiac abnormality.

When a VSD is suspected on routine sonographic examination, a complete fetal echocardiogram should always be performed.

Treatment

There are no known treatment options available in the prenatal period for VSDs. Normal obstetrical management need not be altered when an isolated VSD is identified in utero. However, if a VSD is found in conjunction with other defects that compromise fetal well-being, intervention may be justified.

Because most isolated VSDs will resolve spontaneously before birth (74%) and because VSDs detected in utero do not contribute to significant fetal morbidity and mortality, close prenatal follow-up is unwarranted, and re-evaluation can be performed at birth.[26] This posture should minimize or allay unwarranted anxiety on the part of the parents prenatally. Even with persistent small defects, the risk of surgery is greater than is the natural course of the disease.

After birth, a careful physical evaluation may be helpful in recognizing subtle physical features that are not evident prenatally. Infants with small defects do not require treatment.[14] However, surveillance or intervention may be required in infants with moderate or large defects. Administration of prophylactic antibiotics is often emphasized to protect against endocarditis at times of suspected bacteremia (i.e., during any operative or manipulative procedure).

Neonatal echocardiography is often used to confirm in utero findings. In more complicated heart disease, magnetic resonance imaging or angiography may be warranted.[19]

Treatment may include both medical and surgical options. If heart failure develops in infants with larger defects, effective therapy may often be achieved through a medical course, avoiding early surgical intervention. Medical therapeutic agents may include digoxin, furosemide, and spironolactone. Rarely, primary surgical closure of a VSD is justified. Surgical treatment is necessary only when there is pulmonary hypertension, congestive heart failure or hypoxia, or failure to thrive.[51] In general, these procedures have excellent success rates, but they have been associated with some long-term morbidity. This risk is increased when concomitant abnormalities are present.[16,52] Right bundle-branch block is a common postsurgical complication. It develops in 45% to 60% of patients with surgical muscular defect closure.[53] Complete heart block requiring a pacemaker and aortic or tricuspid injury resulting in insufficiency have also been reported but are rare.[2]

Depending on location, repair of a VSD is usually accomplished by a transatrial approach from the right atrium (Fig. 5–18). The defect is closed with a synthetic patch. Lower defects pose a challenge because they may require surgical opening of the ventricle. Approaching the defect from the left ventricle often results in significant left ventricular dysfunction. However, the coarse trabeculations in the right ventricle also make that approach difficult. For this reason, minimal access

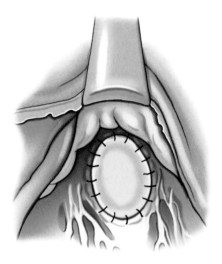

Figure 5–18 Diagram depicting synthetic patch placement to repair a VSD.

surgeries, involving guiding a catheter through a percutaneous or periventicular approach, are being developed.

Transcatheter device closure is also being used to close perimembranous defects. These pose a greater challenge because of their proximity to the aortic and tricuspid valves. An Amplatzer muscular VSD occluder (AAVSDO) has reported success in closing muscular septal defects.[54] The AAVSDO has been especially designed to close perimembranous defects.[55] Its unique design ensures that when properly deployed, it does not encroach on surrounding structures. The reported success rate of this device is approximately 89%.

As with conventional surgery, these procedures are also associated with complications. Larger and longer-term studies are still needed to confirm the safety and efficacy of these devices.

Prognosis

Survival rates for children with VSDs depend on the anatomy and the degree of hemodynamic disturbance caused by the defect.[56–59] Samanek[56] investigated the morbidity and mortality rates resulting from congenital heart disease during a 27-year period. The 1-month and 1-year survival rates for infants with VSD were 92% and 80%, respectively. It should be borne in mind, however, that these numbers "lump together" all cases of VSD, both isolated and complex. Because the

prognoses of small and benign VSDs and cases of VSD that are complicated by significant concomitant congenital heart disease are far different, they should be investigated separately. Small and isolated VSDs usually close spontaneously either before or shortly after birth; therefore those that are usually detected prenatally may represent the largest of defects, and they may be predisposed to fail to close independently. Conversely, Orie et al[27] reported that isolated VSDs detected in utero did not contribute to fetal morbidity and mortality rates. Recent data suggest that the prognosis for infants with an isolated VSD is good. Only rarely do isolated VSDs fail to close spontaneously, and very rarely do they require operative intervention.

In 1993, a long-term follow-up study of almost 1300 patients with VSDs was reported. The authors concluded that although there was a "higher than normal" incidence of serious arrhythmia and sudden death (accounting for 30% of deaths), including patients with small VSDs, these patients had an 87% probability of a 25-year survival.[57] This rising rate of survival is probably attributable to better methods of ascertainment, increased rates of elective termination of the pregnancy because of the diagnosis of heart disease, and more effective methods of medical and surgical management.[46] Improvements in general perinatal and neonatal care have also favorably influenced the outcomes of infants with congenital heart disease.

Because prenatal ultrasonography is notoriously inaccurate for the diagnosis of VSD (high false-positive and false-negative rates plague the diagnosis), it is fortunate that most missed VSDs are inconsequential and spontaneous closure usually occurs before detection. They are not thought to unduly influence childhood development.[29]

There are significantly higher rates of termination of pregnancy (41%), spontaneous intrauterine death (16%), neonatal death (15%), and infant or childhood morbidity and death (3%) in all cases of VSDs compared with fetuses without congenital heart disease.[60,61]

Associated Anomalies

VSDs often occur as part of more complex cardiac disease (Table 5–3).[7,22,61] Cardiac defects associated with VSD include AVSD, tetralogy of Fallot, truncus arteriosus, coarctation of the aorta, interrupted aortic arch, transposition of the great

TABLE 5–3	Conditions Associated with Ventricular Septal Defects			
Maternal		**Fetal**		
Condition	Drug Use	Associated Cardiac Abnormalities	Chromosome Abnormalities	Syndromes
Diabetes	Retinoic acid	Tetralogy of Fallot	Monosomy 1q,	Aase-Smith syndrome
Phenylketonuria	(Accutane)	Transposition of	1q4, 10q2,	Adducted thumb
Rubella	Alcohol	the great vessels	11q, 16q,	Alopecia-anosmia-deafness-hypogonadism,
	Amphetamine	Pulmonic atresia	medial, 2q,	Johnson type
	Cortisone	Atrioventricular	7p2, 8p2	Alopecia, mental retardation
	Phenytoin	septal defect	Trisomy distal	Alpert syndrome
	(Dilantin)	Double-outlet	2q, 5p3, 6p2,	Arthrogryposis multiple congenita
	Penicillamine	right ventricle	7p2, 8, 9, 9p,	Carpenter syndrome
	Primidone	Mitral atresia	12p, 13, 14p1,	Cayler syndrome
	Thalidomide	Coarctation of the	15q2, 18	CHARGE (coloboma of the eye, heart anomaly,
	Trimethadione	aorta	(Edwards	choanal atresia, retardation, and genital and
	Valproic acid	Tricuspid	syndrome),	ear anomalies) syndrome
		insufficiency	20pter → q11,	CHILD (congenital hemidysplasia with
		Aortic arch	21 (Down	ichthyosiform erythroderma and limb
		interruption	syndrome),	defects) syndrome
		Aortic stenosis	22, partial	Choroid plexus cyst
		Complete heart	trisomy 22	Conradi-Hünermann syndrome
		block	Deletions	deLange syndrome
		Ebstein anomaly	4p–,5p–	Eagle-Barrett (prune-belly) syndrome
		Mitral stenosis	(cri-du-chat	Ehlers-Danlos syndrome
		Right aortic arch	syndrome),	DiGeorge syndrome
			13q–, +14q–,	Factor V deficiency
			18q–, 22q11	Fraser syndrome
			Turner	Goldenhar syndrome
			syndrome	Heart-hand syndrome
			(45,X)	Hirschsprung disease
			Triploidy	Holt-Oram syndrome
				Keutel syndrome
				Klippel-Feil sequence
				Laurence-Moon (Bardet-Biedl) syndrome
				Lethal faciocardiomelic dysplasia
				McDonough syndrome
				Meckel-Gruber syndrome
				Mesomelic dysplasia
				Multiple pteryglia
				Neurofibromatosis
				Noonan syndrome
				Opitz-Kaveggia FG
				Osteoporosis-pseudoglioma
				Pentalogy of Cantrell
				Polycystic kidney disease
				Polysyndactyly-cardiac
				Rubinstein-Taybi syndrome
				Scimitar syndrome
				Seckel syndrome
				Shprintzen syndrome
				Siegler syndrome
				Silver syndrome
				Sirenomelia
				Situs inversus
				Smith-Lemli-Opitz syndrome
				Sofer syndrome
				Tar-Williams syndrome
				Treacher Collins syndrome
				VACTERL (vertebral anomalies, anal atresia,
				cardiovascular anomalies, tracheoesophageal
				fistula, esophageal atresia, renal or radial
				anomalies, limb anomalies) syndrome
				Waardenburg syndrome
				Weaver syndrome
				Weill-Marchesani syndrome
				Williams syndrome
				Zellweger syndrome

arteries, double-outlet right ventricle, and aortic stenosis.[11]

The presence of a VSD increases the risk of aneuploidy.[61] Whenever a VSD is diagnosed, fetal karyotyping should be offered. More than 40% of fetuses with a VSD will have a chromosomal anomaly. Commonly, these include trisomies 21, 13, and 18 and 22q11 deletion (DiGeorge syndrome). VSDs are the most common cardiac defect associated with trisomy 18.[12] Fifty percent of inlet defects are seen in cases of trisomy 21, and approximately 56% of malalignment defects occur with trisomy 18.[12,15,62]

References

1. Fontana RS, Edwards JE: Ventricular septal defect. In: Fontana RS, Edwards JE (eds): Congenital Cardiac Disease. A Review of 357 Cases Studied Pathologically. Philadelphia, WB Saunders, 1962, pp 640–669.

2. Mavroudis C, Backer CL, Idriss FS: Ventricular septal defect. In: Mavroudis C, Backer CL (eds): Pediatric Cardiac Surgery, 2nd ed. St Louis, Mosby–Year Book, 1994, pp 201–221.

3. Goor DA, Lillehei CW: Isolated ventricular septal defects. In: Goor DA, Lillehei CW (eds): Congenital Malformations of the Heart. New York, Grune & Stratton, 1975, pp 112–131.

4. Pansky B: Malformations of the heart and great vessels. In: Pansky B (ed): Review of Medical Embryology. New York, Macmillan, 1982, pp 348–351.

5. Moore KL, Persaud TVN: The cardiovascular system. In: Moore KL, Persaud TVN (eds): The Developing Human, 5th ed. Philadelphia, WB Saunders, 1993, pp 304–353.

6. Buyse ML: Ventricular septal defect. In: Buyse ML (ed): Birth Defects Encyclopedia, vol II. Dover, UK, Blackwell Scientific, 1990, pp 1763–1764.

7. Romero R, Pilu G, Jeanty P, et al: Ventricular septal defect. In: Romero R, Pilu G, Jeanty P, et al (eds): Prenatal Diagnosis of Congenital Anomalies. Norwalk, CT, Appleton & Lange, 1988, pp 141–144.

8. Soto B, Becker AE, Moulaert AJ, et al: Classification of ventricular septal defects. Br Heart J 1980; 43:332–343.

9. Peironi DR, Nishimura RA, Bierman FZ: Second natural history study of congenital heart defects: Ventricular septal defects: Echocardiography. Circulation 1993; 87:180–187.

10. Nyberg DA, Emerson DS: Cardiac malformations. In: Nyberg DA, Emerson DS (eds): Diagnostic Ultrasound of Fetal Anomalies: Text and Atlas. Chicago, Year Book Medical, 1990, pp 300–341.

11. Yagel S, Silverman N, Gembruch U: Ventricular septal defect. In: Yagel S, Silversman N, Gembruch U (eds): Fetal Cardiology, Embryology, Genetics, Physiology, Echocardiographic Evaluation, Diagnosis and Perinatal Management of Cardiac Diseases. New York, Martin Dunitz, 2003, pp 207–209.

12. Armstrong WF: Congenital heart disease. In: Feigenbaum H (ed): Echocardiography, 4th ed. Philadelphia, Lea & Febiger, 1986, pp 413–424.

13. Yale University School of Medicine: Anatomy of Ventricular Septal Defects (Web site): http://www.med.yale.edu/intmed/cardio/chd/e-vsd/index.html. Accessed October 29, 2007.

14. Emmanouilides GC: Congenital cardiovascular defects. In: Emmanouilides GC (ed): Heart Disease in Infants, Children, and Adolescents: Including the Fetus and Young Adult, 5th ed. Baltimore, Williams & Wilkins, 1995, pp 707–745.

15. Mahoney LT: Acyanotic congenital heart disease: Atrial and ventricular septal defects, atrioventricular canal, patent ductus arteriosus, pulmonic stenosis. Cardiol Clin 1993; 11:603–616.

16. Kirklin JK, Castaneda AR, Keane JK, et al: Surgical management of multiple ventricular septal defects. J Thorac Cardiovasc Surg 1980; 12:485–493.

17. Ramaciotti C, Vetter JV, Bornemeier RA, et al: Prevalence, relation to spontaneous closure and association of muscular ventricular septal defects with other cardiac defects. Am J Cardiol 1995; 75:61–65.

18. Lincoln C, Jamieson S, Shinebourne E, et al: Transatrial repair of ventricular septal defects with reference to their anatomic classification. J Thorac Cardiovasc Surg 1977; 74:183–190.

19. Tatsuno K, Ando M, Taken A, et al: Diagnostic importance of aortography in conal ventricular septal defects. Am Heart J 1975; 89:171–177.

20. Nadas AS, Flyer DC: Communications between systemic and pulmonary circuits with dominantly left-to-right shunts. In: Nadas AS, Flyer DC (eds): Pediatric Cardiology, 3rd ed. Philadelphia, WB Saunders, 1972, p 348.

21. Meberg A, Otterstad JE, Froland G, et al: Increasing incidence of ventricular septal defects caused by improved detection rate. Acta Paediatr 1994; 83:653–657.

22. Nora JJ, Fraser FC, Bear J, et al: Medical Genetics: Principles and Practice, 4th ed. Philadelphia, Lea & Febiger, 1994.

23. Carlgren LE, Ericson A, Kallen B: Monitoring of congenital cardiac defects. Pediatr Cardiol 1987; 8:247–256.

24. Hiraishi S, Agata Y, Nowatari M, et al: Incidence and natural course of trabecular ventricular septal

defect: Two-dimensional echocardiography and color Doppler flow imaging study. J Pediatr 1992; 120:409–415.

25. Samanek M, Slavik Z, Zobrilova B, et al: Prevalence, treatment and outcome of heart disease in live-born children: A prospective analysis of 91,823 live-born children. Pediatr Cardiol 1989; 10:205–211.

26. Fixler DE, Pastor P, Chamberlin M, et al: Trends in congenital heart disease in Dallas County births 1971–1984. Circulation 1990; 81:137–142.

27. Orie J, Flotta D, Sherman FS: To be or not to be a VSD. Am J Cardiol 1994; 74:1284–1285.

28. Hoffman JIE, Kaplan S: The incidence of congenital heart disease. J Am Coll Cardiol 2002; 39:1890–1900.

29. Axt-Fliedner R, Schwarze A, Smrcek J, et al: Isolated ventricular septal defects detected by color Doppler imaging: Evolution during fetal and first year of postnatal life. Ultrasound Obstet Gynecol 2006; 27:266–273.

30. Ramaswamy R, Anbumani P, Srinivasan K, et al: Ventricular septal defect, general concepts. www.emedicine.com/ped/topic2402.htm. Accessed October 2007.

31. Graham TP Jr, Bender HW Jr, Spach MS: Ventricular septal defect. In: Adams FH, Emmanouilides JC (eds): Moss's Heart Disease in Infants, Children and Adolescents, 4th ed. Baltimore, Williams & Wilkins, 1989, pp 189–209.

32. Paladini D, Palmieri S, Lamberti A, et al: Characterization and natural history of ventricular septal defects in the fetus. Ultrasound Obstet Gynecol 2000; 16:118–122.

33. Allan LD, Sharland GK, Milburn A, et al: Prospective diagnosis of 1,006 consecutive cases of congenital heart disease in the fetus. J Am Coll Cardiol 1994; 23:1452–1458.

34. Hoffman JIE: Congenital heart disease: Incidence and inheritance. Pediatr Clin North Am 1990; 37:25–43.

35. Copel JA, Pilu G, Green J, et al: Fetal echocardiographic screening for congenital heart disease: The importance of the four-chamber view. Am J Obstet Gynecol 1987;157:648–655.

36. Sharland GK, Allan LD: Screening for congenital heart disease prenatally: Results of a 22 year study in the Southeast Thames region. Br J Obstet Gynaecol 1992; 99:220–225.

37. Vergani P, Mariani S, Ghidini A, et al: Screening for congenital heart disease with the four chamber view of the fetal heart. Am J Obstet Gynecol 1992; 167:1000–1003.

38. Jaffe CC, Atkinson P, Raylor JKW: Physical parameters affecting the visibility of small ventricular septal defects using two-dimensional echocardiography. Invest Radiol 1979; 14:149–155.

39. Carrale JM, Sahn DJ, Allen HD, et al: Factors affecting real-time cross-sectional echocardiographic imaging of perimembranous ventricular septal defects. Circulation 1981; 63: 689–697.

40. Paladini D, Russo M, Vassallo M, et al: The "in-plane" view of the inter-ventricular septum: A new approach to the characterization of ventricular septal defects in the fetus. Prenat Diagn 2003; 23:1052–1055.

41. Yagel S, Benachi A, Bonnet D, et al: Rendering in fetal cardiac scanning: the intracardiac septa and the coronal atrioventricular valve planes. Ultrasound Obstet Gynecol 2006; 28:266–274.

42. Hornberger LK, Sahn DJ, Krabill KA, et al: Elucidation of the natural history of ventricular septal defects by serial Doppler color flow mapping studies. J Am Coll Cardiol 1989; 13:1111–1118.

43. Chiba Y, Kanzaki T, Kobayaski H, et al: Evaluation of fetal structural heart disease using color flow mapping. Ultrasound Med Biol 1990; 16:221–229.

44. Stewart PA, Wladimiroff JW: Fetal echocardiography and color Doppler flow imaging. Ultrasound Obstet Gynecol 1993; 3:168–175.

45. Sharland GK, Chita SK, Allan LD: The use of colour Doppler in fetal echocardiography. Int J Cardiol 1990; 28:229–236.

46. Chao RC, Shih-Chu Ho E, Hsieh KS, et al: Fluctuation of interventricular shunting in a fetus with an isolated ventricular septal defect. Am Heart J 1994; 127:955–958.

47. Copel JA, Morotti R, Hobbins JC, et al: The antenatal diagnosis of congenital heart disease using fetal echocardiography: Is color mapping necessary? Obstet Gynecol 1991; 78:1–8.

48. Yagel S, Cohen SM, Messing B: First and early second trimester fetal heart screening. Curr Opin Obstet Gynecol 2007; 19:183–190.

49. Crawford DC, Chita SK, Allan LD: Prenatal detection of congenital heart disease: Factors influencing obstetrical management and survival. Am J Obstet Gynecol 1988; 159:352–356.

50. Benacerraf BR, Pober BR, Sanders SP: Accuracy of fetal echocardiography. Radiology 1987; 165:847–849.

51. Ren JG, Freed MD, Norwood WI: Early and late results of closure of ventricular septal defect in infancy. Ann Thorac Surg 1977; 24:19–26.

52. Fishberger SB, Bridges ND, Keane JF, et al: Intraoperative device closure of ventricular septal defects. Am Heart J 1993; 88:205–209.

53. Okoroma EC, Guller B, Maloney JD, et al: Etiology of right bundle branch block pattern

after surgical closure of ventricular septal defects. Am Heart J 1975; 90:14–18.

54. Diab KA, Cao QL, Mora BN, et al: Device closure of muscular ventricular septal defects in infants less than one year of age using the Amplatzer devices: Feasibility and outcome. Catheter Cardiovasc Interv 2007; 70:90–97.

55. Pinto RJ, Dalvi BV, Sharma S: Transcatheter closure of perimembranous ventricular septal defects using Amplatzer asymmetric ventricular septal defect occluder: Preliminary experience with 18-month follow up. Catheter Cardiovasc Interv 2006; 68:145–152.

56. Samanek M: Children with congenital heart disease: Probability of natural survival. Pediatr Cardiol 1992; 13:152–158.

57. Kidd L, Driscoll DJ, Gersony WM, et al: Second natural history study of congenital heart defects: Results of treatment of patients with ventricular septal defects. Circulation 1993; 87:138–151.

58. Hoffman JIE, Christianson R: Congenital heart disease in a cohort of 19,502 births with long-term follow-up. Am J Cardiol 1978; 42:641–647.

59. Mitchell SC, Korones SB, Berendes HW: Congenital heart disease in 56,109 births. Circulation 1971; 43:323–330.

60. Allan L: Fetal cardiology. Ultrasound Obstet Gynecol 1994; 4:441–444.

61. Allan LD, Crawford DC, Chita SK, et al: Prenatal screening for congenital heart disease. BMJ 1986; 292:1717–1719.

62. Ferencz C, Neill CA, Boughman JA, et al: Congenital cardiovascular malformations associated with chromosomal abnormalities: An epidemiologic study. J Pediatr 1989; 114:79–86.

CHAPTER 6

Atrioventricular Septal Defects

Britt C. Smyth

Definition

Atrioventricular septal defect (AVSD) refers to a spectrum of cardiac malformations that include abnormalities of the interatrial septum, the interventricular septum, and the atrioventricular (AV) (mitral and tricuspid) valves. An AVSD results from the endocardial cushions of the heart failing to fuse properly. AVSDs are also referred to as AV canal defects or endocardial cushion defects. AVSDs are usually categorized as partial, intermediate, or complete (Fig. 6–1). All forms tend to be large defects, and they share many similarities.[1-12]

Complete Atrioventricular Septal Defect

The complete form of AVSD is characterized by a large septal defect involving both the interatrial and interventricular septa and a common AV valve that connects both atria to the ventricles. The deformed AV valve is composed of five leaflets: two that bridge the septal defect, called the anterosuperior bridging leaflet and the posteroinferior bridging leaflet, and three lateral or mural leaflets. Underneath the five commissures are five papillary muscle structures. The two left-sided or mitral papillary muscles are closer together and smaller than those in a normal heart. This usually results in inability of the valve leaflets to coapt, thus becoming regurgitant. Over time the leaflets become thickened and deformed.

Rastelli et al[13,14] and Calabrò and Limongelli[15] have subclassified the complete form of AVSD on the basis of the chordal insertions and the degree of bridging of the anterosuperior bridging leaflet of the common AV valve (Fig. 6–2).

In type A, the anterosuperior bridging leaflet is attached almost entirely to the left ventricle, and its commissure with the anterior tricuspid leaflet lies along the right anterosuperior rim of the ventricular septum. Beneath this commissure, multiple direct chordal insertions into the septum usually exist. Interventricular communication beneath the anterior bridging leaflet is not as significant as that seen in type B or C defects. A type A AVSD usually occurs as an isolated defect or in association with Down syndrome (trisomy 21).

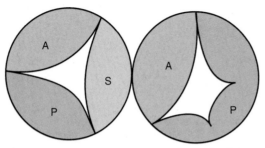

I.　NORMAL TRICUSPID AND MITRAL VALVES

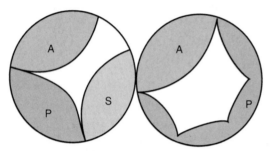

II.　PARTIAL ATRIOVENTRICULAR CANAL

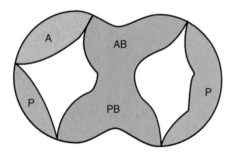

III. INTERMEDIATE ATRIOVENTRICULAR CANAL

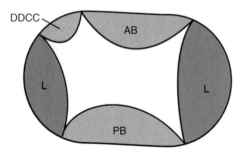

IV.　COMPLETE ATRIOVENTRICULAR CANAL

Figure 6–1　*Valve leaflet morphology.* **I,** Normal tricuspid and mitral valve formation. **II,** Partial AV canal defect. **III,** Intermediate AV canal defect. **IV,** Complete AV canal defect. *A,* Anterior leaflet; *AB,* anterior bridging leaflet; *DDCC,* dextrodorsal conus cushion; *L,* lateral leaflet; *P,* posterior leaflet; *PB,* posterior bridging leaflet; *S,* septal leaflet.

Most type A AVSDs are not associated with other cardiac malformations; however, they have been associated with left-sided obstructions.[10,11,15–18]

Type B AVSD is the rarest form of a complete defect; it consists of a large anterior septal bridging leaflet overhanging the ventricular septum to a greater degree than occurs in type A. The medial papillary muscle is usually attached apically on the septal band or on the moderator band. Because there are no chordal attachments between the anterosuperior bridging leaflet and the underlying ventricular septum, free interventricular communication exists.[15]

Type C AVSD consists of an anterosuperior bridging leaflet that is larger and overhangs the ventricular septum to a greater degree than in either type A or type B. In type C AVSD, the medial papillary muscle attaches to the anterior tricuspid papillary muscle and the anterior tricuspid leaflet is usually very small. Free interventricular communication is also present in type C defects. Type C AVSDs are frequently associated with other congenital cardiac abnormalities such as tetralogy of Fallot, double-outlet right ventricle, complete transposition of the great arteries, and heterotaxic syndromes (asplenia and polysplenia).[1,2,15,18–22] Complete AVSD occurring with tetralogy of Fallot is usually seen in patients with Down syndrome, whereas complete AVSD with double-outlet right ventricle is more commonly seen in the asplenia syndrome.[9,11,17]

AVSD can be further described as either balanced or unbalanced. In most cases of AVSD, the AV junction is connected equally to the right and left ventricles so that each ventricle receives a similar amount of blood and the ventricles are symmetrical in size. This is known as a balanced AVSD. An unbalanced AVSD occurs when the AV junction is predominantly committed to either the right or left ventricle, leading to hypoplasia of the opposing ventricle receiving the smaller amount of blood.[18,23]

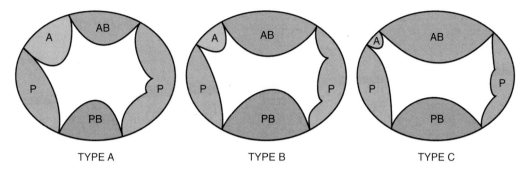

Figure 6–2 Complete AV canal defect, types A, B, and C, according to the Rastelli classification. *A*, Anterior leaflet; *AB*, anterior bridging leaflet; *P*, posterior leaflet; *PB*, posterior bridging leaflet.

In all types of complete AVSDs, the right atrium and pulmonary arteries are usually dilated, with the right ventricular outflow tract bulging anteriorly. The right ventricle may be hypertrophied. The left atrium may also be dilated. Because of the loss of normal AV valve continuity, the left ventricular outflow tract will usually appear as a long, narrow chamber. Dextroposition of the aorta is commonly associated with complete AVSD.[24]

Partial Atrioventricular Septal Defect

The partial form of AVSD differs from the complete form in that the mitral and tricuspid orifices are distinct and separate. It is usually defined by four criteria, which may occur alone or in any combination: (1) primum atrial septal defect, (2) ventricular septal defect, (3) cleft anterior mitral leaflet, and (4) widened anteroseptal tricuspid commissure (cleft septal tricuspid leaflet). The most commonly occurring form of partial AVSD consists of a primum atrial septal defect and a cleft anterior mitral leaflet. A partial AVSD is also known as an ostium primum atrial septal defect.[15,25]

The mitral annulus is displaced apically so that the mitral and tricuspid valves appear to be inserted at the same level. The deficient AV septum is associated with an interatrial communication rather than an interventricular or right atrial-to-left ventricular shunt. The cleft in the anterior mitral leaflet is directed toward the midportion of the ventricular septum, along the anteroinferior rim of the septal defect.

This differs from an isolated mitral cleft (not associated with AVSD), in which the cleft is directed toward the aortic valve annulus. Associated anomalies commonly include secundum atrial septal defects and a persistent left superior vena cava that drains into the coronary sinus. Less commonly associated cardiac defects include pulmonary stenosis, discrete subaortic stenosis, tricuspid stenosis or atresia, coarctation of the aorta, a membranous ventricular septal defect, and hypoplastic left ventricle.[15,21,22,24–26]

Intermediate Atrioventricular Septal Defect

The intermediate type of AVSD occurs least frequently. It is similar to the complete form; however, the anterior and posterior septal bridging leaflets are fused above the ventricular septum, dividing the common AV valve into separate mitral and tricuspid components.[1]

Embryology

Normal embryogenesis of the AV canal consists of two processes: (1) separation of the common AV orifice into mitral and tricuspid valves and (2) closure of the atrial septum (ostium primum) and of the ventricular septum (secondary interventricular foramen).[1] Development of the AV canal occurs by proliferation of the four endocardial cushions (superior, inferior, right lateral, and left lateral) and the dextrodorsal conus cushion. The superior and inferior cushions develop initially, followed by the right and left lateral cushions.

This is followed by a portion of the dextrodorsal conus cushion interposing between the superior and right lateral endocardial cushions. As the superior and inferior cushions grow toward each other, the common AV canal becomes two separate and distinct orifices: mitral and tricuspid (Fig. 6–3).

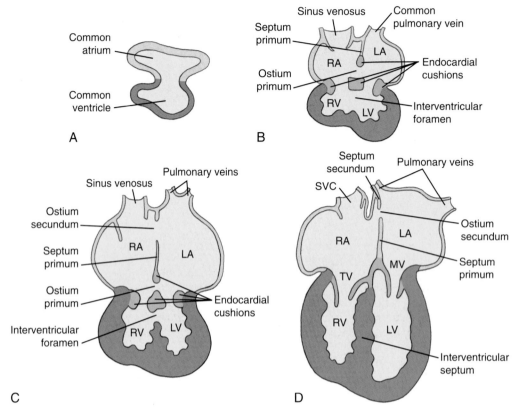

Figure 6–3 Diagram showing normal embryogenesis of the AV canal. **A,** Primitive common atrium and common ventricle. **B,** Four endocardial cushions (superior, inferior, right lateral, left lateral) begin to grow toward each other. **C,** Atrial and ventricular septa continue to form and common AV canal becomes two separate orifices (mitral and tricuspid). **D,** Normal fetal heart. Atrial and ventricular septum formation complete. Separate mitral and tricuspid valves formed. *LA,* Left atrium; *LV,* left ventricle; *MV,* mitral valve; *RA,* right atrium; *RV,* right ventricle; *SVC,* superior vena cava; *TV,* tricuspid valve.

Next, the anterior mitral leaflet forms from the superior cushion and the left half of the inferior cushion. The posterior mitral leaflet arises from the left lateral endocardial cushion, and the anterior tricuspid leaflet arises from the right lateral endocardial cushion and the dextrodorsal conus cushion. Finally, the posterior tricuspid leaflet forms from the right lateral endocardial cushion, and the septal tricuspid leaflet forms from the inferior endocardial cushion.[1-5]

In addition to separating the common AV orifice into mitral and tricuspid components, the superior and inferior endocardial cushions also extend along the perimeter of the ostium primum, resulting in its closure. The anterior mitral valve leaflet eventually becomes positioned more basely than the septal tricuspid leaflet, allowing the AV septum to form between the right atrium and the left ventricle, with the interatrial septum above and the interventricular septum below.

Occurrence Rate

AVSDs account for approximately 2.9% of all congenital heart defects and have an occurrence rate of 0.19 per 1000 live births.[9,15,27–29] The incidence has been reported to be as high as 17% in fetuses with congenital heart disease.[4,27,28] AVSDs are associated with a variety of syndromes and chromosomal abnormalities (Table 6–1). AVSD accounts for 40% of congenital heart malformations in individuals with Down syndrome.[8,10] Complete AVSDs are also prevalent in patients with heterotaxic syndromes such as asplenia (right atrial isomerism) and polysplenia (left atrial isomerism).[11,12,17,20,26]

TABLE 6–1 Conditions Associated with Atrioventricular Septal Defect			
Maternal		**Fetal**	
Condition	**Associated Cardiac Abnormalities**	**Chromosome Abnormalities**	**Syndromes**
Diabetes	Complete heart block	Trisomy 13 (Patau syndrome)	Asplenia
	Total anomalous pulmonary venous connection	Trisomy 18 (Edwards syndrome)	C syndrome
	Mesocardia	Trisomy 21 (Down syndrome)	Cardiofacial syndrome
	Dextrocardia	Turner syndrome (46,XO)	Cayler syndrome
	Coarctation		CHARGE (coloboma of the eye, central nervous system anomalies, heart defects, atresia of the choanae, retardation of growth or development, genital or urinary defects, and ear anomalies or deafness) syndrome
	Tetralogy of Fallot		Cornelia de Lange syndrome
	Hypoplastic left heart syndrome		Duodenal atresia
	Atrial isomerism		Ellis–Van Creveld syndrome
	Secundum atrial septal defect		Goldenhar syndrome
	Double-outlet right ventricle		Hydrocephalus
	Transposition of the great arteries		Hydrolethalus
	Pulmonary stenosis		Malrotation
	Pulmonary atresia		Meningocele
	Subaortic stenosis		Omphalocele
	Additional muscular ventricular septal defects		Polysplenia
			Polysyndactyly
			Smith-Lemli-Opitz syndrome
			VACTERL (vertebral anomalies, anal atresia, cardiovascular anomalies, tracheoesophageal fistula, esophageal atresia, renal or radial anomalies, and limb anomalies) syndrome

They occur slightly more often in females.[8] The incidence of congenital heart defects in the off-spring of mothers with AVSD is 14%, much higher than that of most congenital heart defects.[24,29]

Sonographic Criteria

The four-chamber view (either subcostal or apical) is often the most useful in evaluating an AVSD. Most complete AVSDs are large defects that are easily recognized in a four-chamber view of the fetal heart. Partial AVSDs may be more subtle and require multiple views to make a correct diagnosis. In either the subcostal or apical four-chamber view, the complete form of AVSD appears as a wide opening within the center of the heart (Fig. 6–4). The continuity between the interatrial and interventricular septa and the AV valves is lost. Instead of identifying separate mitral and tricuspid valves, one single multileaflet AV valve is seen (Fig. 6–5).

In a balanced AVSD, both ventricles appear to be of similar size because the blood flows relatively evenly through the single AV valve into each

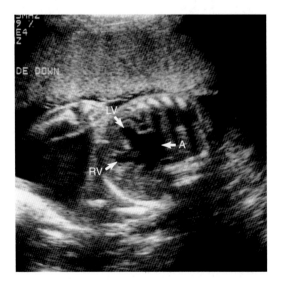

Figure 6–4 Subcostal four-chamber view in a fetus with an AVSD. Defects of the interatrial and interventricular septae and abnormal AV valve results in the AV canal remaining open. *A,* Atria; *LV,* left ventricle; *RV,* right ventricle.

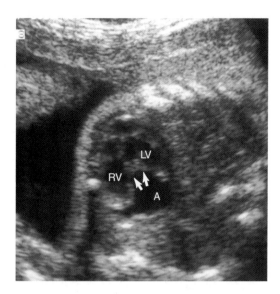

Figure 6–5 Apical four-chamber view showing a single multileaflet AV valve *(arrows)* in a fetus with an AVSD. *A,* Atria; *LV,* left ventricle; *RV,* right ventricle.

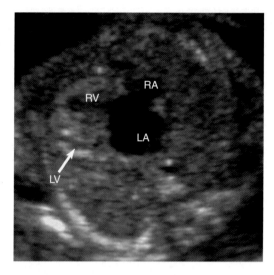

Figure 6–7 Subcostal four-chamber view in a fetus with an unbalanced AVSD. The left ventricle *(LV)* is much smaller than the right ventricle *(RV)* because of an inequity in blood flow. *LA,* Left atrium; *RA,* right atrium.

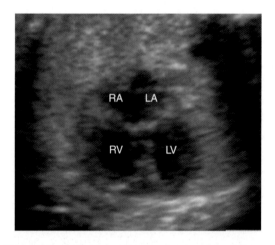

Figure 6–6 Apical four-chamber view in a fetus with a balanced AVSD. The right *(RV)* and left *(LV)* ventricles are of relatively equal size. *LA,* Left atrium; *RA,* right atrium.

ventricle. Either an apical or subcostal four-chamber view can be used to demonstrate the symmetry of the ventricles (Fig. 6–6).

An unbalanced AVSD occurs because the AV junction is primarily connected to one ventricle, resulting in the opposing ventricle becoming hypoplastic as a result of decreased blood flow.

The sonographic appearance of an unbalanced AVSD is to have one dominant ventricle, which receives the majority of the AV junction and therefore the majority of the blood flow. The other ventricle will appear small or hypoplastic (Fig. 6–7).

In the partial form of AVSD, two AV valves are present. Their leaflet formation is abnormal, but this may be difficult to appreciate sonographically. The presence of an atrial and a ventricular septal defect may be the only clue that an abnormality is present (Fig. 6–8). The apical four-chamber view is useful in showing the abnormal insertion of the AV valves (Fig. 6–9). In the normal heart, the tricuspid valve has a more apical insertion compared with the mitral valve. This normal relationship is lost in all forms of AVSD; however, in partial AVSD, this insertion discrepancy may be subtle.

The full extent of the ventricular septal defect associated with an AVSD is important to assess with regard to surgical repair. The best view for this is usually the subcostal four-chamber view (Fig. 6–10).

Another relationship lost in an AVSD is that of the aortic root to the AV junction. The aortic root normally lies within the fold of the two-valve annuli. The "sprung" AV junction leads to elongation of the left ventricular outflow tract. The

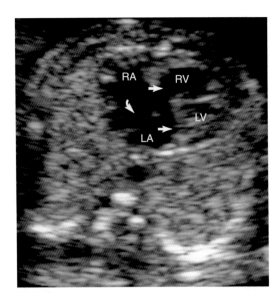

Figure 6–8 Subcostal four-chamber view in a fetus with a partial AVSD. Two separate AV valves *(straight arrows)* are seen in addition to a large atrial septal defect *(curved arrow). LA,* Left atrium; *LV,* left ventricle; *RA,* right atrium; *RV,* right ventricle.

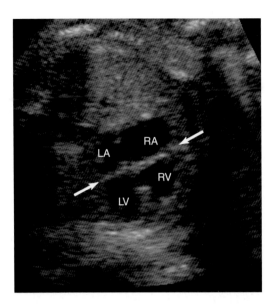

Figure 6–9 Apical four-chamber view in a fetus with a partial AVSD. Although subtle, the tricuspid valve and mitral valve *(arrows)* in this form of AVSD can be inserting at the same level. In a normal heart, the tricuspid valve would have a slightly more apical insertion than would the mitral valve. *LA,* Left atrium; *LV,* left ventricle; *RA,* right atrium; *RV,* right ventricle.

anteriorly and superiorly displaced aortic root, along with the position of the anterior septal bridging leaflet, causes a "goose-neck" deformity or narrowing of the left ventricular outflow tract.[3,18] This may be appreciated in a long-axis view of the aorta (Fig. 6–11).

The short-axis view of the fetal heart is useful for evaluating the AV junction, including the valve leaflets and the annulus. When a complete AVSD is present, a single large AV valve is seen common to both ventricles (Fig. 6–12). If a partial AVSD is present, a right and left orifice will be visualized, with the mitral orifice being triangular rather than elliptical, as in a normal heart, and resembling a mirror-image tricuspid orifice.

Color Doppler imaging is a useful adjunct in the evaluation of an AVSD. Color Doppler imaging confirms the communication occurring among all four cardiac chambers (Fig. 6–13). Color Doppler imaging in the apical four-chamber view is useful for detecting and quantifying valve regurgitation within the atria (Fig. 6–14). The area of the atrium occupied by the regurgitant jet can be determined planimetrically and may have some prognostic significance. Pulsed Doppler imaging can be used

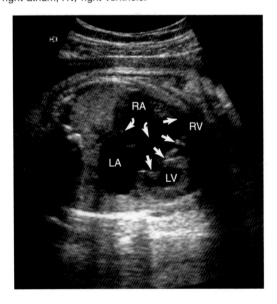

Figure 6–10 Subcostal four-chamber view in a fetus with a complete AVSD. A single multileaflet AV valve is seen *(arrows)* in addition to a large ventricular septal defect and atrial septal defect *(curved arrows). LA,* Left atrium; *LV,* left ventricle; *RA,* right atrium; *RV,* right ventricle.

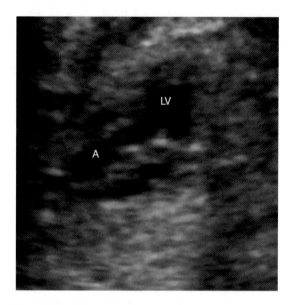

Figure 6–11   Long-axis view of the aorta *(A)* showing the narrowing of the left ventricular outflow tract often seen with an AVSD. *LV,* Left ventricle.

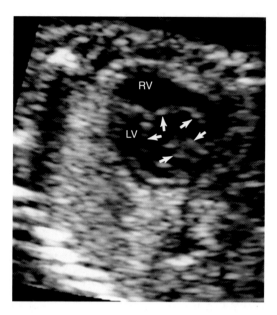

Figure 6–12   Short-axis view of a single multileaflet AV valve *(arrows)* in a fetus with a complete AVSD. *LV,* Left ventricle; *RV,* right ventricle.

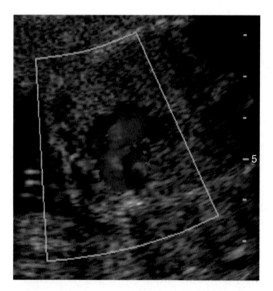

Figure 6–13   Apical four-chamber view in a fetus with a complete AVSD using color Doppler imaging to show the large communication within the center of the heart.

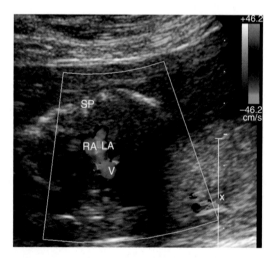

Figure 6–14   Apical four-chamber view in a fetus with a complete AVSD. Color Doppler imaging shows a large regurgitant jet flowing retrograde into the atria. *LA,* Left atrium; *RA,* right atrium; *SP,* spine; *V,* ventricle.

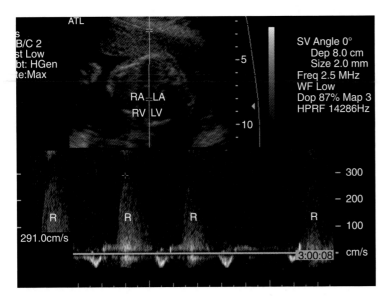

Figure 6–15 Pulsed Doppler imaging showing regurgitant jet *(R)* occurring throughout systole in a fetus with a complete AVSD. *LA*, Left atrium; *LV*, left ventricle; *RA*, right atrium; *RV*, right ventricle.

to assess the duration of the regurgitant jet in systole (Fig. 6–15), which has also been reported to have prognostic value. Pansystolic regurgitation or insufficiency correlates with severe insufficiency and has been associated with nonimmune hydrops fetalis.[13]

Detection of an AVSD requires complete evaluation of the heart to identify associated defects. If an AVSD is found in conjunction with complete heart block, the likelihood of heterotaxy is significant. Therefore fetal abdominal situs should be evaluated. An AVSD occurring in isolation has a higher association with a chromosome anomaly, specifically trisomy 21. In this setting, ultrasound markers for aneuploidy should be evaluated.

Treatment

Most fetuses tolerate AVSDs well. A small number may have congestive heart failure resulting in hydrops as a result of valvular insufficiency or an associated heart block.

With the complete form of AVSD, symptoms usually occur in early infancy, resulting from the large increase in pulmonary blood flow associated with increased pulmonary artery pressure and insufficiency of the common AV valve.[24] Infants often present with heart failure, repeated respiratory infections, and failure to thrive. Children with complete AVSDs are usually small and under-nourished, and virtually all have symptoms by 1 year of age.[15]

All AVSDs require surgical repair. Surgery is usually performed before 6 months of age to prevent the possibility of irreversible pulmonary vascular obstructive disease and Eisenmenger syndrome. In patients with trisomy 21 and complete AVSD, surgery may be appropriate as early as 4 months of age.*

Primary repair is the preferred surgical approach. This includes closure of the interatrial and interventricular communications, construction of two separate incompetent AV valves from the leaflet tissue available, and, if necessary, repair of associated defects. Either a single-patch or two-patch technique may be used to close the septal defects, after which reconstruction of the AV valve is performed.[15,18,30,32–35] Depending on which technique is used, the left AV valve may be left as a trileaflet or bileaflet valve. Most surgeons now opt to repair the cleft mitral valve, leading to improved mortality rates.[18,25,30,36]

Additional surgeries may be required over time because of narrowing of the left ventricular outflow tract or, most commonly, development of valvular insufficiency.[33] Early primary repair mortality rates

---

*References 1, 15, 18, 23, 24, 30, 31.

have been reported to be less than 5% to 10% in infants with isolated complete AVSD. [18,23,30]

Palliative pulmonary artery banding (PAB) may be considered in patients unsuitable for complete repair.* Patients who receive PAB may develop severe pulmonary stenosis and myocardial hypertrophy.[30] Palliative PAB has been reported to carry a 5% mortality rate in infants younger than 1 year of age.[34]

The surgical repair of a partial AVSD is usually not indicated as early in infancy as is repair of a complete AVSD. The mortality risk for the surgical repair of a partial AVSD has been reported to be approximately 3%.[24] Causes of death include congestive heart failure, cyanosis, failure to thrive, and moderate to severe mitral valve insufficiency. Repairing a partial AVSD involves closure of the interatrial septal defect with an autologous pericardial patch and reconstruction of the mitral valve cleft to promote coaptation of the leaflets to correct valvular insufficiency.[31,32,35,37–39]

The surgical repair of either the partial or the complete form of AVSD may be complicated by the association of other cardiac defects. When other defects are present, the surgical technique is modified to correct the associated abnormality, and mortality rates increase.

Postoperative complications include ventricular arrhythmias (33%), right bundle-branch block (22%), and atrial arrhythmias (11%).[24,32,37] Complete heart block after surgery was once common, requiring insertion of a permanent pacemaker, but now is a rare occurrence seen in only 1% to 2% of patients. Other associated complications include right ventricular outflow tract obstruction (11%), residual interventricular shunting (7%), and severe AV valve insufficiency (13% to 24%).[31,32,35,37–39]

Prognosis

In untreated children with complete AVSD not complicated by other associated anomalies, death often occurs before 15 years of age. If other anomalies are present, death usually occurs in infancy. In survivors of surgery, late death is rare, with a reported occurrence rate of 0% to 7%.[24] Failure of the surgical repair itself has been reported to occur approximately 11% to 25% of the time in partial AVSD and 10% of the time in complete AVSD. Long-term survival after surgery has been reported

to be 80% to 90% at 10 years and 65% after 20 years.[18,25,31–33,35,37–39]

It should be taken into consideration, however, that children afflicted with conditions such as Down syndrome, polysplenia, or asplenia may have complications unrelated to the cardiac defect and, therefore, a different prognosis.

Associated Anomalies

Forty to sixty percent of AVSDs are associated with aneuploidy. Down syndrome is the most common chromosomal abnormality, accounting for 40% to 80% of AVSDs.[15,18,23,40–42] Trisomy 13 and trisomy 18 have also been reported.[41] AVSD is also frequently found in infants affected with asplenia or polysplenia. The combination of AVSD with complete heart block is highly suggestive of polysplenia (left atrial isomerism).[2,26] Complete AVSDs are also associated with malposition of the heart, such as mesocardia or dextrocardia.[2] Other cardiac abnormalities associated with AVSD include outflow tract obstruction, coarctation of the aorta, tetralogy of Fallot, double-outlet right ventricle, transposition of the great arteries, pulmonary stenosis, or atresia, and secundum ASDs.[2,19,40,41] Extracardiac abnormalities occurring with AVSD include musculoskeletal, central nervous system, gastrointestinal, and genitourinary tract anomalies.[41] A reanalysis of the Baltimore-Washington Infant Study data found a strong association of isolated complete AVSD with maternal diabetes.[43]

References

1. Feldt RH, Porter CJ, Edwards WD, et al: Atrioventricular septal defects. In: Emmanouilides GC, Riemenschneider RA, Allen HD, et al (eds): Moss and Adams' Heart Disease in Infants, Children, and Adolescents, Including the Fetus and Young Adult, 5th ed, vol I. Baltimore, Williams & Wilkins, 1995, pp 704–723.

2. Romero R, Pilu G, Jeanty P, et al: Atrioventricular septal defects. In: Romero R, Pilu G, Jeanty P, et al (eds): Prenatal Diagnosis of Congenital Anomalies. Norwalk, CT, Appleton & Lange, 1988, pp 144–147.

3. Higgins CB, Silverman NH, Kersting-Sommerhoff B, et al: Atrioventricular septal (canal) defects. In: Higgins CB, Silverman NH, Kersting-Sommerhoff B, et al (eds): Congenital Heart Disease: Echocardiography and Magnetic Resonance Imaging. New York, Raven Press, 1990, pp 135–150.

4. Van Mierop LH, Alley RD, Kausel HW, et al: The anatomy and embryology and endocardial

---

*References 18, 23, 25, 30, 34, 35, 37–39.

cushion defects. J Thorac Cardiovascular Surg 1962; 43:71–83.

5. Wenink AC: Quantitative morphology of the embryonic heart: An approach to development of atrioventricular valves. Anat Rec 1991; 234:129–135.

6. Piccoli GP, Wilkinson JL, Macartney FJ, et al: Morphology and classification of complete atrioventricular defects. Br Heart J 1979; 42:633–639.

7. Bharati S, Lev M: The spectrum of common atrioventricular orifice (canal). Am Heart J 1973; 86:553–561.

8. Van Praagh R: Terminology of congenital heart disease. Circulation 1977; 56:139–143.

9. Marino B: Atrioventricular septal defect anatomic characteristics in patients with and without Down syndrome. Cardiol Young 1991; 2:308–310.

10. DeBiase L, Di Ciommo V, Ballerini L, et al: Prevalence of left-sided obstructive lesions in patients with atrioventricular canal without Down's syndrome. J Thorac Cardiovascular Surg 1986; 91:467–469.

11. Marino B, Papa M, Guccione P, et al: Ventricular septal defect in Down syndrome: Anatomic types and associated malformations. Am J Dis Child 1990; 144:544–545.

12. Akiba T, Becker AE, Neirotti R, et al: Valve morphology in complete atrioventricular septal defect: Variability relevant to operation. Ann Thorac Surg 1993; 56:295–299.

13. Rastelli GC, Kirklin JW, Titus JL: Anatomic observations on complete form of persistent common atrioventricular canal with special reference to atrioventricular valves. Mayo Clin Proc 1966; 41:296–308.

14. Rastelli GC, Ongley PA, Kirklin JW, et al: Surgical repair of the complete form of persistent common atrioventricular canal. J Thorac Cardiovasc Surg 1968; 55:299–308.

15. Calabrò R, Limongelli G: Complete atrioventricular canal. Orphanet J Rare Dis 2006; 1:8.

16. Gembruch U, Knopfle G, Chatterjee M, et al: Prenatal diagnosis of atrioventricular canal malformations with up-to-date echocardiographic technology: Report of 14 cases. Am Heart J 1991; 121:1489–1497.

17. Carmi R, Boughman JA, Ferencz C: Endocardial cushion defect: Further studies of "isolated" versus "syndromic" occurrence. Am J Med Genet 1992; 43:569–575.

18. Craig B: Atrioventricular septal defect: from fetus to adult. Heart 2006; 92:1879–1885.

19. Stamm ER, Drose JA, Thickman D: The fetal heart. In: Rumack CM, Wilson SR, Charboneau JW (eds): Diagnostic Ultrasound, vol 11. St Louis, Mosby–Year Book, 1991, pp 800–827.

20. Machado MV, Crawford DC, Anderson RH, et al: Atrioventricular septal defect in prenatal life. Br Heart J 1988; 59:352–355.

21. Freedom RM, Culham JAG, Moes CAF: Atrioventricular septal defects. In: Freedom RM, Culham JAG, Moes CAF (eds): Angiography of Congenital Heart Disease. New York, Macmillan, 1984, pp 141–159.

22. Crawford DC, Chita SK, Allan LD: Prenatal detection of congenital heart disease: Factors affecting obstetric management and survival. Am J Obstet Gynecol 1988; 159:352–356.

23. Birk E, Silverman NH: Intracardiac shunt malformations. In: Yagel S, Silverman NH, Gembruch U (eds): Fetal Cardiology. London, UK, Martin Dunitz, 2003, pp 205–207.

24. Merrill WH, Hoff SJ, Bender HW: Surgical treatment of atrioventricular septal defects. In: Mavroudis C (ed): Pediatric Cardiac Surgery, 2nd ed. St Louis, Mosby–Year Book, 1994, pp 225–236.

25. Boening A, Scheewe J, Heine K, et al: Long-term results after surgical correction of atrioventricular septal defects. Eur J Cardiothorac Surg 2002; 22:167–173.

26. Nyberg DA, Emerson DS: Cardiac malformations. In: Nyberg J, Mahony DA, Pretorius BS (eds): Diagnostic Ultrasound of Fetal Anomalies. Text and Atlas. Chicago, Year Book Medical, 1990, pp 300–337.

27. Hoffman JI, Christianson R: Congenital heart disease in a cohort of 19,502 births with long-term follow-up. Am J Cardiol 1978; 42:641–647.

28. Mitchell SC, Karones SB, Berendes HW: Congenital heart disease in 56,109 births. Incidence and natural history. Circulation 1971; 43:323–332.

29. Drenthen W, Peiper PG, van der Tuuk K, et al: Cardiac complications relating to pregnancy and recurrence of disease in the offspring of women with atrioventricular septal defects. Eur Heart J 2005; 26:2581–2587.

30. Kobayashi M, Takahashi Y, Ando M: Ideal timing of surgical repair of isolated complete atrioventricular septal defect. Interact Cardiovasc Thorac Surg 2007; 6:24–26.

31. Graham TP Jr: When to operate on the child with congenital heart disease. Pediatr Clin North Am 1984; 31:1275–1291.

32. Bender HW Jr, Graham TP Jr, Hubbard SG: Repair of AV canal malformation in the first year of life. J Thorac Cardiovasc Surg 1982; 84:512–522.

33. Boening A, Scheewe J, Heine K, et al: Long-term results after surgical correction of atrioventricular septal defects. Eur J Cardiothorac Surg 2002; 22:167–173.

34. Leblanc JG, Ashmore PG, Pineda E, et al: Pulmonary artery banding: Results and current indications in pediatric cardiac surgery. Ann Thorac Surg 1987; 44:628–632.

35. Thies WR, Breymann T, Matthies W, et al: Primary repair of complete atrioventricular septal defect in infancy. Eur J Cardiothorac Surg 1991; 5:571–574.

36. Krasemann T, Debus V, Rellensmann G, et al: Regurgitation of the atrioventricular valves after corrective surgery for complete atrioventricular septal defects—Comparison of different surgical techniques. Thorac Cardiovasc Surg 2007; 55:229–232.

37. Samánek M: Children with congenital heart disease: Probability of natural survival. Pediatr Cardiol 1992; 13:152–158.

38. Graham TP Jr, Bender JW Jr: Preoperative diagnosis and management of infants with critical congenital heart disease. Ann Thorac Surg 1980; 29:272–288.

39. Williams WH, Guyton RA, Michalik RE, et al: Individualized surgical management of complete atrioventricular canal. J Thorac Cardiovasc Surg 1983; 86:838–844.

40. Huggon IC, Cook AC, Smeeton NC, et al: Atrioventricular septal defects diagnosed in fetal life: Associated cardiac and extra-cardiac abnormalities and outcome. J Am Coll Cardiol 2000; 36:593–601.

41. Ashok M, Thangavel G, Indrani S, et al: Atrioventricular septal defect-associated anomalies and aneuploidy in prenatal life. Indian Pediatr 2003; 40:659–664.

42. Paladini D, Tartaglione A, Agangi A, et al: The association between congenital heart disease and Down syndrome in prenatal life. Ultrasound Obstet Gynecol 2000; 15:104–108.

43. Loffredo CA, Hirata J, Wilson PD, et al: Atrioventricular septal defects: Possible etiologic differences between complete and partial defects. Teratology 2001; 63:87–93.

CHAPTER 7

Hypoplastic Left Heart Syndrome

Sarah H. Martinez

OUTLINE

Definition

Hypoplastic left heart syndrome (HLHS) refers to a spectrum of cardiac abnormalities that includes underdevelopment of the left ventricle, mitral valve, aorta, and aortic valve.[1-3]

This syndrome is the most severe form of left-sided obstructive lesions, and it is among the most severe forms of congenital heart disease (CHD).[4-8] It consists, in varying degrees, of a small left ventricle associated with aortic atresia, a hypoplastic ascending aorta, mitral valve atresia or hypoplasia, and a small left atrium (Fig. 7–1).

HLHS may be associated with a malaligned atrioventricular canal, although this is much less common than its association with mitral valve atresia or hypoplasia.

Cardiac anomalies resulting in a hypoplastic aorta or coarctation of the aorta with a normally functioning left ventricle are not included in this syndrome.

The terms "aortic atresia" and "HLHS" are often used in reference to the same lesion; however, these two anomalies are not synonymous because a small percentage of patients with aortic atresia have a normal left ventricle.[9]

Embryology

The early developmental changes that result in a hypoplastic left ventricle are not completely understood.[10] Several hypotheses currently exist.[4]

Decreased ventricular size has been achieved in animal models by reducing the blood flow through the foramen ovale.[11] The development of the cardiac chambers is dependent on the flow of blood through them. Therefore decreased perfusion of the left atrium and left ventricle may result in hypoplastic chambers, aortic valve atresia, mitral valve atresia, and hypoplasia of the aortic arch.[4,12]

Malalignment of the interatrial septum toward the left has also been proposed as a mechanism of interfering with left ventricular filling, resulting in poor development of that chamber.[13]

Another explanation for HLHS is that fusion of the endocardial cushions occurs but fails to produce a valve.[12,13]

It may also be due to an overgrowth of the ventral atrioventricular cushion, which deprives the ascending aorta of adequate blood flow.[14] The resultant change in flow leads to the development

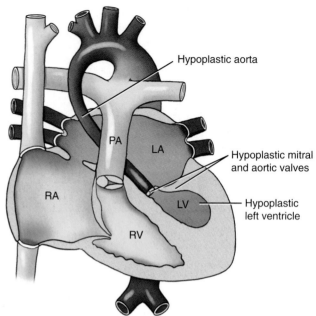

Figure 7-1 Diagrammatic representation of the abnormalities associate with HLHS. Note the small left ventricle (*LV*), an atretic or hypoplastic mitral valve, and the very small aorta. *LA*, Left atrium; *PA*, pulmonary artery; *RA*, right atrium; *RV*, right ventricle.

Labels in figure: Hypoplastic aorta; PA; LA; Hypoplastic mitral and aortic valves; RA; LV; Hypoplastic left ventricle; RV

of the structural cardiac anomalies associated with this syndrome.[12,15]

Normally, the primitive heart tube in the embryo forms three wall layers, becomes elongated, and bends into a loop—the cardiac loop. Expanded portions of the heart tube form the atrioventricular canal.

Endocardial cushions develop at the superior and inferior ends of the atrioventricular canal; lateral endocardial cushions develop on the right and left edges of the canal. Fusion of the superior and inferior atrioventricular cushions divides the canal into right and left atrioventricular orifices. Each orifice is surrounded by mesenchymal tissue that eventually becomes thinned out by the flow of blood over it, thus forming valves that are attached to the ventricular wall. These valves develop into the mitral and tricuspid valves at approximately 6 or 7 weeks' gestation.

Part of the interventricular septum and the ventricular muscle develops from this atrioventricular canal; papillary muscles and chordae tendinae arise from the ventricular muscle.[10]

In the embryo, the aorta and pulmonary artery develop from the division of a common trunk, and small projections or tubercles form within the lumen. These tubercles grow toward the midline and become thinned out by resorption of excess tissue and hollowed out at the site of attachment with the vessel walls, thus giving rise to the semilunar valves.

A third hypothesis is that the causative factor is a rudimentary left atrium and, consequently, diminished blood flow to the mitral portion of the atrioventricular canal. The left ventricle and aorta or aortic valve thus fail to develop properly because of the decreased blood flow through the lumen.[10]

The left ventricle will be small, the aortic valve may be stenotic, and coarctation of the aorta may result.[12,16] Aortic stenosis or atresia may be valvular, subvalvular, or supravalvular. Subvalvular and valvular types often occur together.[14,17]

The position of the heart in HLHS is usually normal. There are also normal atrioventricular and ventriculoarterial connections. The great vessels are normally oriented to one another. The inferior and superior venae cavae drain normally into the right atrium; however, anomalies of pulmonary venous return frequently occur.

The tricuspid valve is structurally normal; however, the right ventricle is often enlarged and in some cases hypertrophic because of the increase in blood volume and blood pressure caused by the obstructive left side. This increase in volume may lead to tricuspid insufficiency. The pulmonary artery and its branches are usually dilated. The pulmonary valve is normal in the majority of cases.

The ductus arteriosus is patent; however, the foramen ovale may close completely in utero with resultant severe hypoplasia of the left ventricle.[18]

The ascending aorta is poorly developed, with normal coronary artery orientation. Coarctation of the aorta is present in the majority of patients with HLHS, and this may result in narrowing of the subclavian artery and left common carotid artery origins. An interrupted aortic arch occurs much less commonly. The aortic valve is either stenotic or atretic in most cases.

An abnormal mitral valve is always present. If the valve is atretic, the left ventricle is severely underdeveloped, appearing as a slitlike cavity. However, if the mitral valve is stenotic but perforate, the left ventricle is somewhat larger with thickened walls.

The ventricular septum is generally intact but may be deviated into a subaortic position.

Conduction disturbances may be present in HLHS because of an interruption in the bundle of His.[12,16,19–21]

Hemodynamically, blood is unable to pass through the left ventricle and aortic valve and therefore is shunted in a retrograde manner from the left atrium, through the foramen ovale, and back into the right atrium (Fig. 7–2). This results in an increase in the size of the right atrium, right ventricle, and main pulmonary artery.

Because of the left heart hypoplasia, the right ventricle supplies both the pulmonary and systemic circulations. The pulmonary veins may be either normal or increased in size. The blood volume and pressure in the right heart are elevated.[22] The left atrium, left ventricle, and aorta are all decreased in size. In severe cases of hypoplasia of the ascending aorta, the coronary arteries are perfused in a retrograde manner by the ductus arteriosus.[6,23]

HLHS results in cardiac function similar to that seen in univentricular hearts. The increased right ventricular pressure, together with inadequate flow out of the left atrium, results in elevated pulmonary venous pressure and pulmonary congestion.[16]

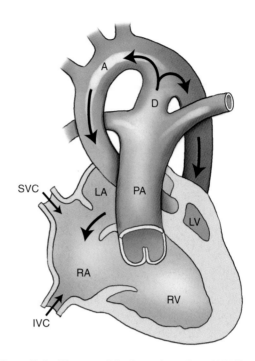

Figure 7–2 Diagram of the hemodynamics of HLHS, showing blood being supplied to the aorta only through the ductus arteriosus *(D)*. Blood flow from the left atrium *(LA)* is shunted in a retrograde fashion to the right atrium *(RA)* as a result of the atretic mitral valve and hypoplastic left ventricle *(LV)*. A, Aorta; *IVC*, inferior vena cava; *PA*, pulmonary artery; *RV*, right ventricle; *SVC*, superior vena cava.

Occurrence Rate

HLHS is the most common cause of death from CHD in the early neonatal period, accounting for 7% to 9% of all structural heart defects and 25% of all cardiac-related deaths.[3,24] HLHS comprises 13% of all prenatally diagnosed CHD. There appears to be a male dominance, especially in the presence of atresia of the aortic valve.[20–22,25,26]

Most cases of HLHS are likely multifactorial. However, multiple studies suggest a genetic basis as the etiology of many cases. Approximately 19% of affected patients with HLHS have a first-degree relative with CHD, reinforcing the case for a genetic link to HLHS.[4,27,28] It is thought to have an autosomal recessive inheritance pattern.

The risk of occurrence has been reported to be 2% in siblings of an affected child.[24,25,28–30]

Sonographic Criteria

HLHS is easily recognized in utero. It should be borne in mind, however, that HLHS is a progressive lesion and may not manifest itself until the late second trimester. Studies show early screening may be advantageous but does not obviate the importance of second-trimester fetal echocardiography.[3,31]

First trimester nuchal translucency screening has increased early detection of HLHS. Studies suggest a stronger correlation between left-sided obstructive lesions and a thickened nuchal translucency. A measurement greater than 2.5 multiples of the median is associated with an increased risk for CHD, including HLHS and should be an considered an indication for fetal echocardiography.[3,32]

The majority of patients with HLHS maintain a normal cardiac axis. An apical (Fig. 7–3) or subcostal (Fig. 7–4) four-chamber view of the heart can be used to show the size discrepancy of the ventricles. It is important to identify the morphological features of the right ventricle, including the moderator band and the tricuspid valve, to confirm it is the left ventricle that is hypoplastic. In HLHS, the right ventricle constitutes the cardiac apex, giving rise to the term "apex-forming ventricle" (Fig. 7–5).[21,22,33]

A short-axis view of the great vessels (Fig. 7–6), a long-axis view of the aorta (Fig. 7–7), or a three-vessel view (Fig. 7–8) can be used to assess the size of the ascending aorta. An atretic aorta can be difficult to visualize because of its small size. On the other hand, the pulmonary artery is often enlarged. Sonographically, an atretic aorta and aortic valve

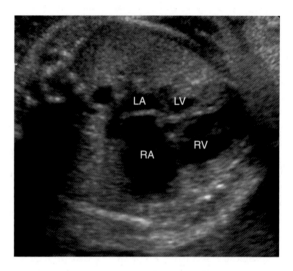

Figure 7–4 Subcostal four-chamber view in a fetus with HLHS showing the small left ventricle *(LV)* and left atrium *(LA)*. The right atrium *(RA)* and right ventricle *(RV)* are enlarged because of the alterations in hemodynamics.

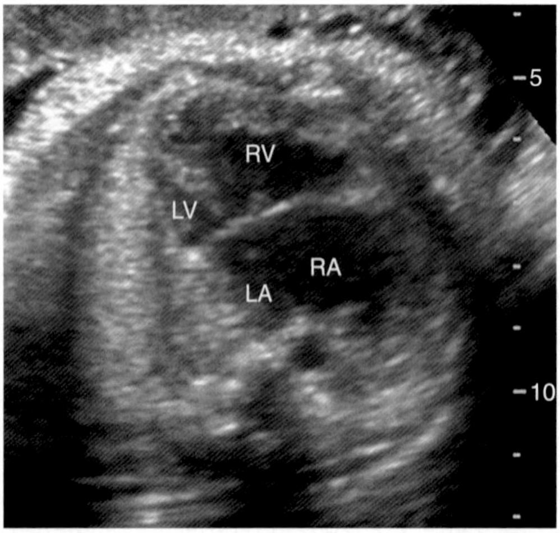

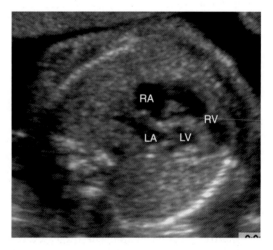

Figure 7–3 Apical four-chamber view in a fetus with HLHS showing the decreased size of both the left ventricle *(LV)* and the left atrium *(LA)*. *RA*, Right atrium; *RV*, right ventricle.

Figure 7–5 Subcostal four-chamber view showing the right ventricle *(RV)* becoming the "apex-forming ventricle" as a result of the decreased size of the left ventricle *(LV)*. *LA*, Left atrium; *RA*, right atrium.

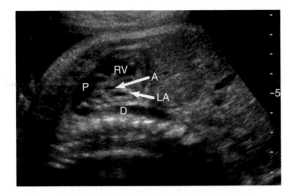

Figure 7-6 Short-axis view of the great vessels in a fetus with HLHS showing the very small size of the aortic root *(A)* and the left ventricle *(LV)*. The pulmonary artery *(P)* and right ventricle *(RV)* are enlarged because of alterations in hemodynamics. *D,* Descending aorta.

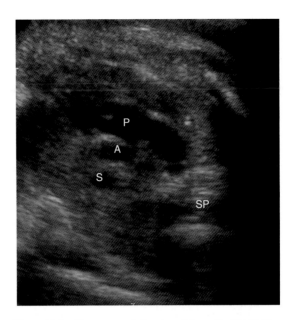

Figure 7-8 Three-vessel view in a fetus with HLHS. The size discrepancy of the enlarged pulmonary artery *(P)* and smaller aorta *(A)* can be appreciated. *S,* Superior vena cava; *SP,* spine.

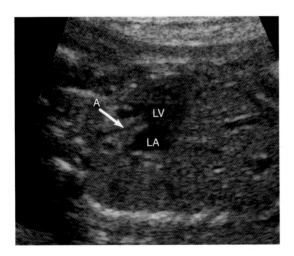

Figure 7-7 Long-axis view of the aorta in a fetus with HLHS. The atretic aorta *(A)* can be seen arising from the small left ventricle *(LV)*. *LA,* Left atrium.

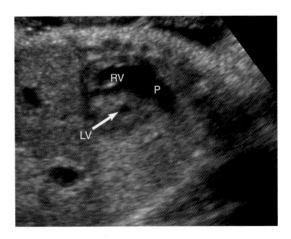

Figure 7-9 Short-axis view of the ventricles in a fetus with HLHS. Left ventricle *(LV)* size is markedly diminished. The right ventricle *(RV)* and the pulmonary artery *(P)* are dilated.

can appear hyperechoic in addition to being small.

The presence and size of the left ventricle can be evaluated in a short-axis view of the ventricles (Fig. 7-9) and either four-chamber view.

Anomalous pulmonary venous connection is not uncommon with HLHS. The connection of the pulmonary veins to the left atrium should be determined in either four-chamber view. The pulmonary veins are often enlarged as a result of

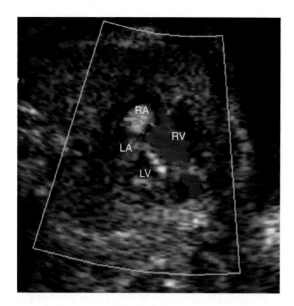

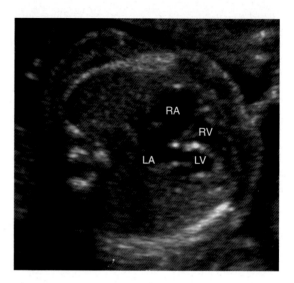

Figure 7–10 Apical four-chamber view in a fetus with HLHS using color Doppler imaging to confirm the presence and direction of blood flow. Color shows retrograde blood flow from the left atrium *(LA)* to the right atrium *(RA)*. Color also shows blood entering the right ventricle *(RV)*, but no flow is appreciated entering the hypoplastic left ventricle *(LV)*.

Figure 7–11 The hyperechoic walls of the left ventricle *(LV)* are indicative of endocardial fibroelastosis in a fetus with HLHS. *LA,* Left atrium; *RA,* right atrium; *RV,* right ventricle.

pulmonary congestion. Color or pulsed Doppler imaging is useful in confirming their normal connection the left atrium.[29]

A restrictive foramen ovale is one of the worst prognostic signs associated with HLHS. Therefore a thorough assessment of the interatrial septum is mandatory. Color or pulsed Doppler imaging should be used to confirm the presence and direction of blood flow through the foramen ovale (Fig. 7–10). If the interatrial septum is seen bowing to the left, either anomalous pulmonary venous drainage or severe tricuspid regurgitation may be present.[29]

Endocardial fibroelastosis of the left ventricle or aorta may be present. Endocardial fibroelastosis results from blood entering a chamber or vessel but being unable to exit efficiently. Therefore fibrin develops and is deposited along the walls of the structure. This produces a hyperechoic endocardium (Fig. 7–11). Regardless of the size of the left ventricle, endocardial fibroelastosis results in a stiff, poorly contracting chamber.

Imaging of the aortic arch usually reveals a hypoplastic ascending aorta, which may be diffi-cult to visualize or enlarged slightly at the sinuses of Valsalva (Fig. 7–12).[8] Blood flow through the aorta is often retrograde from the ductus arteriosus (Fig. 7–13).

The long-axis view of the aorta or the four-chamber views of the heart will demonstrate an atretic or hypoplastic mitral valve. Even if the mitral valve is patent, generally all its components are abnormal, including a hypoplastic annulus; thickened, short chordae tendineae; and small papillary muscles.[9]

In the setting of mitral valve atresia, a membranous band may be apparent, instead of valve leaflets, at the valve orifice (Fig. 7–14).

The majority of patients with HLHS have both aortic valve and mitral valve stenosis, hypoplasia, or atresia. The result is an extremely small, often slitlike, left ventricle. However, if only the aortic valve is atretic and the mitral valve function is not severely affected, the left ventricle can appear somewhat larger than expected.

Ultimately, left ventricular size depends on the degree of mitral valve disease. In addition, mitral valve hypoplasia in association with right-to-left shunting of blood through a ventricular septal defect can result in a normal ascending aorta and normal left ventricular size.

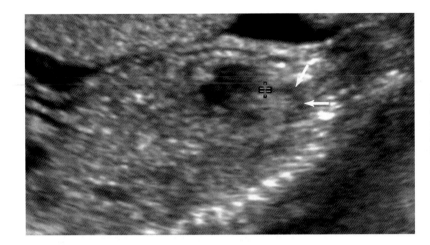

Figure 7–12 A very small atretic aortic arch is barely visualized *(arrows)* in a fetus with HLHS. The aortic root (calipers) measures only 6 mm.

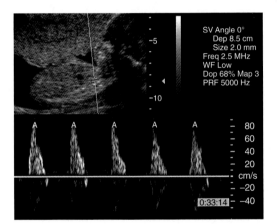

Figure 7–13 Pulsed-wave Doppler imaging of the atretic aortic arch seen in Figure 7–12, showing reversed flow *(A)* from the ductus arteriosus back through the arch.

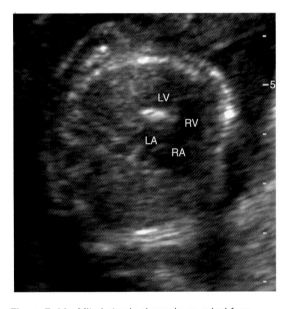

Figure 7–14 Mitral atresia shown in an apical four-chamber view in a fetus with HLHS. The mitral valve orifice appears as a hyperechoic band. *LA,* Left atrium; *LV,* left ventricle; *RA,* right atrium; *RV,* right ventricle.

M-mode diagnostic criteria for HLHS includes a left ventricular end-diastolic diameter less than 9 mm and aortic root diameter less than 6 mm.[9] Regardless of an exact measurement, if the left-sided heart structures appear smaller than expected for gestational age at any time, follow-up examinations are necessary to exclude the development of HLHS.

Pulsed-wave and color Doppler imaging are helpful in evaluating flow through the valves. Additionally, because HLHS is a ductal-dependent lesion after delivery, confirming patency of the ductus arteriosus and foramen ovale is essential.[3] Regurgitation through the tricuspid valve or a common atrioventricular valve occurs in more than 50% of patients with HLHS; therefore this should also be investigated.[29]

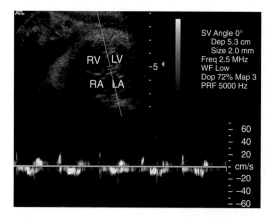

Figure 7–15 Apical four-chamber view using pulsed Doppler imaging distal to the atretic mitral valve in a fetus with HLHS. Virtually no flow is appreciated above the baseline (mitral inflow) or below the baseline (aortic outflow) as a result of the atretic valves. *LA*, Left atrium; *LV*, left ventricle; *RA*, right atrium; *RV*, right ventricle.

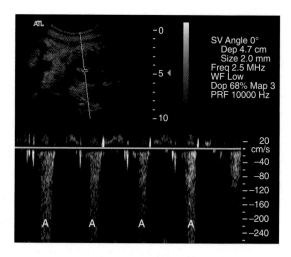

Figure 7–16 Apical four-chamber view using pulsed Doppler imaging distal to the aortic valve in a fetus with HLHS. The aortic velocity *(A)* of greater than 240 cm/second is indicative of aortic stenosis.

The mitral valve (Fig. 7–15) and ascending aorta (Fig. 7–16) should be interrogated with Doppler imaging to determine whether they are stenotic or atretic.

Flow through the ductus arteriosus to the descending aorta during systole should be confirmed. During diastole, a small amount of blood normally flows back through the ductus arteriosus into the pulmonary artery. If this does not occur, there may be elevated pressure in the pulmonary artery, which can be suggestive of a small or absent foramen ovale.[29]

In addition to imaging all cardiac structures, the fetus with HLHS should be evaluated for signs of hydrops fetalis, such as skin thickening, ascites, or pericardial or pleural effusions (Fig. 7–17). Hydrops fetalis is not as common in HLHS as in other congenital cardiac anomalies, but congestive heart failure may result from right ventricular overload. If present, it can be indicative of premature closure of the foramen ovale or endocardial fibroelastosis of the right or left ventricle.[6,34]

Treatment

Historically, HLHS was considered inoperable and therefore a fatal form of CHD because these infants are incapable of sustaining adequate systemic circulation. In the past, the diagnosis was important

only to differentiate this lesion from one that could be surgically repaired.[12,20,29,35] Advancement in surgical treatment options for HLHS have contributed to increased survival.[1]

At birth, an infant with HLHS may appear normal, but within 2 to 5 days cyanosis will develop as a result of the mixing of blood.

HLHS is a ductal-dependent lesion, meaning survival in the early neonatal period depends on the patency of the ductus arteriosus and the foramen ovale. Prostaglandin E should be given at birth to maintain ductal patency. Blood flow is retrograde from the left atrium through the foramen ovale to the right atrium and from the ductus arteriosus into the descending aorta, with the coronary and cerebral circulations supplied by retrograde flow.[3,22]

Cardiomegaly is usually noted on the chest film of the neonate because of increased size of the right heart.[9,15] An electrocardiogram will demonstrate hypertrophy of the right atrium and ventricle.

HLHS infants exhibit a low systemic blood pressure and a decrease in peripheral pulses. The onset of symptoms is attributed to a decrease in pulmonary vascular resistance. If the right ventricle continues to function as a systemic ventricle and pulmonary pressure remains elevated, the systemic vasculature will receive adequate perfusion.

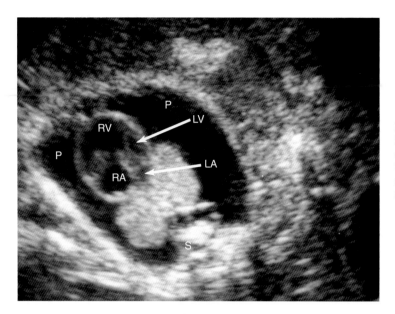

Figure 7–17 Apical four-chamber view in a fetus with HLHS. Massive pleural effusions *(P)* and skin thickening, indicative of hydrops, are also present. *LA,* Left atrium; *LV,* left ventricle; *RA,* right atrium; *RV,* right ventricle.

However, a decrease in pulmonary pressure results in decreased flow through the ductus arteriosus and into the systemic circulation.[20]

On auscultation, a normal first heart sound will be heard; however, the second heart sound will be single, which represents pulmonary valve closure only. Because the right ventricle is acting as a systemic ventricle, the pulmonary valve sound will be increased.[22]

Surgical interventions have evolved and continue to improve the management of HLHS. Currently they include staged surgical reconstruction, hybrid palliation, and orthotopic heart transplant. Hospice care also remains a valid option in some cases of HLHS.[1,2,4]

Medical management of these patients is not generally successful and is currently undertaken only as a supportive maneuver until surgical repair or heart transplantation can be performed. Heart transplantation, first performed in infants with HLHS in 1984, is hampered by the adequate number of donors. The long-term survival of these infants is uncertain. Successful heart transplantation provides the advantage of normal cardiac anatomy after a single surgery but carries significant risks, both surgical and long-term.[1,25,29]

The conventional approach in treating HLHS is a three-stage surgical reconstruction. This consists of a Norwood procedure, the modified Fontan, also called the bidirectional Glenn shunt, and the Fontan procedure.

Stage I, the Norwood procedure, which is performed shortly after birth, attempts to establish communication between the right ventricle and the aorta (Fig. 7–18). The pulmonary artery is ligated and a patch is used to close the pulmonary artery near its branches. The aorta is made larger by opening it from its origin at the ventricle to the descending portion. A graft is sewn in along the aortic opening. This creates a larger and more functional aorta. The aorta is banded to the proximal end of the previously ligated pulmonary artery. The right ventricle is then connected to the aorta, which becomes the pumping chamber. The ductus arteriosus is closed and the interatrial septum removed.[36]

A modified Blalock-Taussig shunt is placed from the right subclavian artery to the right pulmonary artery (Fig. 7–19). This is done to establish pulmonary circulation. A portion of the blood that leaves the aorta is pumped to the lungs, where it is reoxygenated.

An alternative to the Blalock-Taussig shunt is the Sano modification, in which the pulmonary artery is banded directly to the right ventricle (Fig. 7–20).[37]

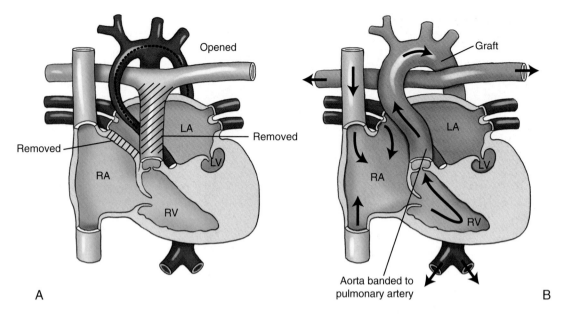

A   B

Figure 7–18 Diagram of the Norwood procedure. The pulmonary artery is ligated and sewn off near its branches. The aorta is opened and a graft is sewn in. The aorta is then banded to the ligated pulmonary artery. The right ventricle is connected to the aorta, the ductus arteriosus is removed, and the interatrial septum is removed. **A,** Sections of cardiac anatomy removed or opened. **B,** Completed procedure. *LA,* Left atrium; *LV,* left ventricle; *RA,* right atrium; *RV,* right ventricle.

Stage II, the bidirectional Glen shunt procedure, is usually performed between 4 and 6 months of age. This procedure connects the superior aspect of the superior vena cava to the right pulmonary artery (Fig. 7–21). The cardiac end of the superior vena cava is oversewn. This allows for reduction in the volume and pressure loads on the right ventricle.

Stage III, the Fontan procedure, is performed between 2 and 4 years of age. During this stage, the right atrium and the inferior vena cava are connected to the pulmonary artery (Fig. 7–22). This results in oxygen-poor blood bypassing the heart and going directly to the lungs.*

Neonates who undergo conventional surgical reconstruction encounter a variety of challenges and face the risk of circulatory arrest as a result of cardiopulmonary bypass. Hybrid palliation involves a spectrum of modifications that include pulmonary artery banding, stenting of the ductus arteriosus, and removal of the atrial septum. All are performed shortly after birth as interim steps to the Norwood procedure. These techniques are less invasive and have been adapted in an attempt to alleviate the morbidity and mortality associated with the Norwood procedure.[1,2,4,38,39]

Tricuspid and pulmonary valve abnormalities adversely affect the outcome of surgical repair.

A right ventricle with thicker muscle mass and better function improves postoperative results. The right ventricle of a fetus will adapt in utero, and the best surgical candidates are infants born with increased right ventricular wall thickness.[40]

Prognosis

Without surgical intervention, HLHS is always lethal. However, recent advances in surgical techniques have drastically improved the prognosis. Although not curative, these procedures have provided a means of survival for patients with HLHS.

Patency of the foramen ovale, the severity of the left-sided lesions, and associated cardiac abnormalities all influence survival rates.

---

*References 1, 2, 4, 5, 20, 25, 29, 33, 36–38.

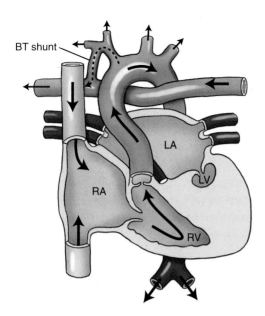

Figure 7–19 Diagram of the modified Blalock-Taussig shunt procedure. The Blalock-Taussig shunt connects the right subclavian artery to the right pulmonary artery. The *arrows* show the directions of blood flow once the procedure is complete. *LA,* Left atrium; *LV,* left ventricle; *RA,* right atrium; *RV,* right ventricle.

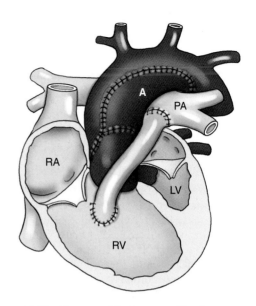

Figure 7–20 Diagram of the Sano modification, an alternative to the Blalock-Taussig shunt. In this setting, the pulmonary artery *(PA)* is banded directly to the right ventricle *(RV)*. *A,* Aorta; *LV,* left ventricle; *RA,* right atrium.

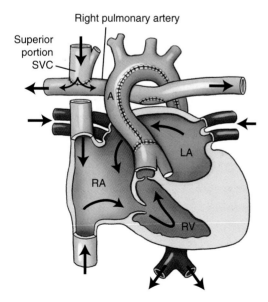

Figure 7–21 Diagram of the bidirectional Glen shunt procedure. This procedure connects the superior portion of the superior vena cava *(SVC)* to the right pulmonary artery. *A,* Aorta; *LA,* left atrium; *RA,* right atrium; *RV,* right ventricle.

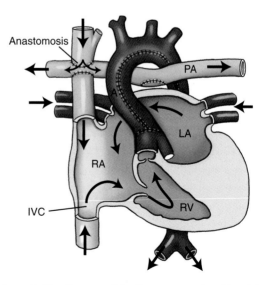

Figure 7–22 Diagram of the Fontan procedure. The right atrium *(RA)* and inferior vena cava *(IVC)* are anastomosed to the pulmonary artery *(PA)*. *A,* Aorta; *LA,* left atrium; *RV,* right ventricle.

The 5-year survival rate after staged surgical repair is approximately 70%. However, significant morbidity can occur, specifically renal failure, hepatic failure, feeding difficulties, and poor growth. Developmental and behavioral abnormalities, compared with healthy control subjects, are also reported.*

Cardiac transplantation carries a lower operative mortality rate; however, 25% of neonates listed for transplantation never receive a donor heart.[44,45] Infants who do undergo transplant surgery are subject to lifetime immunosuppression and increased risk of rejection and infection. The survival rate after cardiac transplant has been reported to be 61% at 1 year and 55% at 5 years.[46] Morbidity is similar to individuals undergoing staged repairs, including decreased renal function and neurological and developmental defects. Transplant-related coronary artery disease is not uncommon.

Associated Anomalies

The association of HLHS with other cardiovascular anomalies is high (Table 7–1). The most frequently associated anomaly is coarctation of the aorta. Although initially thought to be uncommon, it is reported in more than 70% of patients with HLHS.[†]

*References 1, 4, 9, 25, 29, 38, 41–43.
[†]References 7, 21, 33, 36, 38, 47, 48.

Coarctation is more commonly seen when severe mitral valve atresia, rather than mitral valve hypoplasia, is present.[40]

Atresia of the mitral valve is also common, followed by anomalies of the systemic and pulmonary venous connections, abnormal branching of the aorta, and ventricular septal defects. Atresia of both the mitral and aortic valves can coexist but is uncommon.[47] The most commonly associated systemic venous anomaly is a persistent left superior vena cava with venous drainage into the right atrium through the coronary sinus.[19,21] It is uncommon for HLHS to be associated with anomalies of the tricuspid or pulmonary valves.

HLHS is associated with extracardiac anomalies in 28% to 40% of cases, most commonly two-vessel cord, gastrointestinal, genitourinary, central nervous system, and craniofacial abnormalities.[7,14,21,33] Also, intrauterine growth restriction is not uncommon as a result of a decrease in cardiac output.

An association with HLHS has been reported in trisomy 13 and Turner syndrome; in addition, partial chromosome deletions, such as monosomy 7p2, have also been found to occur with HLHS.[29] An abnormal karyotype is reported in 11% to 16% of cases.

After birth, there is an increased incidence of liver ischemia and necrosis in children with HLHS. Abnormal liver function or hepatic vascular thrombosis resulting from congestive heart failure

TABLE 7–1 Conditions Associated with Hypoplastic Left Heart Syndrome			
Maternal		**Fetal**	
Drug Use	**Associated Cardiac Abnormalities**	**Chromosome Abnormality**	**Syndromes**
Trimethadione Valproic acid	Aortic atresia Aortic stenosis Coarctation Interrupted aortic arch Mitral atresia Partial anomalous pulmonary venous connection Total anomalous pulmonary venous connection Arrhythmias Endocardial fibroelastosis Mitral stenosis Ventricular septal defect Persistent left superior vena cava	Monosomy 7p2 Trisomy 13 (Patau syndrome) Turner syndrome (XO)	Bernheim syndrome Hydrolethalus Opitz-Kaveggia FG syndrome Salonen-Herva-Norio syndrome VACTERL (vertebral, anal, cardiac, tracheal, esophageal, renal, and limb anomalies) syndrome

occurs in other cardiac anomalies but seems to be more common in HLHS associated with coarctation of the aorta.[36,40]

Hypoperfusion of the liver occurs more often in the left lobe. In utero, the left lobe receives the majority of its blood supply from the ductus venosus and is better oxygenated. After birth, it is normally deprived of some of its blood flow and diminishes in size; therefore the left lobe may be even less capable of dealing with the hypoxia resulting from a cardiac abnormality.

HLHS is a ductal-dependent lesion; if the ductus closes, the resultant perfusion failure causes significant changes in other organs. This failure is most commonly seen in the liver and the adrenal glands. The brain and kidneys are least affected because of preferential perfusion.[38,43]

References

1. Alsoufi B, Bennetts, J, Verma S, et al: New developments in the treatment of hypoplastic left heart syndrome. Pediatrics 2007; 119:109–117.
2. Tibballs J, Kawahira Y, Carter BG, et al: Outcomes of surgical treatment of infants with hypoplastic left heart syndrome: An institutional experience 1983–2004. J Paediatr Child Health 2007; 43:746–751
3. Tongsong T, Sittiwangkul R, Khunamornpong S, et al: Prenatal sonographic features of isolated hypoplastic left heart syndrome. J Clin Ultrasound 2005; 33:367–371.
4. Grossfield P: Hypoplastic left heart syndrome: New insights. Circ Res 2007; 100:1246–1248.
5. Sinha NS, Rusnak SL, Sommers HM, et al: Hypoplastic left ventricle syndrome: Analysis of thirty autopsy cases in infants with surgical considerations. Am J Cardiol 1968; 21:166–173.
6. Sahn DJ, Shenker L, Reed KL, et al: Prenatal ultrasound diagnosis of hypoplastic left heart syndrome in utero associated with hydrops fetalis. Am Heart J 1982; 104:1368–1372.
7. Norwood WI, Kirklin JK, Sanders SP: Hypoplastic left heart syndrome: Experience with palliative surgery. Am J Cardiol 1980; 45:87–92.
8. Higgins CB, Karsting-Sommerhoff BA, Silverman NH, et al: Left heart obstructive lesions. In: Higgins CB, Karsting-Sommerhoff BA, Silverman NH, et al (eds): Congenital Heart Disease: Echocardiography and Magnetic Resonance Imaging. New York, Raven Press, 1990, pp 285–287.
9. Freedom RM, Benson LN, Smallhorn, JF: Hypoplastic left heart syndrome. In: Freedom RM, Benson LN, Smallhorn JF (eds): Neonatal Heart Disease. London, Springer-Verlag,1992, pp 333–356.
10. Sadler TW: Cardiovascular system. In: Sadler TW (ed): Langman's s Medical Embryology, 6th ed. Baltimore, Williams & Wilkins, 1990, pp 179–227.
11. Harth JY, Paul MH, Gallen WJ, et al: Experimental production of hypoplastic left-heart syndrome in the chicken embryo. Am J Cardiol 1973; 31:51–56.
12. Keith JD: Congenital mitral atresia. In: Keith JD, Rowe RD, Vlad P (eds): Heart Disease in Infancy and Childhood, 3rd ed. New York, Macmillan, 1978, pp 549–553.
13. Chin AJ, Weinberg PM, Barber G: Subcostal two-dimensional echocardiographic identification of anomalous attachment of septum primum in patients with left atrioventricular valve underdevelopment. J Am Coll Cardiol 1990; 15:678–681.
14. Monie IW, DePape AD: Congenital aortic atresia: Report of one case with analysis of 26 similar reported cases. Am Heart J 1950; 40:595–602.
15. Odgers PNB: The development of the atrioventricular valves in man. J Anat 1939; 73:643–656.
16. Friedman S, Murphy L, Ash R: Congenital mitral atresia with hypoplastic non-functioning left heart. Arch Pediatr Adolesc Med 1955; 90:176–188.
17. Friedman S, Murphy L, Ash R: Aortic atresia with hypoplasia of the left heart and aortic arch. J Pediatr 1951; 38:354–368.
18. Lev M, Arcilla R, Rimolde HJA, et al: Premature narrowing or closure of the foramen ovale. Am Heart J 1963; 65:638–647.
19. Freedom RM, Bini M, Rowe RD: Endocardial cushion defect and significant hypoplasia of the left ventricle: A distinct clinical and pathologic entity. Eur J Cardiol 1978; 7:263–281.
20. Saied A, Folger GM: Hypoplastic left heart syndrome: Clinicopathologic and hemodynamic correlation. Am J Cardiol 1972; 29:190–198.
21. Mahowaid JM, Lucas RD Jr, Edwards JE: Aortic valvular atresia: Associated cardiovascular anomalies. Pediatr Cardiol 1982; 2:99–105.
22. Fink BW: Hypoplastic left heart syndrome. In: Fink BW (ed): Congenital Heart Disease: A Deductive Approach to its Diagnosis, 3rd ed. St Louis, Mosby-Yearbook, 1991, pp 193–202.
23. Neill CA, Tuerk J: Aortic atresia, hypoplasia of the ascending aorta and underdevelopment of the left ventricle. In: Watson H (ed): Paediatric Cardiology. St Louis, Mosby–Year Book, 1968, pp 351–360.
24. Romero R, Pilu G, Jeanty P, et al: Hypoplastic left heart syndrome. In: Romero R, Pilu G, Jeanty P, et al (eds): Prenatal Diagnosis of Congenital

Anomalies, Norwalk, CT, Appleton & Lange, 1987, pp 151–154.

25. Freedom RM, Benson LN: Hypoplastic left heart syndrome. In: Emmanouilides GC, Riemenschneider TA, Allen HD, et al (eds): Moss and Adams' Heart Disease in Infants, Children, and Adolescents: Including the Fetus and Young Adults, 5th ed. Baltimore, Williams & Wilkins, 1995, pp 1133–1153.

26. Fyler DC, Rothman KJ, Bulkley LP, et al: The determinants of five year survival of infants with critical congenital heart disease. Cardiovasc Clin 1981; 11:393–405.

27. Hinton R, Martin L, Tabangin M, et al: Hypoplastic left heart syndrome is heritable. J Am Coll Cardiol 2007; 50:1590–1595.

28. Shokeir MHK: Hypoplastic left heart syndrome: An autosomal recessive disorder. Clin Genet 1971; 2:7–14.

29. Barber G: Hypoplastic left heart syndrome. In: Garson A Jr, Bricker T, McNamara DG (eds): The Science and Practice of Pediatric Cardiology, vol II. Philadelphia, Lea & Febiger, 1990, pp 1316–1333.

30. Nora JJ, Nora AH: Genetics and Genetic Counseling in Cardiovascular Diseases. Springfield, IL, Charles C Thomas, 1978, p 181.

31. Yagel S, Cohen S, Baruch M: First and early second trimester fetal heart screening. Curr Opin Obstet Gynecol 2007; 19:183–190.

32. Simpson L, Malon F, Bianchi D, et al: Nuchal translucency and the risk of congenital heart disease. Obstet Gynecol 2007; 109:376–383.

33. Bharati S, Lev M: The surgical anatomy of hypoplasia of the aortic tract complex. J Thorac Cardiovasc Surg 1984; 88:97–101.

34. Silverman NH, Golbus MS: Echocardiographic techniques for assessing normal and abnormal fetal cardiac anatomy. J Am Coll Cardiol 1985; 5:20S–29S.

35. Deely WJ, Ehlers KH, Levin AR, et al: Hypoplastic left heart syndrome: Anatomic, physiologic and therapeutic considerations. Arch Pediatr Adolesc Med 1971; 121:168–175.

36. Norwood WI, Lang P, Castaneda AR, et al: Experience with operations for hypoplastic left heart syndrome. J Thorac Cardiovasc Surg 1981; 82:511–519.

37. Reemtsen B, Pike N, Vaughn S: Stage I palliation for hypoplastic left heart syndrome: Norwood versus Sano modification. Curr Opin Cardiol 2007; 22:60–65.

38. National Institute for Health and Clinical Excellence. (2007). Hybrid procedure for interim management of hypoplastic left heart syndrome (HLHS) in neonates (interventional procedures consultation): http://www.nice.org.uk/guidance/index.jsp?action=article&o=37668. Accessed November 2, 2007.

39. Bacha E: The hybrid stage I operation in hypoplastic left heart syndrome: A new alternative. Heart Views 2006; 7:105–110.

40. Hawkins JA, Doty DB: Aortic atresia: Morphologic characteristics affecting survival and operative palliation. J Thorac Cardiovasc Surg 1984; 88:620–626.

41. da Silva JP, da Fonseca L, Baumgratz JF, et al: Hypoplastic left heart syndrome: The influence of surgical strategy on outcomes. Arq Bras Cardiol 2007; 88:319–324.

42. Mahle WT, Visconti KJ, Freier MC, et al: Relationship of surgical approach to neurodevelopmental outcomes in hypoplastic left heart syndrome. Pediatrics 2006; 17(1):e90–e97.

43. Connor JA, Arons RR, Figueroa M, et al: Clinical outcomes and secondary diagnoses for infants born with hypoplastic left heart syndrome. Pediatrics 2004; 114:e160–e165.

44. Chrisant MR, Naftel DC, Drummond-Webb J, et al: Fate of infants with hypoplastic left heart syndrome listed for cardiac transplantation: A multicenter study. J Heart Lung Transplant 2005; 24:576–582.

45. Jenkins PC, Flanagan MF, Sargent JD, et al: A comparison of treatment strategies for hypoplastic left heart syndrome using decision analysis. J Am Coll Cardiol 2001; 38:1181–1187.

46. Jenkins PC, Flanagan MF, Jenkins KJ, et al: Survival analysis and risk factors for mortality in transplantation and staged surgery for hypoplastic left heart syndrome. J Am Coll Cardiol 2000; 36:1178–1185.

47. Kanjuh VI, Eliot RS, Edwards JE: Coexistent mitral and aortic valvular atresia: A pathologic study of 14 cases. Am J Cardiol 1965; 15:611–621.

48. Norwood WI, Stellin GJ: Aortic atresia with interrupted aortic arch: Reparative operation. J Thorac Surg 1981; 81:239–244.

CHAPTER 8

Hypoplasia of the Right Ventricle

Heidi S. Barrett

Definition

Pulmonary Atresia with Intact Ventricular Septum

Hypoplasia of the right ventricle is uncommon as an isolated entity. It usually results from *pulmonary atresia with intact ventricular septum*.

Pulmonary atresia in this malformation is always valvular[1] and, in conjunction with the intact ventricular septum, severely reduces blood flow to the right ventricular chamber, thus impeding its ability to develop properly (Fig. 8–1).[2,3] Pulmonary atresia with intact ventricular septum may also result in a normal or enlarged right ventricle, but both are less common.[4,5]

Recent data reported a hypoplastic right ventricle in 80% of cases. A normal ventricle is present in 6.5%, and in 13% the ventricle is enlarged.[5,6]

Right ventricular hypoplasia is classified on the basis of the tripartite approach originally described by Goor and Lillehei.[7,8] The normal right ventricle is divided into a sinus (inlet) portion, incorporating the tricuspid valve apparatus; an apical trabecular portion lying beyond the insertion of the papillary muscles of the tricuspid valve toward the apex; and a conus (infundibulum) portion leading to the pulmonary valve.[8]

By use of this sectional definition, it is postulated that variations in muscular hypertrophy account for the presence or absence of any of these components. The degree of attenuation of one or more sections determines the degree of right ventricular hypoplasia associated with pulmonary atresia with intact ventricular septum.

Classifications included the following:
- Tripartite: inlet, trabecular, and outlet components
- Bipartite: inlet and outlet components
- Unipartite: inlet component only

These classifications are useful in determining the surgical treatment to be used as well as the prognosis.

The pulmonary valve tissue in this abnormality is described as a membrane with fused commissures depicted by raphae and with three formed cusps.[8] Rarely is the valve bicuspid or without leaflets.[9,10]

The tricuspid valve is, by definition, patent in all cases of pulmonary atresia with intact ventricular septum, but it is rarely normal.[1] The tricuspid valve orifice is usually proportional to the size of the right ventricular cavity.[9,11,12] The valve leaflets are usually dysplastic and result in varying degrees of insufficiency or stenosis.

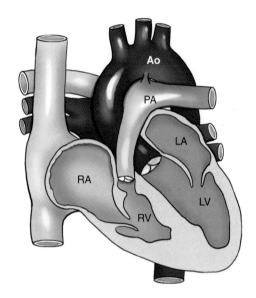

Figure 8–1 Diagram of pulmonary atresia with intact ventricular septum. A hypoplastic right ventricle *(RV)* with a small pulmonary artery *(PA)* is seen. Pulmonary blood flow is maintained through the ductus arteriosus. *AO,* Aorta; *LA,* left atrium; *LV,* left ventricle; *RA,* right atrium.

The right atrium may be dilated, depending on the degree of tricuspid regurgitation, as may the foramen ovale. In some cases of right atrium dilatation, bulging of the interatrial septum can obstruct the mitral valve.[6] Severe restriction of the foramen ovale has been reported in 10% of cases.[13]

The aortic valve is usually normal; however, rare cases of aortic stenosis have been described.[14] The left ventricle is often dilated and hypertrophied secondary to increased blood volume resulting from hemodynamic changes. The left atrium, mitral valve, and pulmonary veins are usually unaffected.

Tricuspid Atresia

Tricuspid atresia also results in a hypoplastic right ventricle but should be considered a separate anomaly from pulmonary atresia with intact ventricular septum. Tricuspid atresia is defined as complete agenesis of the tricuspid valve, resulting in the absence of direct communication between the right atrium and the right ventricle.[15,16]

Tricuspid atresia is divided into three types on the basis of the relationship of the great arteries (Table 8–1). In type I, the relationship of the great vessels is normal; it accounts for approximately 70% of cases of tricuspid atresia at autopsy. In 28% of cases, there is dextro (d)-transposition (complete transposition) of the great arteries (type II), and levo (l)-transposition (corrected transposition) of the great arteries (type III) occurs in 3% of cases.[15] These three types are subclassified on the basis of the presence or absence and size of the

TABLE 8–1   Classification of Tricuspid Atresia Based on Relationship of the Great Arteries (Roman Numerals) and Pulmonary Blood Flow (Capital Letters)

Type	Relationship	Frequency (%)
I	Normal great vessels	69
IA	No VSD, pulmonary atresia	9
IB	Restrictive VSD, pulmonary atresia	51
IC	Nonrestrictive VSD, no pulmonary stenosis	9
II	Dextrotransposition of great arteries	28
IIA	VSD, pulmonary atresia	2
IIB	VSD, pulmonary stenosis	8
IIC	VSD, no pulmonary stenosis	18
III	Levotransposition of great arteries	3

Adapted from Rosenthal A, Dick M: Tricuspid atresia. In: Adams FH, Emmanouilides GC, Riemenschneider TA (eds): Moss' Heart Disease in Infants, Children, and Adolescents, 4th ed. Baltimore, Williams & Wilkins, 1989, p 903.

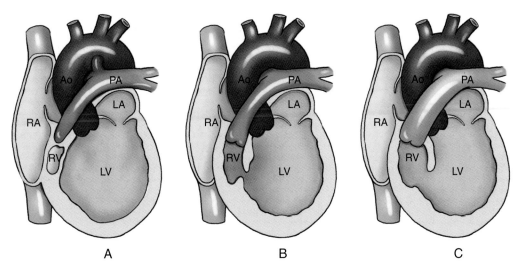

Figure 8–2 Diagram of tricuspid atresia with a normal relationship of the great vessels. **A,** Type IA with normally related great vessels, no VSD, and pulmonary atresia. **B,** Type IB with normally related great vessels, a restrictive VSD, and pulmonic stenosis. **C,** Type IC with normally related great vessels and a large VSD. *Ao,* Aorta; *LA,* left atrium; *LV,* left ventricle; *PA,* pulmonary artery; *RA,* right atrium; *RV,* right ventricle.

associated ventricular septal defect (VSD) and on the presence or absence of pulmonary atresia or stenosis (Figs. 8–2 and 8–3).

Weinberg described five morphological variants of the tricuspid valve associated with tricuspid atresia[17]:

1. Muscular atresia: The most common type, occurring in 76% to 84% of cases. No tricuspid valvular tissue is found, and the floor of the right atrium is muscular.
2. Membranous atresia: The membranous portion of the atrioventricular septum, between the right atrium and the left ventricle, forms the floor of the right atrium. Four percent to 12% of patients have membranous atresia.
3. Valvular atresia: Six percent of cases involve a right atrial floor composed of a thin, imperforate membrane of valvular tissue.
4. Ebstein form: Valvular tissue in the floor of the right atrium is adherent to the right ventricular wall, forming an "atrialized" portion of the right ventricle. Seen in 4% to 6% of cases.
5. Common atrioventricular canal: The rarest form (2%), consisting of a leaflet of a common atrioventricular valve completely sealing the entrance to the right ventricle.

Aneurysmal dilatation of the foramen ovale due to right atrial dilatation occasionally occurs, resulting in obstruction to left atrial blood flow.[18,19] A true atrial septal defect (ostium secundum) is present in about one third of cases. Less commonly, a primum atrial septal defect, or complete absence of the atrial septum, may occur.[20] As with pulmonary atresia with intact ventricular septum, the mitral valve and left atrium are usually normal, and the left ventricle is enlarged and hypertrophied as a result of increased blood volume.

The degree of right ventricular hypertrophy associated with tricuspid atresia is dependent on the anatomical type of atresia and the size of the VSD.[21] However, it is smaller than normal in all cases and is usually described as "slitlike."

Embryology

Pulmonary atresia with intact ventricular septum is postulated to occur after cardiac septation.[1] Kutsche and Van Mierop[10] suggested that this defect might result from a prenatal inflammatory disease rather than being a true congenital malformation. Although little data exist to support this theory, the association of pulmonary artery obstruction with maternal rubella infection has been reported.[22,23]

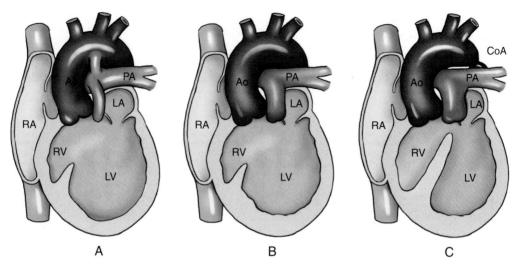

Figure 8–3 Diagram of tricuspid atresia with dextrotransposition (complete) of the great arteries. **A,** Tricuspid atresia with dextrotransposition of the great arteries, a VSD, and pulmonary atresia. **B,** Tricuspid atresia with dextrotransposition of the great arteries, a VSD, and pulmonic stenosis. **C,** Tricuspid atresia with dextrotransposition of the great arteries, a restrictive VSD, and coarctation of the aorta *(CoA)*. Note the large pulmonary artery *(PA)* caused by the left ventricle *(LV)* ejecting preferentially into the pulmonary artery because of a restrictive VSD (subaortic stenosis) and coarctation. *Ao,* Aorta; *LA,* left atrium; *RA,* right atrium; *RV,* right ventricle.

A more plausible explanation is that the decreased blood flow through the right ventricle, resulting from the pulmonary atresia and abnormal tricuspid valve, impedes chamber growth.

Tricuspid atresia is thought to be the result of malalignment of the ventricular septum in relation to the atria and the atrioventricular canal. Failure of the right ventricular chamber to develop results in the ventricular septum shifting toward the right and obliterating the right atrioventricular orifice. This occurs between the twenty-fifth and fifty-fifth days of embryological development.

Occurrence Rate

Pulmonary atresia with intact ventricular septum accounts for 1% to 5% of cases of congenital heart disease.[5,11,24,25] It occurs in 0.1 to 0.4 in 10,000 live births.[26] Pulmonary atresia with intact ventricular septum has been reported to occur slightly more frequently in males.[8]

Tricuspid atresia has been reported in 0.3% to 3.7% of patients with congenital heart disease.[14] The prevalence at autopsy has been reported to be between 2% and 3%.[27-29] Tricuspid atresia occurs in approximately 1 in 15,000 live births.[27,28] There

does not appear to be a sex predilection; however, cases associated with transposition of the great arteries occur more commonly in males.[16,30,31]

Sonographic Criteria

Hypoplasia of the right ventricle can be diagnosed on fetal echocardiography by identifying a small right ventricular chamber. This is best accomplished in an apical (Fig. 8–4) or subcostal four-chamber view (Fig. 8–5). Careful attention is necessary to identify the small right ventricle and avoid confusion with a univentricular heart.

Once a small chamber is identified, the pulmonary artery and tricuspid valve should be evaluated to determine the cause. As stated previously, pulmonary atresia with intact ventricular septum and tricuspid atresia are separate entities. They share many similar features, however, so differentiation may be challenging.

The size and patency of the tricuspid valve should be addressed with use of color and pulsed Doppler imaging. In tricuspid atresia, no flow will be detected on either side of the valve (Figs. 8–6 and Fig. 8–7). The valve and valve orifice appear hyperechoic and thickened (Fig. 8–8). In pulmonary atresia with intact ventricular septum, the

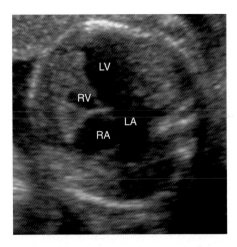

Figure 8–4 Apical four-chamber view in a fetus with a hypoplastic right ventricle *(RV)*. The right ventricle chamber is much smaller than the left ventricle *(LV)*. *LA*, Left atrium; *RA*, right atrium.

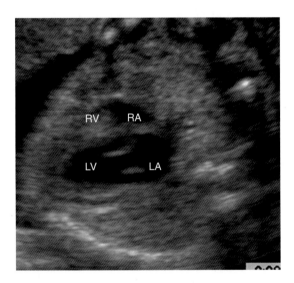

Figure 8–5 Subcostal four-chamber view in a fetus with a hypoplastic right ventricle *(RV)*. The right ventricle and right atrium *(RA)* are very small. The left ventricle *(LV)*, left atrium *(LA)*, and mitral valve orifice are all dilated.

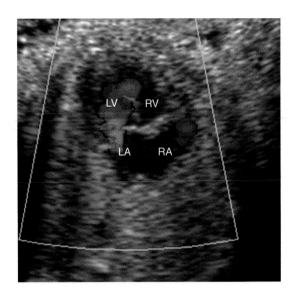

Figure 8–6 Apical four-chamber with color Doppler imaging to show blood flow from the left atrium *(LA)* to the left ventricle *(LV)*. No flow is appreciated entering the right ventricle *(RV)* as a result of tricuspid atresia. *RA*, Right atrium.

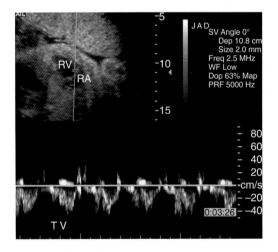

Figure 8–7 Pulsed Doppler cursor placed distal to the tricuspid valve in the right ventricle *(RV)* in a fetus with tricuspid atresia. No flow is appreciated entering the right ventricle (above baseline). *RA*, Right atrium.

tricuspid valve may also appear small and hyperechoic, but some blood flow should be detected. If the tricuspid valve is stenotic, Doppler interrogation distal to the valve shows an increase in velocity and, often, turbulent flow. The tricuspid valve is often insufficient in cases of pulmonary atresia with intact ventricular septum. In this setting, regurgitant flow should be apparent by placing the pulsed Doppler cursor proximal to the valve in the right atrium (Fig. 8–9). Because pulsed

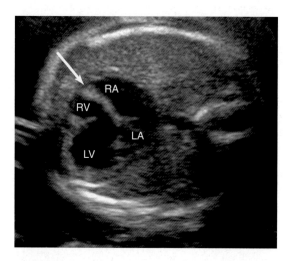

Figure 8–8 Apical four-chamber view in a fetus with tricuspid atresia. The echogenic tricuspid valve *(arrow)* is seen between the small right ventricle *(RV)* and enlarged right atrium *(RA)*. A VSD can also be appreciated. *LA,* Left atrium; *LV,* left ventricle.

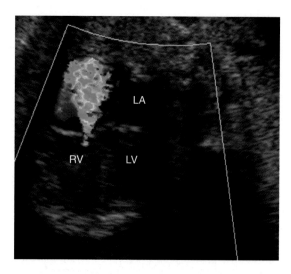

Figure 8–10 Color Doppler imaging showing massive tricuspid regurgitation entering the right atrium in a fetus with hypoplasia of the right ventricle *(RV)*. *LA,* Left atrium; *LV,* left ventricle.

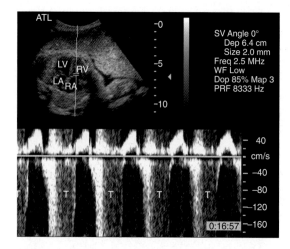

Figure 8–9 Pulsed Doppler cursor placed proximal to the tricuspid valve in the right atrium *(RA)* in a patient with pulmonary atresia with intact ventricular septum. Massive tricuspid regurgitation *(T)* occurring throughout systole can be appreciated. *LA,* Left atrium; *LV,* left ventricle; *RV,* right ventricle.

Doppler tracings of regurgitant flow may be of a velocity high enough to cause aliasing, color Doppler imaging is often a more effective means of quantitating the amount of regurgitant flow present (Fig. 8–10).

The parietal band or supraventricular crest of the tricuspid valve orifice can normally appear hyperechoic (Fig. 8–11). This should not be mistaken for an atretic valve. The differentiation is made by angling the transducer inferiorly and identifying the moving valve leaflets. Normal flow through the valve will also rule out tricuspid atresia. If these features are not apparent, tricuspid atresia should be considered.

The pulmonary artery in pulmonary atresia with intact ventricular septum is, by definition, atretic. A long-axis view of the pulmonary artery (Fig. 8–12) or a short-axis view of the great vessels (Fig. 8–13) demonstrates a small pulmonary artery that is often hyperechoic. In some instances, the pulmonary artery will be of normal echogenicity but will be smaller than normal for gestational age (Fig. 8–14). Pulsed Doppler (Fig. 8–15) or color Doppler (Fig. 8–16) interrogation, or both, should confirm the absence of blood flow across the valve. When severe pulmonary atresia is present, flow through the ductus arteriosus may be reversed (Fig. 8–17).

In tricuspid atresia, the pulmonic valve can be stenotic (27%). Pulsed Doppler imaging distal to the valve may show increased, turbulent flow (Fig. 8–18). The pulmonic valve may also be atretic (18%), with no flow detectable.[5] The pulmonary

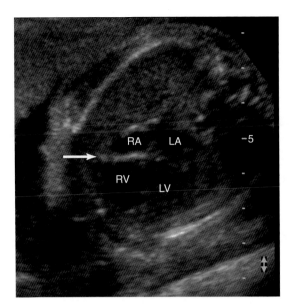

Figure 8–11 Normal parietal band of the tricuspid valve orifice *(arrow)* in a normal fetal heart. This should not be confused with tricuspid atresia. *LA,* Left atrium; *LV,* left ventricle; *RA,* right atrium; *RV,* right ventricle.

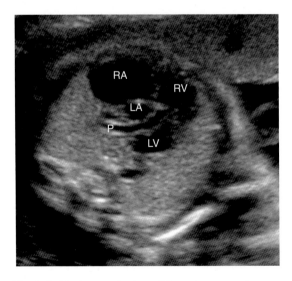

Figure 8–12 Long-axis view of the pulmonary artery *(P)* showing a hyperechoic pulmonary artery resulting from pulmonary atresia with intact ventricular septum. A dilated right atrium *(RA)* and right ventricle *(RV)* are also present. *LA,* Left atrium; *LV,* left ventricle.

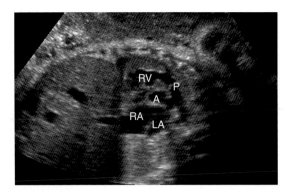

Figure 8–13 Short-axis view of the great vessels showing a small pulmonary artery *(P)* compared with the normal-sized aortic root *(A). LA,* Left atrium; *RA,* right atrium; *RV,* right ventricle.

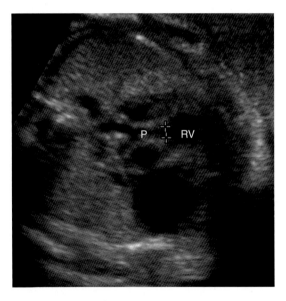

Figure 8–14 Long-axis view of the pulmonary artery *(P)* showing a small pulmonary artery resulting from pulmonary atresia with intact ventricular septum arising from the right ventricle *(RV).*

artery may appear relatively normal in association with tricuspid atresia, although this is rare. Most commonly, the pulmonary artery will be smaller than expected for gestational age. Again, this is a result of decreased blood flow within the right ventricle. If the pulmonary artery is normal or stenotic, a VSD must be present to supply blood to the right ventricle through the left ventricle. If

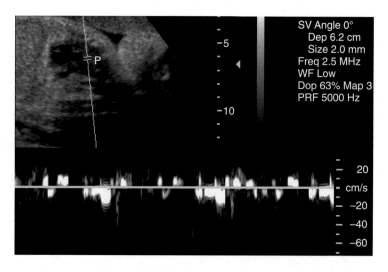

Figure 8–15 Short-axis view of the great vessels with the pulsed Doppler cursor placed distal to the pulmonic valve *(P)*. No flow is appreciated through the pulmonic valve *(below baseline)* as a result of pulmonary atresia.

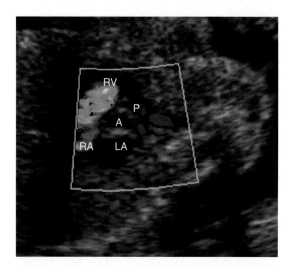

Figure 8–16 Short-axis view of the great vessels with color Doppler imaging to confirm the absence of flow through the pulmonic valve *(P)*. Color imaging also shows massive tricuspid regurgitation entering the right atrium *(RA)*. *A,* Aorta; *LA,* left atrium; *RV,* right ventricle.

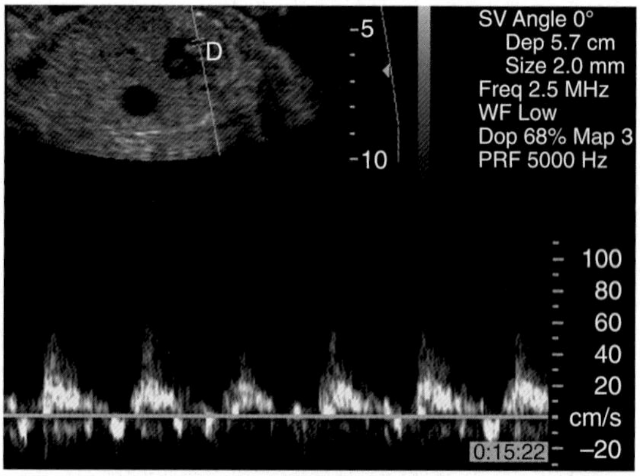

Figure 8–17 Short-axis view of the great vessels with pulsed Doppler imaging to identify reversed flow in the ductus arteriosus *(D) (above baseline)* as a result of pulmonary atresia.

no VSD is present, the pulmonary artery will always be atretic.

Color Doppler imaging is essential for evaluating the interventricular septum for defects. A view aligning the septum in a perpendicular fashion to the transducer is optimal for identifying a VSD. The status of the interatrial septum is also impor-

tant. Color or pulsed Doppler imaging is needed to document the patency of the foramen ovale. At birth, the neonate must rely on right-to-left shunting through the foramen ovale for survival. Therefore diagnosing a restrictive foramen ovale in utero would have a profound effect on postnatal management and prognosis.

The mitral and aortic valves should also be evaluated with Doppler imaging to identify the

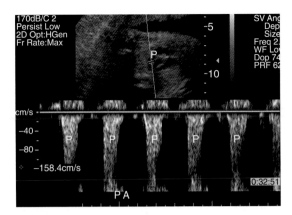

Figure 8–18 Short-axis view of the great vessels with the pulsed Doppler cursor placed distal to the pulmonic valve *(P)* to identify pulmonary stenosis.

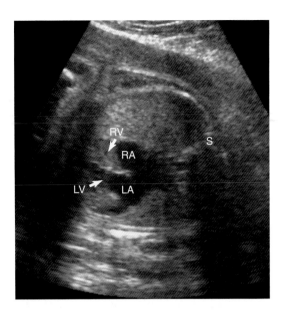

Figure 8–19 Four-chamber view in a fetus with tricuspid atresia showing a small, almost obliterated right ventricle *(RV)* and a hypertrophied left ventricle *(LV)*. *LA,* Left atrium; *RA,* right atrium; *S,* spine.

presence or absence of either stenosis or valvular insufficiency. These valves are usually normal in both conditions; however, abnormalities have been reported.[29] Both tricuspid atresia and pulmonary atresia with intact ventricular septum can be associated with a large left atrium and a dilated hypertrophied left ventricle (Fig. 8–19). Measurements of the atria and the left ventricle may be an important means of monitoring progression of either anomaly throughout gestation. The aortic root may also dilate in either entity (Fig. 8–20). This left-sided enlargement is a result of the majority of blood being forced across the foramen ovale because it is unable to enter the right ventricle. Retrograde flow through the ductus arteriosus and pulmonary artery is also possible, again resulting from the overload to the aorta and the decreased or absent flow of blood through the pulmonary artery. If this occurs, the pulmonary artery may appear larger than expected.

Finally, the orientation of the pulmonary artery and the aorta should be determined. In the majority of cases, pulmonary atresia with intact ventricular septum and tricuspid atresia are associated with normally oriented great vessels. However, both dextrotransposition and levotransposition do occur.[29]

It is important to keep in mind that right ventricular hypoplasia can progress as pregnancy

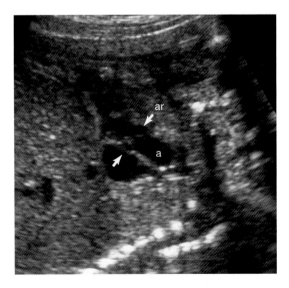

Figure 8–20 Long-axis view of the aorta *(a)* in a fetus with pulmonary atresia with intact ventricular septum. The aortic root *(ar)* is dilated.

progresses; therefore serial examinations should be performed to monitor the severity of abnormalities.[4,5]

Pulsed Doppler interrogation of the inferior vena cava (IVC) and ductus venosus may also provide useful information regarding the progression of the disease. Fetuses with isolated right-sided cardiac lesions have been shown to have increased venous pulsatility in the IVC and increased rates of reversed flow during atrial contraction in the ductus venosus.[32–34] Alterations in flow were dependent on the presence or absence of a ventricular septal defect (which equalizes interventricular pressures).[32] Alterations in venous flow is a definitive sign of cardiac compromise and is associated with an adverse outcome.[29,32–34]

Peterson et al[3] evaluated several fetal echocardiographic characteristics of pulmonary atresia with intact ventricular septum. They found a tricuspid valve annulus of 5 mm or less beyond 30 weeks, a right ventricular–to–left ventricular ratio of <0.5, and the absence of tricuspid regurgitation, all indicative of a poor prognosis.

Treatment

Neonates with *pulmonary atresia with intact ventricular septum* require administration of prostaglandin E at birth to maintain ductal patency until surgery is performed. The type of surgery necessary varies with the type of associated cardiovascular abnormalities.[1,35–38] In the setting of a more normal-sized right ventricle, pulmonary valvulotomy is usually performed. In infants with a small right ventricle but an obvious infundibulum, pulmonary valvulotomy in conjunction with a systemic-to-pulmonary artery anastomosis is performed to maintain pulmonary blood flow. These infants may become candidates for biventricular repair. Most neonates with pulmonary atresia with intact ventricular septum have a unipartite or bipartite right ventricle. Therefore they are unlikely candidates for biventricular repair. In these patients, a balloon atrial septostomy, followed by a systemic-to-pulmonary artery anastomosis, is the treatment of choice. Right ventricular growth after initial pulmonary outflow tract decompression has been reported in some patients.[12,39–41]

Walsh et al[42] attempted radiofrequency perforation of the right ventricular outflow tract as a palliative treatment in children with pulmonary atresia with intact ventricular septum. They encountered a high complication rate but found it to be an effective treatment in augmenting pulmonary blood flow.

In utero treatment is possible in some cases.[43–46] However, because in utero cardiac intervention is still in its infancy, cases are usually limited to those with a very poor chance of survival without intervention and an absence of any major extracardiac abnormality. The goal of fetal cardiac intervention is to promote healthier growth of the right ventricle and vascular system in hopes of improving the postnatal outcome.[47]

Surgical treatment of *tricuspid atresia* is also necessary and is usually accomplished in stages. Immediately after birth, prostaglandin E_1 is given to maintain ductal patency. If the atrial septum is unrestricted and a large VSD is present, palliation may not be required.[48] However, most neonates with tricuspid atresia require some type of palliative surgery to augment or reduce pulmonary blood flow before a Fontan procedure is performed. The indications and type of palliation necessary vary with the anatomical type of defect, the associated cardiovascular anomalies, and the hemodynamic abnormalities produced by the lesion.[49–53]

Usually a Blalock-Taussig systemic-to-pulmonary shunt procedure is performed. Although this type of procedure relieves cyanosis, it produces a continuous volume overload of the left ventricle. Therefore once pulmonary vascular resistance has decreased, an arterial shunt is replaced by a systemic venous-to-pulmonary artery shunt—usually the Fontan procedure, a hemi-Fontan procedure, or a bidirectional Glenn anastomosis.[20,54] The second-stage procedures are usually performed between 6 and 12 months of age, with completion procedures occurring at 2 to 3 years of age.

Complications after palliation of tricuspid atresia include aortic and mitral regurgitation resulting from the inherent volume overload of the left ventricle. Long-standing volume overload may eventually impair ventricular performance, occasionally to the extent that further corrective surgery is contraindicated.[20,54]

After a Fontan procedure, complications may include pericardial and pleural effusions that can affect hemodynamics.[20] Arrhythmias have also been reported in 10% to 46% of patients postoperatively.[55,56] Management of tricuspid atresia with transposed great vessels is more complex and usually requires additional procedures.

TABLE 8–2 Conditions Associated with Pulmonary Atresia with Intact Ventricular Septum				
Maternal		**Fetal**		
Condition	**Drug Use**	**Associated Cardiac Abnormalities**	**Chromosome Abnormality**	**Syndromes**
Rubella	Accutane	Aortic stenosis	Monosomy lq4	Short rib polydactyly
	Amantadine	Atrial septal defect		
	Retinoic acid	Dextrocardia		
	Thalidomide	Endocardial fibroelastosis		
	Valproic acid	Left ventricular hypertrophy		
		Right aortic arch		
		Right ventricular hypoplasia		
		Right atrial dilation		
		Tricuspid insufficiency		
		Tricuspid stenosis		
		Transposition of the great arteries		

Finally, cardiac transplantation may be an option in both of these abnormalities.

Prognosis

Coles et al[57] reviewed their surgical experience with pulmonary atresia with intact ventricular septum from 1965 to 1987. They reported an actuarial survival of 24.7% ± 6% at 13 years postoperatively. In their group of patients, the presence of ventriculocoronary connections, a decreasing ratio between right ventricular and left ventricular pressure at initial cardiac catheterization, and lower weight at initial operation all contributed to a poorer prognosis.

The surgical outcomes of 150 babies younger than 3 months of age with a diagnosis of tricuspid atresia were studied between January 1999 and November 2004.[58] Initial palliation included systemic-pulmonary arterial shunting in 64%, pulmonary artery banding in 11%, and cardiopulmonary anastomosis in 24%.[58] At 2 years of age, 89% of the patients underwent cavopulmonary anastomosis, 6% were deceased, and 4% remained living without cavopulmonary anastomosis. Seventeen total deaths occurred, with the 5-year survival rate equaling 86%.[58]

Humes[59] reviewed 134 patients with tricuspid atresia who underwent a modified Fontan operation at the Mayo Clinic through June of 1985. He reported an operative mortality rate of 10%. The 1-year survival rate was 85% and the 5-year survival rate was 78%. Freedom and Benson[49] reported

80 infants with tricuspid atresia seen between 1970 and 1984. They found a surgical mortality rate related to the Fontan operation of approximately 6% to 7%. However, nearly 40% of their patients either died before a Fontan procedure could be performed or did not meet the criteria necessary to undergo the procedure. They found the highest mortality rate among infants with tricuspid atresia with pulmonary atresia and diminutive pulmonary arteries and among those with tricuspid atresia with transposition of the great arteries and coarctation of the aorta.

A more recent report by Wald et al[29] reviewed 88 cases of tricuspid atresia, seen at three tertiary care centers between 1990 and 2005. They found a 1-year survival rate of 83%, with no subsequent deaths for 13 years. Sittiwangkul et al[60] published similar 1-year survival rates in 2004 at 82% but found a steady increase in mortality over time. A 5-year survival rate of 72% and a 20-year survival rate of 61% was reported.

Associated Anomalies

Pulmonary atresia with intact ventricular septum (Table 8–2) and tricuspid atresia (Table 8–3) are both associated with a variety of cardiac abnormalities in addition to hypoplasia of the right ventricle. Extracardiac anomalies occur in 20% of cases of tricuspid atresia.[25,61] Maternal ingestion of various drugs has been associated with both abnormalities.[57]

TABLE 8–3   Conditions Associated with Tricuspid Atresia

Maternal		Fetal		
Condition	Drug Use	Associated Cardiac Abnormalities	Chromosome Abnormality	Syndromes
Enterovirus	Lithium	Lithium	—	Short rib polydactyly
Rubella		Atrioventricular septal defect		
		Coarctation		
		Dextrocardia		
		Left superior vena cava		
		Left ventricular hypertrophy		
		Pulmonary atresia		
		Pulmonary stenosis		
		Right ventricular hypoplasia		
		Subaortic stenosis		
		Truncus arteriosus		
		Transposition of the great arteries		

Abnormal karyotypes are rare, but have been reported in 2.3% to 5% of cases.[5,29] Additionally, an association between maternal rubella infection and tricuspid atresia or pulmonary atresia, and maternal enterovirus infection with tricuspid atresia, has been reported.[22,23]

References

1. Freedom RM, Burrows PE, Smallhorn JR: Pulmonary atresia and intact ventricular septum. In: Freedom RM, Benson LN, Smallhorn JF (eds): Neonatal Heart Disease. London, Springer-Verlag, 1992, pp 269–303.
2. Mizrahi-Arnaud A, Tworetzky W, Bulich LA: Pathophysiology, management, and outcomes of fetal hemodynamic instability during prenatal cardiac intervention. Pediatr Res 2007; 62:325–330.
3. Peterson RE, Levi DS, Williams RJ, et al: Echocardiographic predictors of outcome in fetuses with pulmonary atresia with intact ventricular septum. J Am Soc Echocardiogr 2006; 19:1393–1400.
4. Roman KS, Fouron JC, Masaki N, et al: Determinants of outcome in fetal pulmonary valve stenosis or atresia with intact ventricular septum. Am J Cardiol 2007; 99:699–703.
5. Todros T, Paladini D, Chiappa E, et al: Pulmonary stenosis and atresia with intact ventricular septum during prenatal life. Ultrasound Obstet Gyneol 2003; 21:228–233.
6. Sahn DJ, Allen JD, Anderson R, et al: Echocardiographic diagnosis of atrial septal aneurysm in an infant with hypoplastic right heart syndrome. Chest 1978; 73:227–230.
7. Goor DA, Lillehei CW: Congenital Malformations of the Heart. New York, Grune & Stratton, 1975.
8. Bull C, de Leval MR, Mercanti C, et al: Pulmonary atresia and intact ventricular septum: A revised classification. Circulation 1982; 66:266–272.
9. Zuberbuhler JR, Anderson RH: Morphological variations in pulmonary atresia with intact ventricular septum. Br Heart J 1979; 41:281–288.
10. Kutsche LM, Van Mierop LHS: Pulmonary atresia with and without ventricular septal defect: A different etiology and pathogenesis for the atresia in the 2 types? Am J Cardiol 1983; 51:932–935.
11. Freedom RM, Keith JD: Pulmonary atresia with normal aortic root. In: Keith JD, Rowe RD, Vlad P (eds): Heart Disease in Infancy and Childhood. New York, Macmillan, 1978, pp 506–515.
12. Freedom RM, Wilson G, Trusler FA, et al: Pulmonary atresia and intact ventricular septum. A review of the anatomy, myocardium, and factors influencing right ventricular growth and guidelines for surgical intervention. Scand J Thorac Cardiovasc Surg 1983;17:1–28.
13. Raghib G, Bloemendaal RD, Kanjuh VI, et al: Aortic atresia and premature closure of the foramen ovale: Myocardial sinusoids and coronary arteriovenous fistula serving as outflow channel. Am Heart J 1965; 70:476–480.
14. Patel RG, Freedom RM, Bloom KR, et al: Truncal or aortic valve stenosis in functionally single arterial trunk: A clinical, hemodynamic and pathologic study of six cases. Am J Cardiol 1978; 42:800–809.

15. Rosenthal A, Dick M: Tricuspid atresia. In: Adams FH, Emmanouilides GC (eds): Moss' Heart Disease in Infants, Children and Adolescents, 3rd ed. Baltimore, Williams & Wilkins, 1983, pp 271–283.
16. Rao PS: Demographic features of tricuspid atresia. In: Rao PS (ed): Tricuspid Atresia. Mt Kisco, Futura, 1992, pp 23–37.
17. Weinberg PM: Anatomy of tricuspid atresia and its relevance to current forms of surgical therapy. Ann Thorac Surg 1980; 29:306–311.
18. Freedom RM, Rowe RD: Aneurysm of the atrial septum in tricuspid atresia: Diagnosis during life and therapy. Am J Cardiol 1976; 38:265–267.
19. Reder RF, Yeh HC, Steinfeld L: Aneurysm of the interatrial septum causing pulmonary venous obstruction in an infant with tricuspid atresia. Am Heart J 1981; 102:786–789.
20. Okanlami O, Nichols DG, Nicolson SC, et al: Tricuspid atresia and the Fontan operation. In: Nichols DG, Cameron DE, Greeley WJ, et al (eds): Critical Heart Disease in Infants and Children. St Louis, Mosby–Year Book, 1995, pp 737–767.
21. Rao RS: Is the term "tricuspid atresia" appropriate? Am J Cardiol 1990; 66:1251–1254.
22. Rowe RD: Letter to the editor. J Pediatr 1966; 68:147.
23. Confino E: Infectious causes of congenital cardiac anomalies. In: Elkayam U, Gleicher N (eds): Cardiac Problems in Pregnancy: Diagnosis and Management of Maternal and Fetal Disease, 2nd ed. New York, Alan R Liss, 1990, pp 569–578.
24. Rowe RD, Freedom RM, Mehrizi A, et al: Pulmonary atresia with intact ventricular septum. In: Rowe RD, Freedom RM, Mehrizi A, Bloom KR (eds): The Neonate with Congenital Heart Disease. Philadelphia, WB Saunders, 1981, pp 328–349.
25. Flyer DC, Buckley LP, Hellenbrand WE et al: Report of the New England and Regional Infant Cardiac Program. Pediatrics 1980; 65(Suppl):375–461.
26. CDC Report: Congenital malformations surveillance report, April 1976–March 1977. Atlanta, Centers for Disease Control and Prevention, September, 1977.
27. Behrendt DM, Rosenthal A: Cardiovascular status after repair by Fontan procedure. Ann Thorac Surg 1980; 29:322–330.
28. Case CL, Gillette PC: Automatic atrial and junctional tachycardias in the pediatric patient: Strategies for diagnosis and management. Pacing Clin Electrophysiol 1993; 16:1323–1335.
29. Wald RM, Tham EB, McCrindle BW, et al: Outcome after prenatal diagnosis of tricuspid atresia: A multicenter experience. Am Heart J 2007; 153:772–778.
30. Dick M, Fyler DC, Nadas AS: Tricuspid atresia: Clinical course in 101 patients. Am J Cardiol 1975; 36:327–337.
31. Taussig HB, Keinonen R, Momberger N, et al: Long-time observations on the Blalock-Taussig operation. IV: Tricuspid atresia. Johns Hopkins Med J 1973; 132:135–140.
32. Berg C, Kremer C, Geipel A, et al: Ductus venosus blood flow alterations in fetuses with obstructive lesions of the right heart. Ultrasound Obstet Gynecol 2006; 28:137–142.
33. Wald RM, Tham EB, McCrindle BW, et al: Outcome after prenatal diagnosis of tricuspid atresia: A multicenter experience. Am Heart J 2007; 153:772–778.
34. Galindo A, Gutierrez-Larraya F, Velasco JM, et al: Pulmonary balloon valvuloplasty in a fetus with critical pulmonary stenosis/atresia with intact ventricular septum and heart failure. Fetal Diagn Ther 2006; 21:100–104.
35. Alboliras ET, Julsrud R, Danielson GK, et al: Definitive operation for pulmonary atresia with intact ventricular septum: Results in 20 patients. J Thorac Cardiovasc Surg 1987; 93:454–464.
36. Cobanoglu A, Metzdorff MT, Pinson CW, et al: Valvotomy for pulmonary atresia with intact ventricular septum. J Thorac Cardiovasc Surg 1985; 89:482–490.
37. DeLeval M, Bull C, Stark J, et al: Pulmonary atresia and intact ventricular septum: Surgical management based on a revised classification. Circulation 1982; 66:272–280.
38. DeLeval M, Bull C, Hopkins R, et al: Decision making in the definitive repair of the heart with a small right ventricle. Circulation 1985; 72(Suppl):52–60.
39. Graham TPJ, Bender JW, Atwood GF, et al: Increase in right ventricular volume following valvulotomy for pulmonary atresia or stenosis with intact ventricular septum. Circulation 1974; 49–50(11 Suppl):69–79.
40. Lewis AB, Wells W, Lindesmith FF: Right ventricular growth potential in neonates with pulmonary atresia and intact ventricular septum. J Thorac Cardiovasc Surg 1986; 91:835–840.
41. Patel RG, Freedom RM, Moes CAF, et al: Right ventricular volume determinations in 18 patients with pulmonary atresia and intact ventricular septum: Analysis of factors influencing right ventricular growth. Circulation 1980; 61:428–440.
42. Walsh MA, Lee KJ, Chaturvedi R, et al: Radiofrequency perforation of the right ventricular outflow tract as a palliative strategy for pulmonary atresia with ventricular septal defect. Cathet Cardiovasc Interv 2007; 69:1015–1020.

43. Gardiner HM, Kumar S: Fetal cardiac interventions. Clin Obstet Gynecol 2005; 111:736–741.

44. Tulzer G, Arzt W, Franklin RC, et al: Fetal pulmonary valvuloplasty for critical pulmonary stenosis or atresia with intact septum. Lancet 2002; 360:1567–1568.

45. Duabeney PE, Wang D, Delany DJ, et al: UK and Ireland collaborative study of pulmonary atresia with intact ventricular septum. J Thorac Cardiovasc Surg 2005; 130:1071: e1–e9.

46. Galindo A, Gutierrez-Larraya F, Velasco JM, et al: Pulmonary balloon valvuloplasty in a fetus with critical pulmonary stenosis/atresia with intact ventricular septum and heart failure. Fetal Diagn Ther 2006; 21:100–104.

47. Gardiner HM: Progression of fetal heart disease and rationale for fetal intracardiac interventions. Semin Fetal Neonatal Med 2005; 10:578–585.

48. Tongsong T, Sittiwangkul R, Wanapirak C, et al: Prenatal diagnosis of isolated tricuspid valve atresia. J Ultrasound Med 2004; 23:945–950.

49. Freedom RM, Benson LN: Tricuspid atresia. In: Freedom RM, Benson LN, Smallhorn JF (eds): Neonatal Heart Disease. London, Springer-Verlag, 1992, pp 270–284.

50. Björk VC, Olin CL, Bjarke BB, et al: Right atrial-right ventricular anastomosis for correction of tricuspid atresia. J Thorac Cardiovasc Surg 1979; 77:452–458.

51. Fontan F, Baudet E: Surgical repair of tricuspid atresia. Thorax 1971; 26:240–248.

52. Gago O, Salles CA, Stern AM, et al: A different approach for the total correction of tricuspid atresia. J Thorac Cardiovasc Surg 1976; 72:209–214.

53. Alwi M: Management algorithm in pulmonary atresia with intact ventricular septum. Cath Cardiovasc Interven 2006; 67:679–686.

54. Tanoue Y, Kado H, Boku N, et al: Three hundred and thirty-three experiences with the bidirectional Glenn procedure in a single institute. Interact Cardiovasc Thorac Surg 2007; 6:97–101.

55. Chen SC, Nouri S, Pennington DG: Dysrhythmias after the modified Fontan procedure. Pediatr Cardiol 1988; 9:215–219.

56. Kurer CC, Tanner CS, Norwood WI, et al: Perioperative arrhythmias after Fontan repair. Circulation 1990; 82:IV190–IV194.

57. Coles JG, Freedom RM, Lightfoot NE, et al. Long-term results in neonates with pulmonary atresia and intact ventricular septum. Ann Thorac Surg 1989; 47:213–237.

58. Karamlou T, Ashburn DA, Caldarone CA, et al: Matching procedure to morphology improves outcomes in neonates with tricuspid atresia. J Thorac Cardiovasc Surg 2005; 130:1503–1510.

59. Humes RA: Intermediate follow up and predicted survival after the modified Fontan procedure for tricuspid atresia and double inlet ventricle. Circulation 1987; 76:III67–III71.

60. Sittiwangkul R, Azakie A, Van Arsdell GS, et al: Outcomes of tricuspid atresia in the Fontan era. Ann Thorac Surg 2004; 77:889–894.

61. Buyse ML: Birth Defects Encyclopedia. Cambridge, Blackwell Scientific, 1990.

CHAPTER 9

Univentricular Heart

Kristin E. McKinney

Definition

The diagnosis and study of the univentricular heart is a complex issue, given the debate over the definition. This would seem to be an easy task on the basis of the simple name, "univentricular," indicating one ventricle. A straightforward definition such as *a univentricular heart is a three-chambered organ composed of two atria and one ventricle connected by one or two atrioventricular valves (cor triloculare biatriatum)*[1] is a good starting point. It is also generally agreed that the atrioventricular (AV) connection is central in defining the univentricular heart in which a single, double, or common inlet may exist. However, the controversy stems from the morphologically heterogeneity present and that recognition that truly solitary ventricles are quite rare. The complexity of these lesions has prompted debate over which abnormalities should be included in the univentricular heart syndrome; the debate continues.[2–7]

For the fetal echocardiographer charged with making the diagnosis, this debate is of more than academic interest. It is necessary to understand the most common as well as the variant lesions associated with the anatomy of a single ventricle to make accurate and complete diagnoses and to counsel the parents about the treatment options and outcome.

In general, it is agreed that only one functional ventricle is present within the ventricular mass. Often there is also an incomplete, rudimentary, or hypoplastic ventricle that lacks an AV connection. Only the well-developed ventricular chamber receives inflow from the atria through one or two AV valves and has an outlet portion to a great artery. The physiological result is that the systemic and pulmonary circulations are arranged in parallel fashion rather than in series as in the normal heart.[8] The nomenclature debate focuses primarily on whether hearts with atretic tricuspid or mitral valves should[3,4,6] or should not[2,5] be included in the univentricular heart syndrome.

The classic and most commonly used description follows Hallermann's modification of Van Praagh's classification, in which one or two AV valves empty into a single ventricle.[2] Van Praagh used the terms "single," "common," and "univentricular" interchangeably in his description. Tricuspid and mitral valve atresias are specifically excluded from this definition of the univentricular heart complex. Van Praagh's classification system is depicted in Figure 9–1 and is described in detail further on.

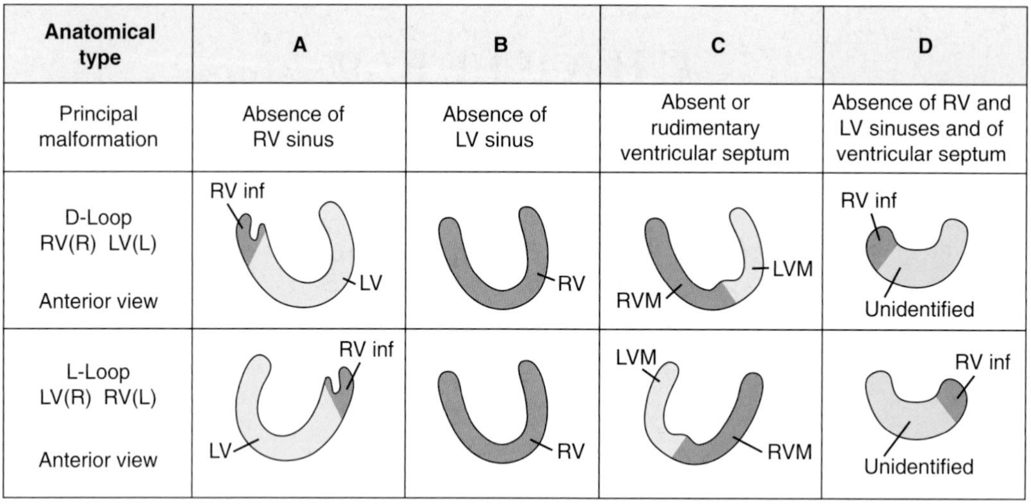

Anatomical type	A	B	C	D
Principal malformation	Absence of RV sinus	Absence of LV sinus	Absent or rudimentary ventricular septum	Absence of RV and LV sinuses and of ventricular septum
D-Loop RV(R) LV(L) Anterior view	RV inf ... LV	RV	RVM ... LVM	RV inf ... Unidentified
L-Loop LV(R) RV(L) Anterior view	RV inf ... LV	RV	LVM ... RVM	RV inf ... Unidentified

Figure 9–1　Diagram showing Van Praagh's classification of the univentricular heart, anatomic types A, B, C, and D. Note the different position of the right ventricular infundibulum (rudimentary chamber) in type A hearts that are associated with different bulboventricular loops. *Inf,* Infundibulum; *LV,* left ventricle; *LVM,* left ventricular myocardium; *RV,* right ventricle; *RVM,* right ventricular myocardium.

If a broader definition is used, namely, that all atrial input goes into one ventricle, other anatomical abnormalities not originally included in Van Praagh's classification can be considered.[3,4] A classification scheme relevant to surgery was proposed by Jacobs in which a "single ventricle" was characterized as lacking two well-developed ventricles. Hypoplastic left heart was recognized as a common form of univentricular heart but was classified independently. The proposed definition encompassed double inlet AV connections, absence of one AV connection (mitral or tricuspid atresia), common AV valve and only one well-developed ventricle, and only one well-developed ventricle and heterotaxy syndrome, which describes a constellation of defects characterized by malposition of cardiac and abdominal visceral structures. By these criteria, univentricular heart becomes a broader category of congenital malformations characterized by both atria relating entirely or almost entirely to one functionally single ventricular chamber.[7,8] This new scheme incorporated aspects of both Van Praagh's and Anderson's classification systems.

Anderson et al[3] stressed that "univentricular heart" should include the tricuspid and mitral atresias because the primary definition for univen-tricular heart was satisfied regardless of whether one of the AV valves was absent or atretic. Although the debate continues, most authors still separate the valve atresias from univentricular heart complex as a matter of tradition.[2,5,9–13] However, the classification of Anderson et al is helpful when trying to understand the embryological and anatomical characteristics of the univentricular heart syndrome, which is described with that of Van Praagh further on.

For purposes of documenting occurrence rates in siblings, other authors have classified the univentricular heart into four groups:
- Double-inlet single ventricle with left ventricular morphology
- Complex univentricular heart with a single or common inlet or with a ventricle of common or right ventricular morphology
- Complex univentricular heart with asplenia
- Complex univentricular heart with polysplenia[14]

Embryology

A univentricular heart is thought to be caused by failure of development at the bulboventricular loop stage.[15] At this stage, the bulbus cordis moves ventrally and to the right of the common ventricle. The folding of the heart tube causes a spur to be formed, the bulboventricular spur. It projects between the common ventricle and the bulbus cordis and is normally absorbed into the ventral wall of the ventricle. At the same time, the bulbus cordis shifts and grows to the left to form the right ventricle and the muscular portion of the interventricular septum. If developmental arrest occurs at this stage, the morphological characteristics of a single ventricle result.

The hemodynamic consequences of developmental arrest (i.e., decreased or obstructed blood flow) result in other findings associated with single ventricles, such as rudimentary chambers and great vessel abnormalities.[16]

Anatomy

To understand the anatomy of univentricular heart disease, it is useful to review the classification schemes that have been proposed.[2,3] The Van Praagh classification of the univentricular heart is detailed and particularly useful for cardiac surgeons, but it is complex.

According to Hallermann's modification of the Van Praagh classification[2] depicted in Figure 9–1, the ventricle is designated by the letters A, B, C, or D, depending on whether the morphological characteristics are left, right, a combination of left and right, or indeterminate and depending on whether a left or a right sinus (rudimentary chamber) is present.

Each ventricular configuration (A, B, C, or D) can be formed from a levo or a dextro bulboventricular loop, each of which results in different ventricular anatomy. The lesions are further subdivided on the basis of the positions of the great vessels, which may be as follows:
• Normally related (subtype 1)
• The aorta anterior and to the right (subtype 2)
• The aorta anterior and to the left (subtype 3)

Note that the position of the great vessels is determined at the level of the semilunar valves. The most common type of univentricular heart diagnosed in children is Van Praagh's A3, accounting for nearly 60% of cases.[2,9]

The ventricle has the morphological characteristics of the left ventricle with, most commonly, a levorotated right rudimentary chamber. The great vessels demonstrate malposition, with the aorta anterior and to the left of the pulmonary artery.

The second most common defect is type A2, with morphological characteristics of the left ventricle and a rudimentary chamber having morphological characteristics of the right ventricle, but with the aorta anterior and to the right of the pulmonary artery.

Next is A1, with morphological characteristics of the left ventricle and a right rudimentary chamber and normally related great vessels, followed by lesions of the C category.

In one series of affected children diagnosed between the ages of 4 and 10 years at the Mayo Clinic,[9] 67% of lesions were type A and 16% were type C. However, selection bias occurred in this sample because diagnoses were generally made later in childhood and the patients represent a subset who had survived past infancy with univentricular hearts. Therefore these data do not include neonates and infants with early-onset symptoms resulting from more severe, life-threatening lesions and may be skewed toward type A ventricles.

The univentricular heart categorization of Anderson et al[3,4] is helpful because it simplifies the anatomical variations in the univentricular heart syndrome diagrammatically. These authors stress that univentricular heart means a main ventricular chamber with morphological characteristics of the left or right ventricle or indeterminate characteristics, with or without a rudimentary chamber within a single ventricular mass (Fig. 9–2). Left ventricles have relatively smooth walls, fine trabeculations, and lack septal chordal attachments of the AV valve. In contrast, right ventricles are more coarsely trabeculated and commonly have chordal attachments of the AV valve to the septal surface.[7]

The ventricle and the rudimentary chamber most commonly have discordant morphological features, that is, a left ventricle with a right rudimentary chamber. By definition, the rudimentary chamber does not have an inlet, but it may have an outlet. If the chamber does have an outlet and supports a great vessel, it is called an outlet chamber; if not, the term *trabecular pouch* is used (Fig. 9–3).

In most cases of univentricular heart disease, the exact cause is not known. Univentricular heart recurrence risks suggest a multifactorial cause in which polygenic factors and unspecified environmental factors interact in the developing fetus early in the embryonic period.[14] For the subgroup

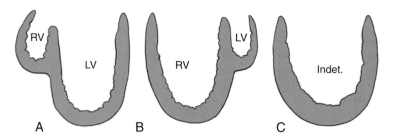

Figure 9–2 Diagram showing Anderson's classification of ventricles and rudimentary chambers in univentricular hearts. **A,** A unventricular heart of left ventricular *(LV)* type with rudimentary chamber of right ventricular *(RV)* type. **B,** A univentricular heart of right ventricular type with rudimentary chamber of left ventricular type. **C,** A univentricular heart of indeterminate *(Indet.)* type without rudimentary chamber.

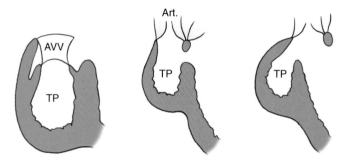

Figure 9–3 Ventricular and rudimentary chamber anatomy according to the classification of Anderson and associates. *Left,* Ventricle. *Middle,* Outlet chamber. *Right,* Trabecular pouch. *Art.,* Arterial outflow vessel; *AVV,* atrioventricular valve; *TP,* trabecular portion of ventricle.

of patients who have associated polysplenia, autosomal recessive inheritance is a strong possibility,[14,17–20] but rare reports also exist of familial cases that apparently occur in the absence of splenic abnormalities.[15]

Because of the significantly increased risk of familial associations when univentricular heart disease is associated with polysplenia, it is crucial to rule out splenic abnormalities in all fetuses with the univentricular heart syndrome.[14]

At least one case has been reported linking a univentricular heart to in utero myocardial infarction in the area of the right ventricle and interventricular septum.[11] In this case, maternal cocaine use was suspected on the basis of metabolic products in the fetal urine. Fetal echocardiography identified a large single ventricle. Another much smaller contractile cavity, described as appearing like a "peach pit," was identified adjacent to the single ventricle. These findings were confirmed at autopsy after termination of pregnancy. The

autopsy also demonstrated scarring in the area of the interventricular septum and the right ventricular remnant consistent with left coronary artery thrombosis. Other studies of cocaine-exposed neonates report increases in ventricular and atrial septal defects[21] and one case of hypoplasia of the right ventricle.[22]

Although the majority of fetuses with univentricular heart disease are affected because of multifactorial events associated with bulboventricular loop development, these data suggest that on rare occasions vascular interruption in utero may cause a univentricular syndrome—especially in fetuses exposed to cocaine. These disruptions may occur later in gestation, well after the embryonic period.

An epidemiological study by Steinberger et al[23] evaluating infants with a single ventricle with respect to infant and family characteristics and maternal and paternal exposures found an association with paternal smoking (2.4%) and alcohol consumption (2.0%) in all cases of single ventricle. These associations were even stronger in infants who also had abnormal situs. Paternal marijuana use was associated with single ventricle in cases of normal situs (2.2%). These results highlight the need for future studies to consider environmental factors in the pathogenesis of this cardiac defect.

Occurrence Rate

There is a relatively wide range of reported occurrence rate in the literature, probably as a result of the continued debate over the nomenclature and classification of lesions.

Kaulitz and Hofbeck[24] reported that nearly 10% of congenital heart defects belong to the group of functionally univentricular hearts, which encompassed a broader definition than included here, namely, hypoplastic left heart. Not including that entity, univentricular heart is a rare cardiac anomaly that occurs in 2.5% of infants born with congenital heart disease.[25,26] A similar rate was found by the New England Regional Infant Cardiac Program, which identified a prevalence of 54 cases per 1 million live births (2.4%).[7,27] Data from the Toronto Hospital for Sick Children revealed that "common ventricle" accounted for 1.65% of all congenital heart defects. Other sources report the incidence as low as 1.25%.[27]

Weigel et al[14] studied the occurrence of congenital heart defects in siblings of patients with univentricular heart and tricuspid atresia. For siblings of patients with a univentricular heart, the occurrence rate is 2.8% overall. The risk is increased if the affected family member has a more complex form of univentricular heart disease (5%) compared with the simple form, that is, a double-inlet left ventricle (0.5%). For lesions associated with asplenia, the occurrence risk in siblings is 3.4% compared with 28.6% for polysplenia. The high occurrence risk for siblings of patients with univentricular heart disease and polysplenia emphasizes the possibility of autosomal recessive inheritance in some families.[14]

Sonographic Criteria

The apical and subcostal four-chamber views are the most useful in diagnosing a univentricular heart.

From either four-chamber view, three chambers are usually apparent (two atria and one large ventricle) in the classic form of a univentricular (Figs.

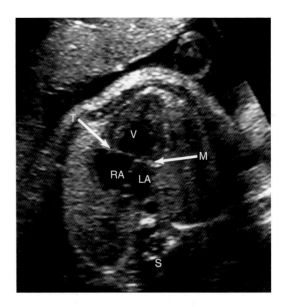

Figure 9–4 Apical four-chamber view in a fetus with a univentricular *(V)* heart with two AV valves. *LA,* Left atrium; *M,* mitral valve; *RA,* right atrium; *S,* spine; *T,* tricuspid valve.

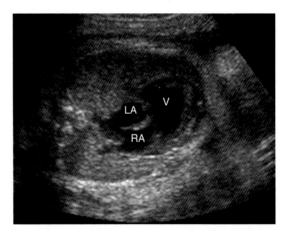

Figure 9–5 Subcostal four-chamber view in a fetus with a univentricular *(V)* heart with two AV valves. *LA,* Left atrium; *RA,* right atrium.

9–4 and 9–5). It should be kept in mind that a rudimentary ventricular chamber is often contained within the single ventricular mass and may be visible (Fig. 9–6).[11]

It is possible to have one AV valve with a univentricular heart (Fig. 9–7). Pulsed or color Doppler

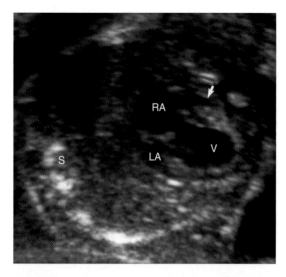

Figure 9–6 Subcostal four-chamber view in a fetus with a univentricular *(V)* heart. A rudimentary chamber *(arrow)* is also visualized. *LA*, Left atrium; *RA*, right atrium; *S*, spine.

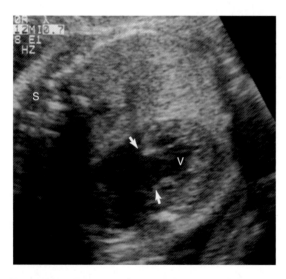

Figure 9–7 Subcostal four-chamber view in a fetus with a univentricular *(V)* heart that has only one multileaflet atrioventricular valve *(arrows)*. *S*, Spine.

imaging, or both, is essential to document flow into the single ventricle from one or both AV valves.

If one AV valve is atretic, the most likely diagnosis is tricuspid or mitral valve atresia, which is most commonly considered a defect separate from

a univentricular heart.[2] Again, Doppler evaluation would be important to document flow through the functioning valve and to document the absence of flow through the atretic valve.

The great vessels are most commonly malpositioned, with the aorta anterior and to the left of the pulmonary artery, but other combinations are possible. The aorta may be anterior and to the right of the pulmonary artery, or the great vessels may have a normal relationship. To determine the orientation of the great vessels, the ascending vessel should be followed cephalad to determine whether it connects with the aortic arch or bifurcates into the pulmonary arteries. A three-vessel view is also useful. In the normal setting the aorta and pulmonary/ductus arteriosus confluence should form a "V" configuration from the spine. If the vessels are transposed, the vessels will be oriented in a more parallel fashion. By sliding the transducer cephalad into a three-vessel trachea view, malpositioned great vessels will result in only the aorta and superior vena cava being visualized.

Aortic arch interruptions and coarctation are associated with univentricular heart syndrome. Therefore a comparison of size of the great vessels is warranted, as well as Doppler evaluation for increased velocity at the site of a coarctation or absent flow in the setting of an interrupted aortic arch.

It is common for the pulmonary artery to be stenotic or atretic, and it is important to determine this on the prenatal evaluation because pulmonary outflow obstruction affects the prognosis and the treatment of univentricular heart.

Pulmonary stenosis should be apparent with pulsed Doppler imaging on either a short-axis view of the great vessels or a long-axis view of the pulmonary artery.

The morphological characteristics of the single ventricle, whether right or left, may also be evaluated by echocardiography. If the ventricular trabecular pattern appears coarse, especially if a moderator band is seen, the morphological features are likely to be right sided. However, the most common morphological pattern is left sided, which may be difficult to determine by sonographic examination, particularly in the fetus.

Finally, because of the association of the univentricular heart with the cardiosplenic syndromes, a thorough evaluation of all fetal extracardiac anatomy is also warranted.

Treatment and Prognosis

Treatment options for univentricular heart disease as described in the literature run the gamut from no therapy to palliative surgery only to more definitive corrective procedures to heart transplantation.

If no surgical correction is performed, the long-term outlook for patients with univentricular heart disease is grim. Even in the most optimistic series,[9,10] which followed patients diagnosed in middle to late childhood (admittedly a group of patients who had already withstood a process of natural selection), progressive deterioration and death characterize the disorder.

Fifty percent of patients with type A ventricles die within 14 years of diagnosis, whereas 50% of patients with type C ventricles die within 4 years of diagnosis. This suggests that the ventricular morphological features, and whether a rudimentary chamber exists (type A) or not (type C), have prognostic significance, with type C being more lethal.

Traditionally, palliative surgery in infancy has been recommended, regardless of whether a corrective procedure will be performed later.[6,10] The treatment strategy is to band the pulmonary artery in patients in whom pulmonary blood flow is excessive, thus preventing the development of pulmonary vascular disease, and to create shunts when severe pulmonary stenosis is present, thereby maintaining adequate pulmonary perfusion. The shunts connect the pulmonary artery to the systemic circulation and vary depending on the surgeon performing the procedure and the defects present at surgery.[6] When significant subaortic stenosis is present, the pulmonary artery may be transected and connected to the aorta in an end-to-side manner, allowing all blood flow from the heart to enter the systemic circulation. A systemic-to-pulmonary shunt is then placed for pulmonary blood flow.

The outcome for patients undergoing palliative treatment only varies, depending on the series. Villani et al[6] reported good results early on, with a hospital mortality rate of only 7.4%, although long-term significant mortality rates may occur in the absence of definitive surgical correction.

Moodie et al[10] reported that 30% of patients with type A ventricles and 46% of patients with type C ventricles died within 5 years of palliative surgery. The most common causes of death were arrhythmias, congestive heart failure, and sudden unexplained death.[7]

These data suggest that the best course is to proceed with a more definitive surgical procedure as soon as possible. Yet there are some patients who have chosen to live with moderate cyanosis and defer additional palliation or corrective therapy indefinitely. In fact, several review studies have found that the risk of cardiovascular death and the need for heart transplant after initial palliative shunt procedure were not significantly reduced by more definitive treatments.[28] Thus these decisions regarding appropriate treatment must be tailored to an individual case by use of an integrated, multidisciplinary approach. The traditional options for more definitive therapy are a modified Fontan procedure or heart transplantation.

With a univentricular heart, the primary problem is that the systemic and the pulmonary circulations are supplied by output from a single ventricle. The Fontan procedure with its many modifications allows the ventricle to pump blood to the systemic circulation, whereas the pulmonary blood flow is not dependent on ventricular contraction. The most common current surgical approach is the total cavopulmonary anastomosis. This is a staged procedure in which the first operation, a bidirectional Glenn shunt, is usually performed at 4 to 6 months of age to provide more pulmonary blood flow. In this procedure, the superior vena cava is connected to the right pulmonary artery and allows desaturated blood to flow to the right and left pulmonary arteries.

The second stage of the procedure is usually carried out at 18 months and 4 years of age with the creation of a lateral intra-atrial tunnel that reroutes the inferior vena cava systemic flow to the orifice of the superior caval vein and the cavopulmonary anastomosis, completing the separation of pulmonary from systemic circulation. The lateral tunnel is created by insertion of a polytetrafluoroethylene baffle or may be created by autologous material from the interatrial septum. In addition, Fontan pathways may be "fenestrated" by creation of an atrial septal defect in the baffle or patch to provide an escape valve that allows right-to-left shunting, which may be beneficial early after the surgical procedure in a subgroup of patients with low cardiac output by increasing systemic ventricular preload.[7,24] These fenestrations can be closed later by a transcatheter approach if hemodynamics are favorable. One study suggested that fenestration of the atrial baffle is associated with reduced Fontan failure rate and decreased occurrence of pleural effusion and that subsequent closure of the fenestration was usually not required.[29,30] An extracardiac tunnel procedure is a recent modification that may better preserve ventricular and pulmonary function because it can be performed with minimal cardiopulmonary bypass. In addition, it avoids right atrial incisions that can reduce the risk of injury to the sinus node and incidence of post-operative arrythmias.[24] Early surgical results are encouraging for this approach to the single ventricle, with an early mortality rate as low as 4%.[31] Fontan palliation has an actuarial survival rate of 91% at 10 years.[7]

There is concern about the long-term fate of the circulation produced with the Fontan procedure. Fontan physiology is paradoxical in that it imposes systemic venous hypertension with concomitant pulmonary arterial hypotension. As a consequence, potential complications are numerous and include arrhythmias, thromboemboli, hepatic dysfunction, protein-losing enteropathy, exercise intolerance, and worsening cyanosis from pulmonary venous compression, systemic venous collateralization, or pulmonary arteriovenous malformations. In cases of failing Fontan circulations, surgical revision may be considered. However, experience in Fontan take-down surgery is limited and the procedure was found to carry a high mortality rate, but it may provide a brief delay before definitive rescue therapy with orthotopic heart transplantation.[7,24,32] Infant heart transplantation has been a successful approach to hypoplastic left heart syndrome, with a 91% 1-month survival rate and a 70% 7-year survival rate.[33] For some patients with a univentricular heart, heart transplantation may be a reasonable

TABLE 9-1   Conditions Associated with Univentricular Heart

Fetal		
Associated Cardiac Abnormalities	**Chromosome Abnormality**	**Syndromes**
Aortic atresia	Trisomy 18 (Edward syndrome)	Asplenia
Aortic stenosis		Polysplenia
Atrioventricular septal defect		Polysyndactyly
Bicuspid aortic valve		
Bicuspid pulmonic valve		
Coarctation		
Common atrium		
Common left pulmonary vein		
Common right pulmonary vein		
Complete heart block		
Complete transposition of the great arteries		
Congenitally corrected transposition of the great arteries		
Dextrocardia		
Double-outlet right ventricle		
Interrupted aortic arch		
Left superior vena cava		
Mitral atresia		
Mitral insufficiency		
Pulmonary atresia		
Pulmonic stenosis		
Right aortic arch		
Subaortic stenosis		
Total anomalous pulmonary venous connection		
Triatrial heart		
Tricuspid atresia		
Tricuspid insufficiency		
Truncus arteriosus		
Unicuspid aortic valve		

alternative to other surgical options. The long-term results with heart transplantation in children remain unknown.

Associated Anomalies

Univentricular heart has been associated with various cardiac and extracardiac malformations. The most common cardiac anomalies associated with univentricular heart are AV valve atresias, pulmonic stenosis, aortic arch interruptions and coarctation, and the heterotaxic syndromes (Table 9–1). Chromosome abnormalities in infants born with a univentricular heart have also been reported.

References

1. Arey JB: Cardiovascular Pathology in Infants and Children. Philadelphia, WB Saunders, 1984, pp 104–105.
2. Hallermann FJ, Davis GD, Ritter DG, et al: Roentgenographic features of common ventricle. Radiology 1966; 87:409–423.
3. Anderson RH, Tynan M, Freedom RM, et al: Ventricular morphology in the univentricular heart. Herz 1979; 4:184–197.
4. Anderson RH, Macartney FJ, Tynan M, et al: Univentricular atrioventricular connection: The single ventricle trap unsprung. Pediatr Cardiol 1983; 4:273–280.
5. Bharati S, Lev M: The concept of tricuspid atresia complex as distinct from that of the single ventricle complex. Pediatr Cardiol 1979; 1:57–62.
6. Villani M, Crupi G, Locatelli G: Experience in palliative treatment of univentricular heart including tricuspid atresia. Herz 1979; 4:256–261.
7. Khairy P, Poirier N, Mercier LA: Univentricular heart. Circulation 2007; 115:800–812.
8. Jacobs ML, Mayer JE Jr: Congenital heart surgery nomenclature and database project: Single ventricle. Ann Thorac Surg 2000; 69:S197–S204.
9. Moodie DS, Ritter DG, Tajik AJ, et al: Long-term follow-up in the unoperated univentricular heart. Am J Cardiol 1984; 53:1124–1128.
10. Moodie DS, Ritter DG, Tajik AH, et al: Long-term follow-up after palliative operation for univentricular heart. Am J Cardiol 1984; 53:1648–1651.
11. Shepard TH, Fantel AG, Kapur RP: Fetal coronary thrombosis as a cause of single ventricular heart. Teratology 1991; 43:113–117.
12. Doty DB, Schieken RM, Lauer RM: Septation of the univentricular heart. J Thorac Cardiovasc Surg 1979; 78:423–430.
13. Doty DB, Marvin WJ, Lauer RM: Modified Fontan procedure: Methods to achieve direct anastomosis of right atrium to pulmonary artery. J Thorac Cardiovasc Surg 1981; 81:470–475.
14. Weigel TJ, Driscoll DJ, Michels VV: Occurrence of congenital heart defects in siblings of patients with univentricular heart and tricuspid atresia. Am J Cardiol 1989; 64:768–771.
15. Stevenson C, Franken EA, Ha-Upala S: Familial occurrence of single ventricle. Arch Dis Child 1971; 46:730–731.
16. Harley HR: The embryology of cor triloculare biatriatum with bulbar (rudimentary) cavity. Guys Hosp Rep 1958; 107:116–143.
17. McKusick VA: Mendelian Inheritance in Man: Catalogs of Autosomal Dominant, Autosomal Recessive, and X-Linked Phenotypes. Baltimore: Johns Hopkins University Press, 1989, pp 826–827.
18. Rose V, Izukawa T, Moes CAF: Syndromes of asplenia and polysplenia: A review of cardiac and non-cardiac malformations in 60 cases with special reference to diagnosis and prognosis. Br Heart J 1975; 37:840–852.
19. Ruttenberg HD, Neufeld HN, Lucas RV: Syndrome of congenital cardiac disease with asplenia: Distinction from other forms of congenital cyanotic cardiac disease. Am J Cardiol 1964; 13:387–406.
20. Ivemark BI: Implications of agenesis of the spleen on the pathogenesis of cono-truncus anomalies in childhood: An analysis of the heart malformations in the splenic agenesis syndrome, with fourteen new cases. Acta Paediatr Scand 1955; 104(Suppl):1–110.
21. Neerhoff MG, MacGregor SN, Retzky SS, et al: Cocaine abuse during pregnancy: Peripartum prevalence and perinatal outcome. Am J Obstet Gynecol 1989; 161:633–638.
22. Bingol N, Fuchs M, Diaz V, et al: Teratogenicity of cocaine in humans. J Pediatr 1987; 110:93–96.
23. Steinberger E, Ferencz C, Loffredo C: Infants with single ventricle: a population-based epidemiological study. Teratology 2002; 65:106–115.
24. Kaulitz R, Hofbeck M: Current treatment and prognosis in children with functionally univentricular hearts. Arch Dis Child 2005; 90:757–762.
25. Fontana RS, Edwards JE: Congenital Cardiac Disease: A Review of 357 Cases Studied Pathologically. Philadelphia, WB Saunders, 1962, pp 13–20.
26. Belloc NB: An estimate of the prevalence of congenital cardiovascular malformations based on mortality rates. Hum Biol 1968; 40:473–483.
27. Freedom RM, Mikailian H: The Natural and Modified History of Congenital Heart Disease. Blackwell Publishing, 2004, pp. 408–415.

28. Day RW, Etheridge SP, Veasy LG, et al: Single ventricle palliation: Greater risk of complications with the Fontan procedure than with the bidirectional Glenn procedure alone. Int J Cardiol 2006; 106:201–210.

29. Airan B, Sharma R, Choudhary SK, et al: Univentricular repair: Is routine fenestration justified? Ann Thor Surg 2000; 69:1900–1906.

30. Krishnan U: Univentricular heart: management options. Ind J Pediatr 2005; 72:519–524.

31. Cetta F, Mair DD, Feldt RH, et al: Improved early mortality after modified-Fontan operation for complex congenital heart disease. Am J Cardiol 1993; 72:499–502.

32. Gajarski RJ, Towbin JA, Garson S: Fontan palliation versus heart transplantation: A comparison of charges. Am Heart J 1996; 131:1169–1174.

33. Razzouk AJ, Chinnock RE, Gundry SR, et al: Transplantation as a primary treatment for hypoplastic left heart syndrome: Intermediate-term results. Ann Thorac Surg 1996; 62:1–8.

CHAPTER 10

Aortic Stenosis and Pulmonary Stenosis

Teresa M. Bieker

Aortic Stenosis

Definition

Congenital aortic stenosis may be caused by a variety of lesions that obstruct outflow from the left ventricle. Aortic stenosis occurs in approximately 3% to 6% of neonates with congenital heart disease.[1,2] In utero, aortic stenosis may be an isolated lesion; however, associated cardiac malformations are seen in approximately 30% of cases.[2–7] These malformations most commonly include hypoplastic left heart syndrome, coarctation of the aorta, endocardial fibroelastosis, ventricular septal defects, pulmonary stenosis, and mitral stenosis.[3–5,8,9] Congenital aortic stenosis can be classified into three types, depending on the site of obstruction: valvular, subvalvular, or supravalvular stenosis.

Types

Valvular stenosis is the most common type of aortic stenosis, occurring in 0.25 of 1000 live births and in 60% to 75% of patients with aortic stenosis.[10–13] It results from an abnormal formation of the valve cusps. In pediatric patients with valvular stenosis, 10% to 15% have symptoms in infancy. These patients usually have a more severe form of stenosis than do those in whom symptoms develop later in childhood.[3,14,15] Neonates with valvular aortic stenosis frequently have severe mitral stenosis, endocardial fibroelastosis, hypoplastic left heart syndrome, and coarctation of the

169

aorta. Atrial and ventricular septal defects are also seen.[16,17] A fetus with valvular aortic stenosis has an increased risk for becoming hydropic in utero.[18,19] Congenital valvular stenosis is three to four times more common in males than in females.[20]

Subvalvular stenosis is considered the second most common form of aortic stenosis, occurring in 8% to 30% of patients with congenital left outflow track obstructions.[21,22] As with valvular stenosis, males are affected two to three times as often as females.[23] Unlike valvular stenosis, severe subvalvular stenosis resulting from a fixed lesion (i.e., a membrane or fibromuscular tunnel) is rarely seen in newborns or infants.[22,24,25] It usually occurs later in childhood as a result of associated congenital heart defects. However, the dynamic form of this lesion has been reported in utero.[26] Dynamic forms include the inherited disorders of asymmetric septal hypertrophy (ASH), idiopathic hypertrophic subaortic stenosis, and hypertrophic obstructive cardiomyopathy.[27]

Infants of diabetic mothers in whom the diabetes is not well controlled are often found to have a transient form of dynamic obstruction of the left ventricular outflow tract.[28] Associated cardiac lesions are common in subvalvular stenosis, occurring in 50% to 65% of patients.[23] They most commonly include ventricular septal defect, interruption of the aortic arch, and coarctation.[29,30] Progressive subvalvular aortic stenosis can also lead to damage of the aortic valve, resulting in aortic regurgitation.[31]

It is also common to detect aortic stenosis caused by an obstructive cardiomyopathy in the recipient twin of a pregnancy affected with twin-twin transfusion syndrome (TTTS). In TTTS, the recipient twin's heart is likely to become hypertrophic as a result of increased preload. As the septum and heart walls hypertrophy, they obstruct the left ventricular outflow tract, resulting in a stenosis.[32] Pulmonary stenosis usually develops in these fetuses before the onset of aortic stenosis.

Supravalvular stenosis is the least common of the three types. It may be an isolated anomaly but is often associated with peripheral pulmonary stenosis.[33] Supravalvular stenosis is described as a narrowing of the ascending aorta that may be localized or diffuse, originating at the superior margin of the sinuses of Valsalva just above the level of the coronary arteries.[1,34]

Three forms of supravalvular stenosis have been described. Fifty percent to 75% of patients have an "hourglass" deformity, with a constricting ridge at the superior margin of the sinuses of Valsalva caused by extreme thickening and disorganization of the aortic media.[33,35]

Approximately 25% of patients have a more diffuse type of narrowing extending along the ascending aorta.[36]

A discrete membrane above the valve has also been reported.[35] In 1961, Williams et al[37] described the association of supravalvular aortic stenosis, mental retardation, and elfin facies. This constellation of findings now bears the name "Williams syndrome," which is a microdeletion of 7q11.23 involving the elastin gene.[33,38] A total of 28% to 50% of patients with supravalvular aortic stenosis have Williams syndrome.[39] The finding of supravalvular aortic stenosis along with peripheral pulmonary artery stenosis is nearly exclusive to patients with Williams syndrome.[38] Neonates with Williams syndrome also have hypercalcemia, narrowing of peripheral systemic and pulmonary arteries, strabismus, auditory hyperacusis, gastrointestinal problems, and urinary tract abnormalities.[1,33,38,40]

Severe or critical aortic stenosis is associated with high mortality and morbidity rates. A critical stenosis is characterized by decreased left ventricular function and ductal dependence.[41] Without intervention, critical aortic stenosis is likely to progress to hypoplastic left heart syndrome.[42,43]

Embryology

The etiology of congenital aortic stenosis is unknown but is thought to be multifactorial. De la Cruz et al[44] and Grant[45] have suggested that aortic valve stenosis may be the result of overgrowth of endocardial cushion tissue. Mechanical interference with blood flow, hypoxia, and pharmacological agents such as thalidomide have all been reported to produce experimental aortic stenosis or a hypertrophic left heart, or both.[46–48] These factors presumably cause cellular death or abnormal differentiation of cells, thus interfering with normal blood flow through the developing heart. This reduction of flow results in underdevelopment of cardiac structures. Some forms of aortic stenosis are known to have an autosomal dominant transmission with variable expression, whereas other forms are thought to be spontaneous mutations.[1]

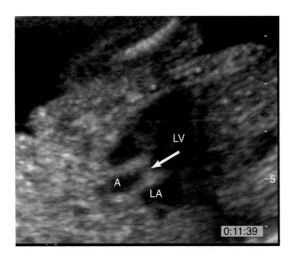

Figure 10–1 Long-axis view of the aorta in a fetus with aortic stenosis showing a thickened and echogenic aortic valve *(arrow)*. *A*, Aorta; *LA*, left atrium; *LV*, left ventricle.

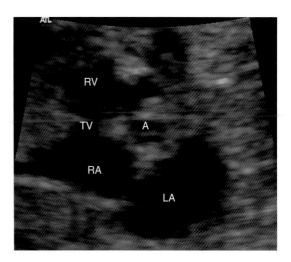

Figure 10–2 Short-axis view of the aorta showing a bicuspid aortic valve with the two leaflets coapting in the center of the aortic annulus. *A*, Aorta; *LA*, left atrium; *RA*, right atrium; *RV*, right ventricle; *TV*, tricuspid valve.

Occurrence Rate

Aortic stenosis has been reported to have a frequency of approximately 5% in live births.[2,49] The suggested risk of occurrence for a fetus with an affected father is approximately 3%. If the mother is affected, the risk of occurrence in the fetus rises to 13% to 18%. The occurrence risk if a sibling is affected is approximately 2%; it is 6% if two siblings are affected.[50]

Sonographic Criteria

The prenatal diagnosis of aortic stenosis may be difficult, depending on the type of obstruction involved.[50–52] In valvular stenosis, a structural abnormality of the aortic valves cusps is present. The aortic valve may appear thickened, immobile, fused or dysplastic (Fig. 10–1). The valve may also be bicuspid or unicuspid or in rare cases have more than three leaflets (Fig. 10–2). These findings can be extremely subtle in a fetus. Poststenotic dilation of the aorta may provide a clue to proximal stenosis. Pulsed and color Doppler imaging are essential in diagnosing stenosis. Flow distal to the aortic valve is increased and turbulent (Fig. 10–3); however, in some cases of critical aortic stenosis, no flow may be appreciated. Severe stenosis may lead to myocardial dysfunction and ventricular enlargement.[34,53] In the setting of severe early-onset aortic stenosis, the decrease in blood flow is likely to result in a hypoplastic left ventricle.[42,43]

Endocardial fibroelastosis resulting from aortic valvular stenosis has been demonstrated prenatally.[54] Sonographically, endocardial fibroelastosis appears as a hyperechoic rim around the affected chamber (Fig. 10–4). It is thought to result from blood stagnating within a chamber because of an outflow obstruction, causing fibrin deposits within the heart wall. Endocardial fibroelastosis has the potential to restrict chamber filling, hence impeding chamber growth.[55] Retrograde flow in the aortic arch (Fig. 10–5) and left-to-right flow across the foremen ovale are also seen with critical aortic stenosis.[42,43]

In the subvalvular form of stenosis, ASH or concentric hypertrophy of the left ventricle may be seen.[56] The ventricular heart wall and the interventricular septum should be measured and compared with gestational age–related nomograms. In the case of ASH, which is often seen in fetuses of diabetic mothers, only the septum will be hypertrophied. With concentric hypertrophy, the interventricular septum and posterior heart walls will both be thickened, possibly reducing chamber size (Figs. 10–6 and 10–7). When ASH or concentric hypertrophy are identified in any fetal heart, serial fetal echocardiograms should be performed to detect the onset of valvular stenosis.

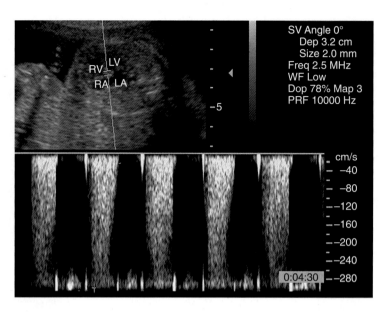

Figure 10–3   Pulsed Doppler imaging through the aortic valve from an apical five-chamber view in a fetus with aortic stenosis. The velocity is well over 120 cm/second, and the waveform shows the spectral broadening indicative of stenosis. *LA,* Left atrium; *LV,* left ventricle; *RA,* right atrium; *RV,* right ventricle.

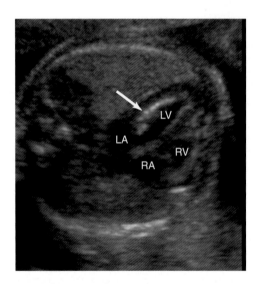

Figure 10–4   Subcostal four-chamber view in a fetus with aortic stenosis. Endocardial fibroelastosis *(arrow)* is seen within the heart wall of the left ventricle *(LV).* *LA,* Left atrium; *RA,* right atrium; *RV,* right ventricle.

Supravalvular stenosis will have pulsed Doppler characteristics similar to valvular or subvalvular stenosis, specifically an increase in blood flow velocity distal to the stenosis and decreased blood flow velocity proximally. The hourglass configuration or diffuse narrowing described previously may also be appreciated.

In all forms of aortic stenosis, the mitral, tricuspid, and pulmonic valves should also be investigated with pulsed or color Doppler imaging for evidence of stenosis or insufficiency. The aortic arch should be evaluated thoroughly because interruption of the aortic arch or coarctation is frequently associated with aortic stenosis. Although difficult in the fetus because of resolution limitations, an attempt should be made to image the aortic valve leaflets in a short-axis view to evaluate for bicuspid or unicuspid valve (see Fig. 10–2). A unicuspid unicommissural aortic valve is commonly seen in infants with aortic stenosis.[57] Congestive heart failure may occur in utero; therefore signs of hydrops fetalis, such as pericardial or pleural effusions or ascites, should be investigated.

Treatment

Neonates with critical aortic stenosis display signs of circulatory collapse, cyanosis, and congestive heart failure. Without surgical intervention, the symptomatic neonate with severe aortic stenosis will not survive. Critically ill neonates require urgent intervention. At birth, prostaglandin E_1 is usually given to maintain ductal patency, thereby relieving pulmonary hypertension and maintaining systemic perfusion.[20,58] Surgical intervention for valvular aortic stenosis usually consists of balloon valvuloplasty, transventricular valvotomy,

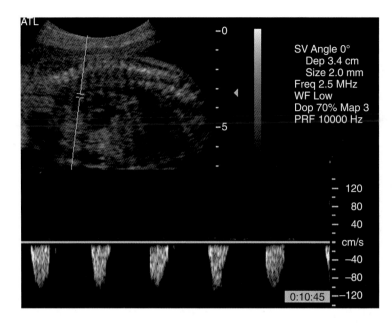

Figure 10–5 Reversed flow in the aortic arch. Pulsed Doppler imaging shows retrograde flow through the aortic arch from the ductus arteriosus. This occurs because of the lack of flow through the aorta as a result of critical aortic stenosis.

or open repair.[2,29] Patch aortoplasty is used to treat supravalvar aortic stenosis, whereas fibrous membrane or muscular resections are performed with subvalvular stenosis. Typically, these types of surgeries are palliative. The majority of children with valvular stenosis will need valve replacements.[2] Critical aortic stenosis requires eventual aortic valve or even aortic root replacement in many, if not all, cases.[59,60]

In cases of critical aortic stenosis, in utero balloon valvoplasty continues to be refined. Under ultrasound guidance, a cannula and needle are passed through the maternal abdomen, uterus, and fetal chest wall into the left ventricle. A guidewire and coronary balloon 10% are placed at the level of the aortic annulus.[61] A balloon is then inflated within the aortic ring. Tierney et al[42] reported 42 patients who underwent this procedure. Of the 30 cases evaluated (12 patients were lost to follow-up), aortic valvuloplasty was a technical success in 26 patients. Success was determined by a decrease in mitral regurgitation, bidirectional flow across the foramen ovale, and the return to antegrade flow in the aortic arch. Postnatally, eight achieved biventricular circulation and 18 had a functional single ventricle palliation. Significant aortic stenosis did not reoccur within the 26 successful procedures. Long-term

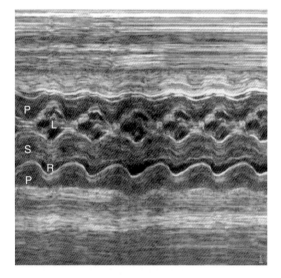

Figure 10–6 M-mode tracing of a fetal heart with concentric hypertrophy. The interventricular septum *(S)* and posterior heart walls *(P)* are hypertrophied, resulting in a diminished chamber size of the right *(R)* and left *(L)* ventricles.

outcomes of this relatively new procedure have not been established.

Prognosis

The prognosis in the various forms of congenital aortic stenosis varies with the severity of the

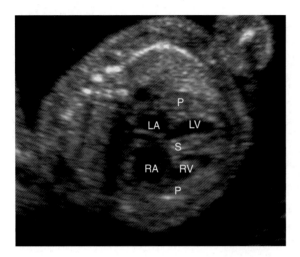

Figure 10–7 Subcostal four-chamber view in a fetal heart with concentric hypertrophy, resulting in subvalvular stenosis. Both the posterior heart walls *(P)* and interventricular septum *(S)* are hypertrophied. *LA,* Left atrium; *LV,* left ventricle; *RA,* right atrium; *RV,* right ventricle.

obstruction and the associated abnormalities. Isolated or mild stenosis has a good prognosis. A mortality rate of 11% in the first 5 years of life has been reported. Surgical mortality rates for aortic valvotomy range from 9% to 67%.[2] Rates can be higher depending on the severity of the stenosis, associated abnormalities. and the type of intervention necessary.[14,29,61] With critical aortic stenosis, aortic valvuloplasty success rates are improving. However, the majority of fetuses will develop hypoplastic left heart syndrome in utero and require a Norwood procedure or heart transplant. In multiple studies, only a handful are born with a functioning biventricular heart. However, fetal hydrops was not identified in any of the live-born fetuses.[42,43,53,61] A report by Brown et al[2] suggested that 25% of patients with aortic stenosis will require reoperation within 10 years, and reoperation is necessary in 38% of patients within 40 years. Untreated aortic stenosis has historically been one of the most common causes of sudden death from heart disease in the pediatric population, with an incidence between 4% and 20%.[62–64] In utero identification of aortic stenosis has helped to reduce this occurrence. Endocardial fibroelastosis, a small left ventricle, and a small mitral or aortic annulus are all considered poor prognostic indicators for children with aortic stenosis. Conversely, ASH resulting in outflow obstruction, which, as discussed previously, is seen in infants of diabetic mothers, is invariably transient and as such carries an excellent prognosis. Concentric hypertrophy seen in TTTS may also regress after birth. However, TTTS pregnancies treated conservatively have a very poor prognosis regardless of the cardiac abnormalities present. Interestingly, in utero treatments of TTTS, including serial amniotic fluid reductions, amniotic septostomy, or anastomoses ablations, do not improve cardiac consequences.[32]

Cases of aortic stenosis diagnosed in utero are usually severe; therefore, they are usually associated with a high mortality rate.[58]

Associated Anomalies

Endocardial fibroelastosis is common in the fetus or neonate with aortic stenosis. Dyck and Freedom[29] reported 23 cases of aortic stenosis seen at autopsy. Of these, 18 (78%) had endocardial fibroelastosis. Other commonly associated lesions include coarctation of the aorta (11%) and mitral stenosis (25%) (Table 10–1).[29] Subvalvular aortic stenosis may be associated with various inheritable disorders or with maternal diabetes. Valvular aortic stenosis has an association with chromosome abnormalities such as Turner syndrome.[27] Supravalvular stenosis occurs commonly in Williams syndrome and has also been reported in cases of maternal rubella.[20,65]

Pulmonary Stenosis

Definition

Congenital pulmonary stenosis is defined as the obstruction of the right ventricular outflow tract by either an abnormal pulmonary valve or narrowing of the infundibulum. It represents approximately 7.4% of structural cardiac anomalies in the newborn population.[49] Obstruction most commonly occurs because of an abnormality of the pulmonary valve (bicuspid or quadricuspid), with various degrees of fusion of the valve leaflets. This forms a diaphragm with a small hole through which blood must exit the right ventricle. Less commonly, a dysplastic pulmonary valve with three thickened, but unfused, cusps may be present. Dysplastic pulmonary valves are frequently found in patients with Noonan syn-

TABLE 10–1 Conditions Associated with Aortic Stenosis				
Maternal		**Fetal**		
Condition	**Drug Use**	**Associated Cardiac Abnormalities**	**Chromosome Abnormalities**	**Syndromes**
Diabetes	Phenytoin	Atrial septal defect	Ring 14	Arthrogryposis multiplex
Rubella	Thalidomide	Atrioventricular septal defect	Trisomy 2q	Bernheim syndrome
	Trimethadione	Coarctation	Turner syndrome (XO)	Cayler syndrome
	Valproic acid	Double-inlet left ventricle		Elfin facies syndrome
		Hypoplastic left heart syndrome		Noonan syndrome
		Interrupted aortic arch		Williams syndrome
		Mitral stenosis		Williams-Beuren syndrome
		Transposition of the great vessels		
		Univentricular heart		
		Ventricular septal defect		

drome.[66] Pulmonary stenosis can progress to pulmonary atresia in utero.[67]

Alternatively, pulmonary stenosis may occur at the level of the infundibulum of the right ventricular outflow tract because of either a thick fibrous ring or thickened muscle tissue. In this type of stenosis, the pulmonary valve may be normal.[68] Interestingly, although there does not appear to be a sex predilection related to pulmonary stenosis, an unusual seasonal variation, with affected males being born in the fall and affected females being born in the spring, has been reported.[69,70]

Obstructive or valvular pulmonary stenosis may also found in the recipient twin of TTTS. The recipient develops biventricular hypertrophy from an increase in pressure and volume. The thickening of the right ventricular wall leads to obstruction of the outflow tract. It has been postulated that the thickening of the right ventricle may be caused by abnormal levels of rennin, aldosterone, catecholamines, or other molecules received from the donor twin.[71] Another theory suggests the imbalance of blood flow between the twins leads to abnormal development of the heart structures. In addition to stenosis, recipients of TTTS may develop pulmonary atresia or obstructive cardiomyopathy.[72]

Embryology

A maldevelopment of the distal part of the bulbus cordis from which the pulmonary valve develops is believed to be the most likely embryological basis for the valvular type of obstruction.[73] It has also been postulated that valvular pulmonary stenosis or atresia may be the result of fetal endocarditis.[74] The known association with maternal rubella infection would support this theory.[64] The common finding of pulmonic stenosis is infants with Noonan syndrome and trisomy 18, in addition to a reported familial occurrence, would imply that genetic factors also likely play an important role.[66]

From a physiological standpoint, pulmonary stenosis obstructs the ejection of blood from the right ventricle. This obstruction leads to an increase in right ventricular pressure, which, in turn, results in an increase in right ventricular muscle mass. In mild or moderate stenosis, the hypertrophic right ventricle may be able to maintain normal output. In severe stenosis, however, right ventricular output falls, resulting in a pattern of circulation in the fetus similar to that in pulmonary atresia.[74]

Occurrence Rate

Isolated pulmonary valve stenosis occurs in approximately 5% to 7.8% of live births with cardiac defects.[33,75] The familial occurrence of pulmonary stenosis has been reported. In an examination of the siblings of 125 patients with pulmonic stenosis, Campbell[76] found that 2.2% had a cardiac defect, usually pulmonary stenosis. Nora et al[50] reported that the probability of occurrence in siblings of pulmonary stenosis was approximately 2% with one affected sibling and 6% when two siblings were affected. The occurrence risk for a fetus with an affected father is about 2%, which rises to 4% to 6.5% when the mother is the affected parent.[50] Right ventricular hypertrophy resulting in obstructive pulmonary stenosis has been reported in up to 58% of recipient twins in the setting of TTTS.[32]

Sonographic Criteria

Antenatal diagnosis of pulmonic stenosis can be difficult because the stenotic region is often not apparent. Poststenotic dilation of the pulmonary artery (Fig. 10–8) and right ventricular hypertrophy with a small right ventricular chamber (Fig. 10–9) should suggest the possibility of pulmonic stenosis. It should be borne in mind, however, that the degree of poststenotic dilation is not always proportional to the severity of the stenosis. Frequently, mild cases of valvular stenosis are associated with the most profound dilation of the main pulmonary artery.[64] Dilation of the pulmonary artery is not present with isolated infundibular stenosis. Copel et al[77] looked at 1022 fetuses at risk for congenital heart disease and correctly identified six cases of pulmonic stenosis. The consistent finding in all cases was an abnormal right atrium and ventricle in the four-chamber view. Pulsed and color Doppler imaging may be extremely valuable in assessing the presence of valvular stenosis. An increase in velocity distal to the valve should be appreciated (Fig. 10–10). The right atrium often appears dilated, whereas the right ventricular walls may be thickened. Reversal of flow within the ductus arteriosus is also likely to be present (Fig. 10–11).[67] The ductus venosus can show pulsatile flow with reversal of flow during atrial contraction.[78] Tricuspid regurgitation may also be present (Fig. 10–12).[79] In the majority of cases, a patent foramen ovale and, less commonly, an atrial septal defect is present.[64] Color and pulsed Doppler imaging should also be used to look for associated ventricular septal defects and obstruction or insufficiency of the tricuspid and mitral valves. It is not unusual for pulmonary stenosis to be detected by pulsed Doppler imaging, even when the right heart chambers appear normal.

Aortic stenosis has also been found in conjunction with pulmonary stenosis, as has a right-sided aortic arch. The pulmonary veins should be identified entering the left atrium to rule out the association of total anomalous pulmonary venous connection. When the stenosis is severe, congestive heart failure and hydrops fetalis may develop

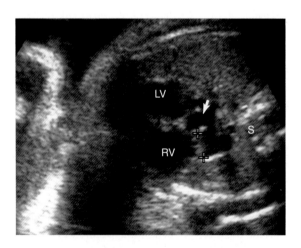

Figure 10–8 Poststenotic dilation of the pulmonary artery *(calipers)* in a fetus with pulmonic stenosis. The normal-sized aorta *(arrow)* can be seen above the large pulmonary artery. *LV,* Left ventricle; *RV,* right ventricle; *S,* spine.

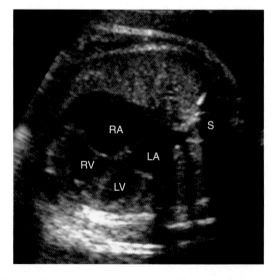

Figure 10–9 Right ventricular hypertrophy in a fetus with pulmonary stenosis. *LA,* Left atrium; *LV,* left ventricle; *RA,* right atrium; *RV,* right ventricle; *S,* spine.

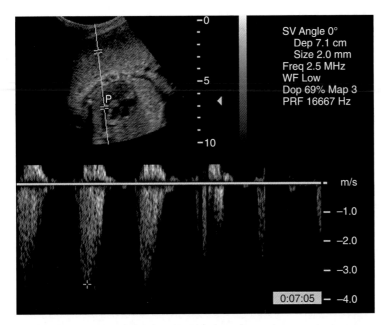

Figure 10–10 Pulsed Doppler imaging through the pulmonic valve in a fetus with pulmonary stenosis. The velocity is well over 120 cm/second and the waveform shows the spectral broadening indicative of stenosis. *P,* Pulmonary artery.

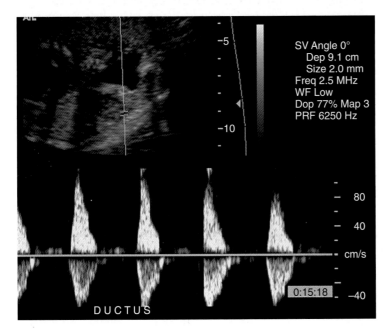

Figure 10–11 Retrograde flow *(above the baseline)* through the ductus arteriosus in a fetus with pulmonary atresia secondary to severe pulmonary stenosis. Blood flow from the left side of the heart travels through the aorta and then into the ductus because of the lack of forward flow through the pulmonary artery.

in utero. Therefore a thorough search for pericardial and pleural effusions, as well as other signs of hydrops fetalis, is also warranted.

With TTTS, the recipient's heart may also exhibit cardiomegaly, biventricular hypertrophy, mitral regurgitation, tricuspid regurgitation, and aortic stenosis.[32] As stated previously, pulmonary stenosis usually occurs before aortic stenosis is identified. Both tend to progress in severity as pregnancy progresses.[79]

Treatment

In cases of pulmonary stenosis, prostaglandin is given to maintain patency in the ductus arterio-

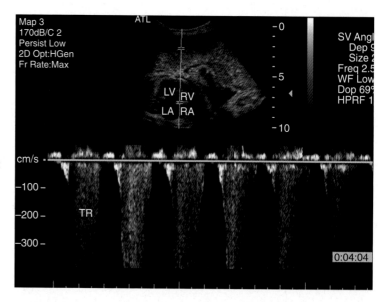

Figure 10–12 Pulsed Doppler imaging proximal to the tricuspid valve in the right atrium, showing massive tricuspid regurgitation *(TR)*. The flow is below the baseline, into the right atrium throughout systole. *LA,* Left atrium; *LV,* left ventricle; *RA,* right atrium; *RV,* right ventricle.

sus.[79] Various surgical interventions have been used to treat pulmonary stenosis. Open transpulmonary valvotomy has been attempted in infants, with variable degrees of success.[80,81] Srinivasan et al[80] and Milo et al[81] reported a low operative mortality rate of 12.5% and 0%, respectively. Flyer[82] found that between 1968 and 1974 the 30-day mortality rate of 10 infants undergoing open valvotomy for pulmonic stenosis was 40%, whereas that for 35 infants undergoing closed valvotomy was significantly lower at 14%. More current data suggest that most neonates can be managed effectively with a closed transventricular valvotomy, producing an acceptably low mortality rate.[83,84] Additionally, percutaneous balloon valvuloplasty has resulted in significant palliation in pulmonic stenosis.[85] Stanger et al[86] published the combined results of the Valvuloplasty and Angioplasty of Congenital Anomalies Registry on the use of balloon valvuloplasty to treat pulmonary valve stenosis.

They reported the results of balloon pulmonary valvuloplasty in 822 children and found only five major complications (0.6%), including two deaths, one cardiac perforation with tamponade, and two new occurrences of tricuspid insufficiency. There are, however, two groups of children in whom balloon valvuloplasty has not been uniformly successful. These include children with dysplastic pulmonary valves and neonates with critical pulmonary stenosis.[86] When pulmonary valvular dysplasia is present, valvuloplasty is suggested. Valvuloplasty in neonates with critical pulmonary stenosis has been reported as successful in 45% to 95% of cases.[87–89] Complications reported after neonatal valvuloplasty include retroperitoneal hematoma, iliofemoral venous occlusion, rupture of the right ventricular infundibulum, and death.[87–89] In utero valvuloplasties have also been performed. Valvuloplasty in utero can decrease the risk for development of hydrops and prevent fetal death; however, this procedure is still in its early stages, and long-term follow-up is needed. All fetal interventions should be considered palliative.[77,83]

From an obstetrical standpoint, all cases of aortic and pulmonic stenosis diagnosed in utero warrant genetic counseling because of the familial recurrence associated with these lesions.

Prognosis

The majority of patients with mild pulmonary stenosis are asymptomatic and have a favorable prognosis. Infant deaths are most often related to associated malformations and not to the pulmonary stenosis itself. Unfortunately, those cases detected in utero are usually severe and accompanied by other cardiac malformations and therefore carry a poorer prognosis. Severe pulmonary stenosis has a mortality rate of approximately 50%.[90] Todros et al[67] reported a survival rate of 67%

when pulmonary stenosis was diagnosed before 24 weeks' gestation. As with other structural lesions, hydrops fetalis in the setting of pulmonic stenosis is an ominous sign.[91] As with aortic stenosis, untreated congenital pulmonic stenosis is a cause of sudden death in children and adults.[64] As stated earlier, survival rates for fetuses with TTTS are dismal regardless of their cardiac abnormalities. In utero treatments do not appear to improve cardiac outcomes.[92]

Associated Anomalies

Pulmonary artery stenosis rarely occurs in isolation. In the majority of cases, the stenosis occurs along with other congenital defects or syndromes.[33] Pulmonary stenosis is associated with several other cardiac abnormalities, including right ventricular hypoplasia, aortic or tricuspid stenosis, and total anomalous pulmonary venous connection (Table 10–2). In Noonan syndrome, approximately 50% of affected infants have congenital cardiac malformations, most commonly pulmonary stenosis.[38,93–95] Approximately 15% to 20% of fetuses born with pulmonary valve abnormalities have dysmorphic features or chromosomal abnormalities.[96] Pulmonary stenosis is also seen with atrial septal defects, ventricular septal defects, and truncus arteriosus that have yet to be repaired.[65] The recipient in TTTS has an increased risk for development of pulmonary stenosis.[71,72] Pulmonary stenosis, like aortic stenosis, has been reported to occur in cases of maternal rubella.[65]

TABLE 10–2   Conditions Associated with Pulmonic Stenosis

Maternal		Fetal		
Condition	Drug Use	Associated Cardiac Abnormalities	Chromosome Abnormalities	Syndromes
Rubella	Alcohol	Aortic stenosis	Partial trisomy 22	Alagille syndrome
	Azathioprine	Atrioventricular septal defect	Ring 14	Cardiofacial syndrome– asymmetric facies
	Dilantin (phenytoin)	Endocardial fibroelastosis	9p	Cat-eye syndrome
	Trimethadone	Mitral stenosis	Turner syndrome (XO)	Dermofaciocardioskeletal syndrome
		Right aortic arch	Monosomy l0q2	Eagle-Barrett syndrome
		Right ventricular hypertrophy	Monosomy 8p2	Femoral-facial syndrome
		Tetralogy of Fallot	Monosomy lq4	Friederich ataxia
		Transposition of the great arteries	Trisomy 18	Geleophysic dwarfism
		Tricuspid insufficiency		Hand-heart syndrome
		Tricuspid stenosis		Keutel syndrome
				LEOPARD (lentigines, electrocardiographic abnormalities, ocular hypertelorism, pulmonary stenosis, abnormalities of genitalia, retardation of growth, deafness) syndrome
				Mcdonough syndrome
				Meckel-Gruber syndrome
				Neurofibromatosis
				Noonan syndrome
				Pentalogy of Cantrell
				Prune-belly syndrome
				TTTS
				Weill-Marchesani syndrome
				Williams syndrome
				Williams-Beuren syndrome

References

1. Friedman WF: Aortic stenosis. In: Emmanouilides GC, Riemenschneider TA, Allen HD, et al (eds): Moss and Adams' Heart Disease in Infants, Children, and Adolescents: Including the Fetus and Young Adult, 5th ed, vol II. Baltimore, Williams & Wilkins, 1995, pp 1087–1110.

2. Brown JW, Ruzmetov M, Vijay P, et al: Surgery for aortic stenosis in children: A 40-year experience. Ann Thorac Surg 2003; 76:1398–1411.

3. Serratto M, Hastreiter AR, Miller RA: Management of congenital aortic stenosis in children and young adults. Prog Cardiovasc Dis 1965; 8:78–80.

4. Braunwald E, Goldblatt A, Aygen MM, et al: Congenital aortic stenosis. I: Clinical and hemodynamic findings in 100 patients. Circulation 1963; 27:426–462.

5. Marrow AG, Goldblatt A, Aygen MM: Congenital aortic stenosis. II: Surgical treatment and results of operation. Circulation 1963; 27:426–462.

6. Bernhard WF, Keane JF, Fellows KE, et al: Progress and problems in the surgical management of congenital aortic stenosis. J Thorac Cardiovasc Surg 1973; 66:404–419.

7. Mulder DB, Katz RD, Moss AJ, et al: The surgical treatment of congenital aortic stenosis. J Thorac Cardiovasc Surg 1968; 55:786–796.

8. Trinkle JK, Norton JV, Richardson JD, et al: Closed aortic valvotomy and simultaneous correction of associated anomalies in infants. J Thorac Cardiovasc Surg 1975; 69:758–762.

9. Paladini D, Russo M, Palmieri S, et al: Prenatal diagnosis of aortic insufficiency. Ultrasound Obstet Gynecol 1998; 12:355–357.

10. Campbell M: The natural history of congenital aortic stenosis. Br Heart J 1968; 30:514–520.

11. Frank S, Johnson A, Ross J: Natural history of valvular aortic stenosis. Br Heart J 1973; 35:41–45.

12. Mody MR, Mody GT: Serial hemodynamic observations in congenital valvular and subvalvular aortic stenosis. Am Heart J 1975; 89:137–140.

13. McLean KM, Lorts A, Pearl JM: Current treatments for congenital aortic stenosis. Curr Opin Cardiol 2006; 21:200–204.

14. Moller JH, Nakib A, Eliot RS, et al: Symptomatic congenital aortic stenosis in the first year of life. J Pediatr 1966; 69:728–730.

15. Harstreiter AR, Oshima M, Miller RA, et al: Congenital aortic stenosis syndrome in infancy. Circulation 1963; 28:1084–1095.

16. Karl TR, Sano S, Brawn WJ, et al: Critical aortic stenosis in the first month of life: Surgical results in 26 infants. Ann Thorac Surg 1990; 50:105–109.

17. Kirklin JW, Barratt-Boyes BG: Aortic valve disease. In: Kirklin JW, Barratt-Boyes BG (eds): Cardiac Surgery. New York, Churchill Livingstone, 1993, pp 491–500.

18. Strasburger JF, Kugler JD, Cheatham JP, et al: Nonimminologic hydrops fetalis associated with congenital aortic valvular stenosis. Am Heart J 1984; 108:1380–1382.

19. Jouk PS, Rambaud P: Prediction of outcome by prenatal Doppler analysis in a patient with aortic stenosis. Br Heart J 1991; 65:53–54.

20. Ungerleider RM: Congenital aortic stenosis. In: Nichols DG, Cameron DE, Greeley WJ, et al (eds): Critical Heart Disease in Infants and Children. St Louis, Mosby, 1995, pp 649–668.

21. Doty DB, Polansky DB, Jenson GB: Supravalvular aortic stenosis: Repair by extended aortoplasty. J Thorac Cardiovasc Surg 1977; 74:362–365.

22. Babaoglu K, Eroglu AG, Oztunç F, et al: Echocardiographic follow-up of children with isolated discrete subaortic stenosis. Pediatr Cardiol 2006; 27:699–706.

23. Newfeld EA, Muster AJ, Paul MH, et al: Discrete subvalvular aortic stenosis in childhood: Study of 51 patients. Am J Cardiol 1976; 38:53–61.

24. Freedom RM, Fowler RS, Duncan WJ: Rapid evolution from "normal" left ventricular outflow tract to fatal subaortic stenosis in infancy. Br Heart J 1981; 45:605–610.

25. Freedom RM, Dische MR, Rowe RD: Pathologic anatomy of subaortic stenosis and atresia in the first year of life. Am J Cardiol 1977; 39:1035–1040.

26. Stamm ER, Drose JA, Thickman D: The fetal heart. In: Rumack CM, Wilson SR, Charbonneau JW (eds): Diagnostic Ultrasound, vol 2. St Louis, Mosby–Year Book, 1991, pp 800–827.

27. Clark CE, Henry WL, Epstein SE: Familial prevalence and genetic transmission of idiopathic hypertrophic subaortic stenosis. N Engl J Med 1973; 289:709–711.

28. Wright GB, Keane JF, Nadas AS, et al: Fixed subaortic stenosis in the young: Medical and surgical course in 83 patients. Am J Cardiol 1983; 52:830–835.

29. Dyck JD, Freedom RM: Aortic stenosis. In: Freedom RM, Benson LN, Smallhorn JF (eds): Neonatal Heart Disease. London, Springer-Verlag, 1992, 357–373.

30. Nathan M, Rimmer D, del Nido PJ, et al: Aortic atresia or severe left ventricular outflow tract obstruction with ventricular septal defect: Results of primary biventricular repair in neonates. Ann Thorac Surg 2006; 82:2227–2232.

31. Karamlou T, Gurofsky R, Bojcevski A, et al: Prevalence and associated risk factors for

intervention in 313 children with subaortic stenosis. Ann Thorac Surg 2007; 84:900–906.

32. Barrea C, Alkazaleh R, Ryan G, et al: Prenatal cardiovascular manifestations in the twin-to-twin transfusion syndrome recipients and the impact of therapeutic amnioreduction. Am J Obstet Gynecol 2005; 192:892–902.

33. Marino B, Digilio MC: Congenital heart disease and genetic syndromes: Specific correlation between cardiac phenotype and genotype. Cardiovasc Pathol 2000; 9:303–315.

34. Marshall AC, Tworetzky W, Bergersen L, et al: Aortic valvuloplasty in the fetus: Technical characteristics of successful balloon dilation. J Pediatr 2005; 147:535–539.

35. O'Conner WN, Davis JB, Geissler R, et al: Supravalvular aortic stenosis. Arch Pathol Lab Med 1985; 109:179–185.

36. Flaker G, Teske D, Kilman J: Supravalvular aortic stenosis: A 20-year clinical perspective and experience with patch aortoplasty. Am J Cardiol 1983; 51:256–260.

37. Williams JCP, Barratt-Boyes BG, Lowe JB: Supravalvular aortic stenosis. Circulation 1961; 24:1311–1315.

38. Piacentini G, Digilio MC, Sarkozy A, et al: Genetics of congenital heart diseases in syndromic and non-syndromic patients: New advances and clinical implications. J Cardiovasc Med (Hagerstown) 2007; 8:7–11.

39. Latson LA: Aortic stenosis: Valvular, supravalvular, and fibromuscular subvalvular. In: Garson A, Bricker JT, McNamara DG (eds): The Science and Practice of Pediatric Cardiology, vol II. Philadelphia, Lea & Febiger, 1990, pp 1334–1351.

40. Prasad C, Chudley AE: Genetics and cardiac anomalies: the heart of the matter. Indian J Pediatr 2002; 69:321–332.

41. Baram S, McCrindle BW, Han RK, et al: Outcomes of uncomplicated aortic valve stenosis presenting in infants. Am Heart J 2003; 145:1063–1070.

42. Tierney ES, Wald RM, McElhinney DB, et al. Changes in left heart hemodynamics after technically successful in-utero aortic valvuloplasty. Ultrasound Obstet Gynecol 2007; 30:715–720.

43. Wilkins-Haug LE, Tworetzky W, Benson CB, et al: Factors affecting technical success of fetal aortic valve dilation. Ultrasound Obstet Gynecol 2006; 28:47–52.

44. de la Cruz MV, Munoz-Castellanos L, Nadal-Ginard B: Extrinsic factors in the genesis of congenital heart disease. Br Heart J 1971; 33:203–213.

45. Grant RP: The morphogenesis of transposition of the great vessels. Circulation 1962; 26:818–840.

46. Harh JY, William JG, Friedberg DZ, et al: Experimental production of hypoplastic left heart syndrome in the chick embryo. Am J Cardiol 1973; 31:51–56.

47. Haring OM: Cardiac malformations in the rat induced by maternal hypercapnia with hypoxia. Circ Res 1966; 195:445–451.

48. Giloni SH: Cardiac malformations in the chick embryo induced by thalidomide. Toxicol Appl Pharmacol 1973; 25:77–83.

49. Hoffman JIE, Christianson R: Congenital heart disease in a cohort of 19,502 births with long term follow-up. Am J Cardiol 1978; 42:641–647.

50. Nora JJ, Fraser FC, Bear J, et al: Medical Genetics: Principles and Practice, 4th ed. Philadelphia, Lea & Febiger, 1994, p 371.

51. Huhta JC, Carpenter RJ, Moise KJ, et al: Prenatal diagnosis and postnatal management of critical aortic stenosis. Circulation 1987; 75:573–576.

52. Robertson MA, Byrne PJ, Penkoske PA: Perinatal management of critical aortic valve stenosis diagnosed by fetal echocardiography. Br Heart J 1989; 61:365–367.

53. Mäkikallio K, McElhinney DB, Levine JC, et al: Fetal aortic valve stenosis and the evolution of hypoplastic left heart syndrome: patient selection for fetal intervention. Circulation 2006; 113:1401–1405.

54. Achiron R, Malinger F, Zaidel L, et al: Prenatal sonographic diagnosis of endocardial fibroelastosis secondary to aortic stenosis. Prenat Diagn 1988; 8:73–77.

55. Tworetzky W, del Nido PJ, Powell AJ, et al: Usefulness of magnetic resonance imaging of left ventricular endocardial fibroelastosis in infants after fetal intervention for aortic valve stenosis. Am J Cardiol 2005; 96:1568–1570.

56. Stewart PA, Buis-Liem T, Verwey RA, et al: Prenatal ultrasonic diagnosis of familial asymmetric septal hypertrophy. Prenat Diagn 1986; 6:249–250.

57. Paladini D, Russo MG, Vassallo M, et al: Ultrasound evaluation of aortic valve anatomy in the fetus. Ultrasound Obstet Gynecol 2002; 20:30–34.

58. Kawamata K, Watanabe K, Chiba Y, et al: Functional aortic stenosis diagnosed in fetal period. Fetal Diagn Ther 2004; 19:106–110.

59. Brown JW, Robison RC, Waller BF: Transventricular balloon catheter aortic valvotomy in neonates. Ann Thorac Surg 1985; 39:376–378.

60. Dobell AR, Bloss RS, Gibbons JE, et al: Congenital valvular aortic stenosis: Surgical management and long term results. J Thorac Cardiovasc Surg 1981; 81:916–920.

61. Tworetzky W, Wilkins-Haug L, Jennings RW, et al: Balloon dilation of severe aortic stenosis in the fetus: Potential for prevention of hypoplastic left heart syndrome: Candidate selection, technique, and results of successful intervention. Circulation 2004; 110:2125–2131.

62. Lambert EC, Menon VA, Wagner HR, et al: Sudden unexpected death from cardiovascular disease in children. Am J Cardiol 1974; 34:89–90.

63. Glew RH: Sudden death in congenital aortic stenosis: A review of eight cases with an evaluation of premonitory clinical features. Am Heart J 1969; 78:615–625.

64. Pelech AN, Neish SR: Sudden death in congenital heart disease. Pediatr Clin North Am 2004; 51:1257–1271.

65. Rocchini AP, Emmanouilides GC: Pulmonary stenosis: In: Moss and Adams' Heart Disease in Infants, Children, and Adolescents: Including the Fetus and Young Adult, 5th ed, vol 2. Baltimore, Williams & Wilkins, 1995, pp 930–959.

66. Rodriguez-Fernandez HL, Char F, Kelly DT, et al: The dysplastic pulmonic valve and the Noonan syndrome. Circulation 1972; 46(2 Suppl):98–100.

67. Todros T, Paladini D, Chiappa E, et al: Pulmonary stenosis and atresia with intact ventricular septum during prenatal life. Ultrasound Obstet Gynecol 2003; 21:228–233.

68. Kink BW: Pulmonary stenosis. In: Congenital Heart Disease: A Deductive Approach to Its Diagnosis, 2nd ed. Chicago, Year Book Medical, 1985, pp 61–73.

69. Campbell M: Factors in the aetiology of pulmonary stenoses. Br Heart J 1962; 24:625–632.

70. Rose V, Hewitt D, Milner J: Seasonal influences on the risk of cardiac malformations: Nature of the problem and some results from a study of 10,007 cases. Int J Epidemiol 1972; 1:235–244.

71. Nizard J, Bonnet D, Fermont L, et al: Acquired right heart outflow tract anomaly without systemic hypertension in recipient twins in twin-twin transfusion syndrome. Ultrasound Obstet Gynecol 2001; 18:669–672.

72. Herberg U, Gross W, Bartmann P, et al: Long term cardiac follow up of severe twin to twin transfusion syndrome after intrauterine laser coagulation. Heart 2006; 92:95–100.

73. Keith A: The Hunterian lectures on malformations of the heart. Lancet 1990; 2:359–363.

74. Oka M, Angrist GM: Mechanism of cardiac valvular fusion and stenosis. Am Heart J 1967; 74:37–40.

75. Galindo A, Gutierrez-Larraya F, Velasco JM, et al: Pulmonary balloon valvuloplasty in a fetus with critical pulmonary stenosis/atresia with intact ventricular septum and heart failure. Fetal Diagn Ther 2006; 21:100–104.

76. Campbell M: Factors in the aetiology of pulmonary stenosis. Br Heart J 1962; 24:625–632.

77. Copel JA, Gianluigi P, Green J, et al: Fetal echocardiographic screening for congenital heart disease: The importance of the four chamber view. Am J Obstet Gynecol 1987; 157:648–655.

78. Berg C, Kremer C, Geipel A, et al: Ductus venosus blood flow alterations in fetuses with obstructive lesions of the right heart. Ultrasound Obstet Gynecol 2006; 28:137–142.

79. Tulzer G, Arzt W, Franklin RC, et al: Fetal pulmonary valvuloplasty for critical pulmonary stenosis or atresia with intact septum. Lancet 2002; 360:1567–1568.

80. Srinivasan V, Konyer A, Broda JJ, et al: Critical pulmonary stenosis in infants less than 3 months of age: A reappraisal of closed transventricular pulmonary valvotomy. Ann Thorac Surg 1982; 34:46–50.

81. Milo S, Yellin A, Smolinsky A, et al: Closed pulmonary valvotomy in infants under 6 months of age: Report of 14 consecutive cases without mortality. Thorax 1980; 35:814–818.

82. Flyer DC: Report of the New England Regional Infant Cardiac Program. Pediatrics 1980; 65(Suppl):377–461.

83. Galindo A, Gutiérrez-Larraya F, Velasco JM, et al: Pulmonary balloon valvuloplasty in a fetus with critical pulmonary stenosis/atresia with intact ventricular septum and heart failure. Fetal Diagn Ther 2006; 21:100–104.

84. Merrill WH, Shuyman TA, Graham TP, et al: Surgical intervention in neonates with critical pulmonary stenosis. Ann Surg 1987; 205:712–718.

85. Marantz PM, Huhta JC, Mullins CE, et al: Results of balloon valvuloplasty in typical and dysplastic pulmonary valve stenosis: Doppler echocardiographic follow-up. J Am Coll Cardiol 1988; 12:476–479.

86. Stanger P, Cassidy SC, Girod DA, et al: Balloon pulmonary valvuloplasty: Results of the Valvuloplasty and Angioplasty of Congenital Anomalies Registry. Am J Cardiol 1990; 65:775–783.

87. Caspi J, Coles JG, Benson LN, et al: Management of neonatal critical pulmonic stenosis in the balloon valvotomy era. Ann Thorac Surg 1990; 49:273–278.

88. Robida A, Pavcnik D: Perforation of the heart in a newborn with critical valvar pulmonary stenosis during balloon valvuloplasty. Int J Cardiol 1990; 26:111–112.

89. Ladusans EJ, Qureshi SA, Parsons JM, et al: Balloon dilation of critical stenosis of the pulmonary valve. Br Heart J 1990; 49:273–278.

90. Rudolph AM: Congenital Diseases of the Heart. Chicago, Year Book Medical, 1974, pp 360–427.
91. Allan LD, Crawford DC, Sheridan R, et al: Etiology of non-immune hydrops: The value of echocardiography: Br J Obstet Gynaecol 1986; 93:223–225.
92. Fisk N, Galea P: Twin-twin transfusion—As good as it gets. N Engl J Med 2004; 35:182–185.
93. Nora JJ, Torres FG, Sinha AK, et al: Characteristic cardiovascular anomalies of XO Turner's syndrome: XX and XY phenotype and XO/SS Turner mosaic. Am J Cardiol 1970; 25:639–640.
94. Noonan JA: Hypertension with Turner phenotype: A new syndrome with associated congenital heart disease. Arch Pediatr Adolesc Med 1968; 116:373–380.
95. Van Der Havwaert LF, Fryns JP, Dumoulin M, et al: Cardiovascular malformations in Turner's and Noonan's syndrome. Br Heart J 1978; 40:500–505.
96. Maeno YV, Boutin C, Hornberger LK, et al: Prenatal diagnosis of right ventricular outflow tract obstruction with intact ventricular septum, and detection of ventriculocoronary connections. Heart 1999; 81:661–668.

CHAPTER 11

Coarctation of the Aorta

Marisa R. Lydia
Julia A. Drose

Definition

Coarctation of the aorta is a narrowing of a segment of the aortic lumen along the aortic arch, which results in an obstruction to blood flow. In more than 90% of cases, this narrowing is located between the origin of the left subclavian artery and the ductus arteriosus, also known as the aortic isthmus.[1] The severity of the coarctation can range from a slight narrowing of the distal end of the arch to severe hypoplasia of the entire arch.[2]

Three types of coarctation are described according to the location of the aortic narrowing in relation to the ductus arteriosus (Fig. 11–1):

- Preductal coarctation: narrowing occurring proximal to the ductus arteriosus
- Ductal coarctation: narrowing occurring at the level of the ductus arteriosus
- Postductal coarctation: narrowing occurring distal to the ductus arteriosus

Preductal coarctation accounts for approximately 2% of all coarctations. They are seen most commonly in infants and are usually associated with other intracardiac abnormalities. Preductal coarctations occur early in embryological development and are thought to result from decreased blood flow through the left side of the fetal heart.

Ductal and postductal coarctations account for the remaining 98% of coarctations. They are usually an isolated finding, but an association with aortic valve abnormalities has been reported.[3] Ductal and postductal coarctations occur as a result of the presence of abnormal muscular-ductal tissue. This type of coarctation occurs after birth when the ductus arteriosus closes.

A surgical classification system of coarctation, based on the presence or absence of hypoplasia and the association of other intracardiac defects, was developed by Amato et al[4] (Table 11–1).

The most severe form of coarctation is termed "interruption of the aortic arch," carrying a mortality rate of greater than 90% in the neonatal period if left untreated.[5,6] Interruption of the aortic arch is usually classified into three types (Fig. 11–2)[7]:

- Type A: interruption of the arch distal to the left subclavian artery

- Type B: interruption of the arch between the left carotid artery and the left subclavian artery
- Type C: interruption of the arch between the innominate artery and the left carotid artery

The most commonly occurring form of aortic arch interruption is type B, with type C being the least common.[7–10]

Interruption of the aortic arch is also associated with numerous intracardiac defects.

Embryology

Coarctation is a primary developmental defect that results from abnormal development of the embryological left fourth and sixth aortic arches.[11]

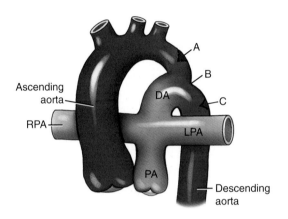

Figure 11–1 Diagram illustrating the different types of coarctation of the aorta. *A,* Preductal; *B,* ductal; *C,* postductal; *DA,* ductus arteriosus; *LPA,* left pulmonary artery; *PA,* main pulmonary artery; *RPA,* right pulmonary artery.

TABLE 11–1 **Surgical Classification of Coarctation of the Aorta**	
Type I	Coarctation with or without patent ductus arteriosus
IA	With ventricular septal defect
IB	With other major cardiac defects
Type II	Coarctation with isthmus hypoplasia, with or without patent ductus arteriosus
IIA	With ventricular septal defect
IIB	With other major cardiac defects
Type III	Coarctation with hypoplasia of isthmus and segment between left carotid and subclavian arteries, with or without patent ductus arteriosus
IIIA	With ventricular septal defect
IIIB	With other major cardiac defects

Adapted from Amato JJ, Galdieri RJ, Cotroneo JV: Role of extended aortoplasty related to the definition of coarctation of the aorta. Ann Thorac Surg 1991; 52:615–620.

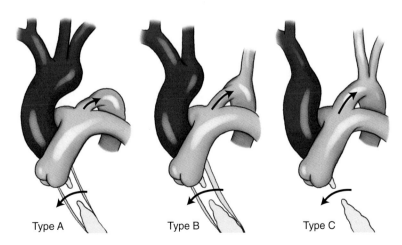

Figure 11–2 Diagram illustrating the different types of interrupted aortic arch. *Type A,* Interruption of the arch distal to the left subclavian artery; *Type B,* interruption of the arch between the left carotid artery and the left subclavian artery; *Type C,* interruption of the arch between the innominate artery and the left carotid artery.

Two theories have been proposed to explain the different types of coarctation. A preductal coarctation is thought to result from decreased blood flow through the left side of the fetal heart, resulting in impaired growth of the isthmus.[12,13] This alteration in hemodynamics can occur as the result of an associated cardiac abnormality or from extracardiac impingement on the ascending aorta.

In a fetus or neonate, the arch normally has a gradual tapering, with the smallest diameter of the arch occurring at the level of the isthmus.[14] In utero, the diameter of the isthmus is approximately two thirds smaller than that of the ascending and descending portions of the aorta. After birth, the ductus arteriosus closes and the isthmus usually enlarges.[15] The smaller size of the isthmus results from the fact that it is the segment of the arch through which the least amount of the combined cardiac output traverses.[16] If blood flow is altered, resulting in the aorta receiving less blood than the ductus arteriosus and pulmonary artery, there may be even further reduction of flow through the isthmus, causing greater tapering of the arch.

One example of this would be a decrease in left ventricular function because of premature narrowing of the foramen ovale. The resulting decrease in left ventricular size would lead to a decrease in left ventricular output and less blood traversing the region of the isthmus, thereby stunting its growth.[17]

A ductal or postductal coarctation is the result of the presence of aberrant ductal tissue in the aortic arch. This extra tissue causes a narrowing of the arch at the time of ductal closure, which results in decreased blood flow to the lower body.[12] In utero, because of the presence of a patent ductus arteriosus, this aberrant tissue is usually inconsequential.

Externally, a coarctation has a localized concavity on its posterolateral surface. Internally, the lumen is smaller because of asymmetry of the aortic wall. This eccentric shelf narrows the lumen from the superior wall opposite the orifice of the ductus arteriosus. As the ductus arteriosus closes, it increases the aortic obstruction by constricting the aortic orifice. There can be thickening of the wall within this area of narrowing. Proximal to the coarctation, the size of the arch may be normal or tubular hypoplasia may be present. Distal to the coarctation, the aortic wall is usually thin and dilated.[7,15]

Occurrence Rate

Coarctation of the aorta accounts for 7% of all congenital heart defects.[18] Coarctation as the primary cardiac lesion has a reported incidence of 6% prenatally. The incidence in stillbirths is 9%.[18,19] These numbers may underestimate the true frequency because coarctations are common components of many types of complex congenital heart disease. Males are affected with coarctation two to three times as frequently as females.[20-22]

In 32% of cases, coarctation is an isolated anomaly. Sixty-eight percent of patients with coarctation have additional anomalies (Table 11–2). These anomalies involve the cardiovascular system (24%), genitourinary system (20%), central nervous system (12%), and skeletal system (6%).[21,23,24] Familial coarctation has been reported in families and siblings. Siblings of an affected child have an occurrence risk estimated at 2%. This risk increases to 6% when two siblings are affected.[24] A woman with a history of coarctation has a 4% chance of having an affected fetus. The risk is 2% when the father is the affected parent. Three percent to 5% of infants of diabetic mothers have coarctation.

Sonographic Criteria

When the diagnosis of coarctation is made in utero or in early infancy, it is easily correctable, but if it goes undetected, irreversible heart failure and acidosis can develop in the neonate.[14,17] Unfortunately, the in utero diagnosis of coarctation can be extremely difficult because of the presence of the ductus arteriosus and the parallel circulation that exists before birth.[13,25-27]

Subtle changes associated with coarctation, such as a narrowing of the aortic arch, may not be apparent even when the arch is well visualized (Fig. 11–3).[14,28]

Indirect signs, such as discrepant ventricular size, with the right ventricle being larger than the left ventricle, are potentially useful for identifying fetuses at risk.[13,14,29,30] However, as pregnancy progresses, the right heart becomes normally larger than the left. Therefore this finding is not as useful in the third trimester.[30] Jung et al[30] reported that 60% of fetuses with right heart enlargement in the second trimester, without clear evidence of coarctation, were found to have a coarctation after birth. In contrast, 86% of fetuses identified as having right heart enlargement in the third trimester had normal hearts at birth.

TABLE 11–2 Conditions Associated with Coarctation and Interrupted Aortic Arch

Maternal		Fetal		
Condition	Drug Use	Associated Cardiac Abnormalities	Chromosome Abnormalities	Syndromes
Diabetes Phenylketonuria Rubella	Alcohol Barbiturates Phenytoin (Dilantin) Primidone	Anomalous origin of contralateral subclavian artery Aortic insufficiency Aortic stenosis Atrial septal defect Atrioventricular septal defect Bicuspid aortic valve Double outlet right ventricle Mitral insufficiency Transposition of the great arteries Wolfe-Parkinson-White syndrome	Monosomy medial 2Q Monosomy 5Q interstitial Monosomy 9 (mosaic) Trisomy 13 (Patau syndrome) Trisomy 18 (Edward syndrome) Trisomy 18P Trisomy 21 (Down syndrome) 45 XO (Turner syndrome)	Achondroplasia Acrocephalosyndactyly, type I Anencephaly Arthrochalasis-multiplex congenital Bernheim syndrome Bourneville-Pringle syndrome Cardiofacial syndrome Cardiofacial syndrome–asymmetric facies Cayler syndrome Chondrodysplasia punctata Crouzon syndrome de Lange syndrome Diaphragmatic hernia DiGeorge syndrome Ehlers-Danlos syndrome Elfin facies syndrome Goldenhar syndrome Halarz syndrome Hirschsprung disease Idiopathic hypercalcemia–supravalvular aortic stenosis Neurofibromatosis Noonan syndrome Oculoauriculo-vertebral anomaly Oropalatal-digital syndrome Pena-Shokeir syndrome Poland syndrome Polycystic kidney disease Polycystic syndrome Pulmonary venolobar syndrome Renal agenesis Scimitar syndrome Shone syndrome Short umbilical cord Thanatophoric dysplasia Tuberous sclerosis Varadi syndrome Venolobar syndrome Williams syndrome Williams-Beuren syndrome

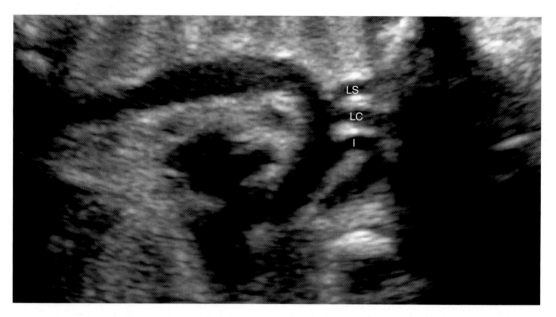

Figure 11–3   Sagittal image of the aortic arch in a fetus diagnosed at birth with coarctation of the aorta. The arch appears normal with no area of narrowing identified. *I,* Innominate artery; *LC,* left carotid artery; *LS,* left subclavian artery.

A fetal echocardiogram should begin with an apical or subcostal four-chamber view to evaluate ventricular size and symmetry. A discrepancy in ventricular size, with the left ventricle appearing smaller than the right ventricle, may be the only sonographic clue that a coarctation is present (Figs. 11–4 and 11–5). In 1994, Hornberger et al[19] studied the prenatal sonograms of 20 infants with coarctation and compared them with 92 normal fetuses (gestational age at initial study ranged from 18 to 36 weeks) to establish criteria that would be helpful in the diagnosis of coarctation. They found a statistically significant difference between right and left ventricular diameter ratios and a difference in ratios when pulmonary artery size was compared with the diameter of the ascending aorta. In their normal group, the mean ratio of right ventricle diameter to left ventricle diameter was around 1.25. In the group with coarctation, this ratio was as high as 2.25. When pulmonary artery diameter was compared with the diameter of the ascending aorta, the mean ratio in the normal controls was again around 1.25. In the group with coarctation, the mean ratio approached 2.[19]

Comparison of pulmonary artery size to that of the ascending aorta can be made in either

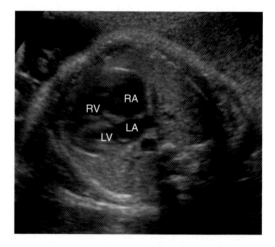

Figure 11–4   Subcostal four-chamber view of the heart in a fetus with coarctation of the aorta showing the right ventricle *(RV)* and right atrium *(RA)* to be larger than the left ventricle *(LV)* and left atrium *(LA).*

a short-axis view of the great vessels or a long-axis view of the aorta and pulmonary artery (Fig. 11–6).

Right ventricular hypertrophy has also been associated with a coarctation, possibly as a result

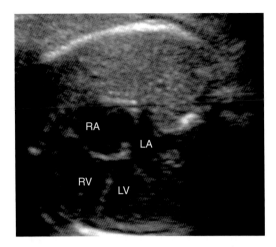

Figure 11–5 Apical four-chamber view in a fetus with coarctation of the aorta showing the right ventricle *(RV)* and right atrium *(RA)* to be larger than the left ventricle *(LV)* and left atrium *(LA)*.

of restricted blood flow through the ductus arteriosus (Fig. 11–7).

Although the aortic arch diameter may appear normal throughout gestation in a fetus with coarctation, it should be evaluated for subtle areas of narrowing (Fig. 11–8). A sagittal view of the fetus through the aortic arch provides visualization of the ascending aorta, transverse arch, isthmus, and descending aorta distal to the ductus (Fig. 11–9). Fetal aortic arch ratios comparing the diameters of normal arches with those of fetuses with coarctation have been established at these levels. The diameters of the transverse aorta and isthmus ratios compared with the ascending aorta were less in fetuses with coarctations. The ratio of the descending aorta to ascending aorta diameter was larger. This is due to the small ascending aorta and possible poststenotic dilation seen with coarctation.

Hornberger et al[19,31] also established normal values for the aortic arch dimensions at different gestational ages (Fig. 11–10). They studied 92 normal fetuses and five fetuses with coarctations. All studies were performed between 16 and 38 weeks' gestation. The largest internal diameter of the aorta was measured at five different levels between the aortic root and the descending aorta. The mean diameter measured at each segment,

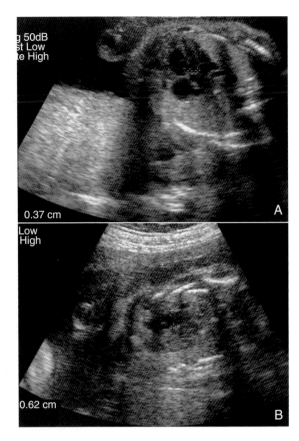

Figure 11–6 Measurements of the ascending aorta **(A)** and pulmonary artery **(B)** in a fetus with coarctation. The pulmonary artery–to–ascending aorta ratio is abnormal at 1.67.

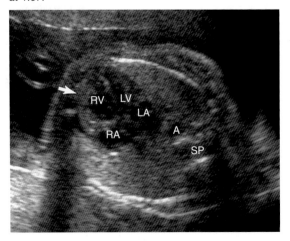

Figure 11–7 An apical four-chamber view of the fetal heart showing right ventricular hypertrophy *(arrow)* in a fetus with coarctation. *A*, Aorta; *LA*, left atrium; *LV*, left ventricle; *RA*, right atrium; *RV*, right ventricle; *SP*, spine.

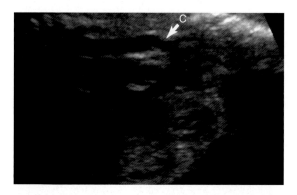

Figure 11–8 View of the aortic arch in a fetus with coarctation of the aorta. A subtle area of narrowing (C) just distal to the left subclavian artery can be appreciated.

regardless of gestational age, for the entire population were as follows:

1. Aortic root: 5 mm
2. Ascending aorta: 4.4 mm
3. Transverse arch: 4.1 mm
4. Isthmus: 3.6 mm
5. Descending aorta: 4.2 mm

These measurements demonstrated a tapering of the aortic arch, with the aortic root diameter being the largest and the isthmus having the smallest diameter. Their results showed that all segments of the aortic arch appeared to grow in a linear fashion.

Beam-width artifact may create the appearance of narrowing in some settings. If a narrowing is seen, pulsed Doppler imaging should be used to confirm an increase in velocity.

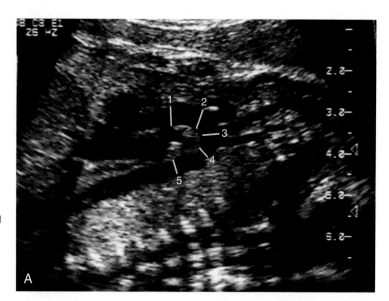

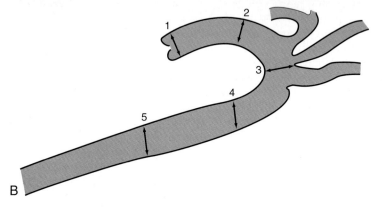

Figure 11–9 Sagittal image of the fetal aortic arch **(A)** and corresponding diagram **(B)** showing sites of measurement of internal diameter. *1*, Aortic root; *2*, ascending aorta; *3*, transverse aorta; *4*, isthmus; *5*, descending aorta.

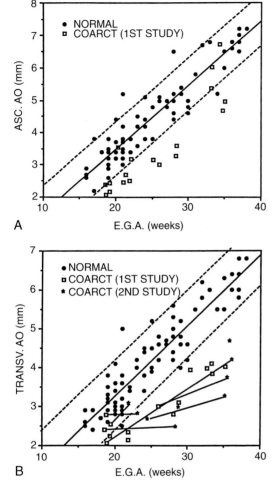

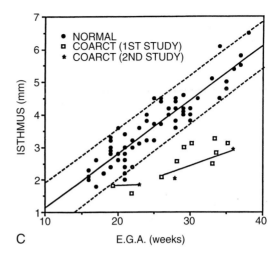

Figure 11–10 Aortic arch dimension versus gestational age. Plots of ascending aorta diameter *(ASC. AO)* **(A),** transverse aortic diameter *(TRANSV. AO)* **(B),** and isthmus diameter **(C)** versus estimated gestational age *(E.G.A.)* in normal fetuses, with line of best fit and the 3rd and 97th percentiles. Superimposed on the graphs are the measurements obtained from 20 fetuses with coarctation *(COARCT).* For the transverse arch and isthmus, measurements from the initial *(open box)* or follow-up *(asterisk)* antenatal studies, or both, are shown. (From Hornberger LK, Sahn DJ, Kleinman CS, et al: Antenatal diagnosis of coarctation of the aorta: A multicenter experience. Reprinted with permission from the American College of Cardiologists. J Am Coll Cardiol 1994; 23:417–423.)

A short-axis view through the great vessels may be helpful in comparing the size of the aortic root with the ductus arteriosus. It is also the appropriate view to evaluate for a bicuspid aortic valve, which can be associated with coarctation (Fig. 11–11).[28,32]

The three-vessel trachea view is also advocated as helping to make the diagnosis of coarctation.[27] This allows a side-by-side comparison of the aortic and ductal arch diameters.

Abnormal levorotation of the heart (>57 degrees) has also been reported in fetuses with coarctation.[33]

In utero identification of an interrupted aortic arch may be more straightforward.[9] The normal arch follows a continuous, smooth curvature from its ascending to its descending portion. When the arch is interrupted, however, the ascending aorta has a straight course to its branches (Fig. 11–12). Type B interruptions (between the left carotid and left subclavian arteries) present with the straight ascending aorta bifurcating into the innominate and left carotid arteries, with the carotid artery pointing toward the neck.[34] When the arch is interrupted distal to the left subclavian artery (type A), the ascending aorta exhibits a slight curvature and has three branches arising from it—the innominate, left carotid, and left subclavian arteries. Also, with an interrupted aortic arch, the ascending aorta and aortic root are consistently small. A short-axis view through the great vessels allows comparison between the aortic root and the pulmonary artery (Fig. 11–13). One final two-dimensional feature of an interrupted aortic arch (as with preductal coarctations) is that a ventricular septal defect is almost always present,

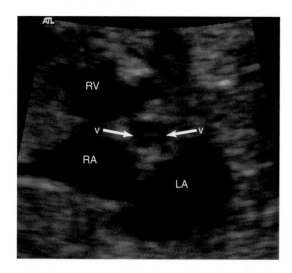

Figure 11–11   Appearance of a bicuspid aortic valve *(v)* in a short-axis view of the great vessels. The two leaflets of the valve can be seen coapting, forming a straight line *(arrows)*. *LA,* Left atrium; *RA,* right atrium; *RV,* right ventricle.

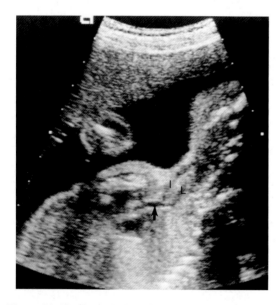

Figure 11–12   Sagittal view of a fetus with a type B interruption of the aortic arch. The interrupted arch follows a straight course *(arrow)* bifurcating into the innominate *(I)* and left carotid *(L)* arteries.

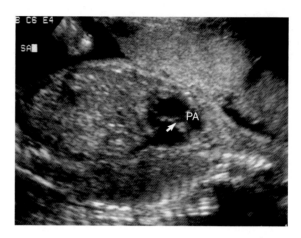

Figure 11–13   Short-axis view of the great vessels in a fetus with an interrupted aortic arch. The aortic root *(arrow)* is very small compared with the pulmonary artery *(PA)*.

occurring in about 50% of type A and more than 90% of type B interruptions.[35-38]

Prominence of the head and neck vessels arising from the aortic arch may be appreciated in cases of severe coarctation or in type A aortic arch interruptions, as a result of blood flow taking the path of least resistance.

Use of pulsed and color Doppler imaging may also be helpful. In fetuses with coarctation, Doppler velocities may be increased distal to the coarctation (Fig. 11–14).[5] In some cases, flow may be retrograde.[16] Decreased velocities may be seen just proximal to the lesion. If a high velocity is seen, it is very important to confirm that the sample volume is in the aortic arch and not the ductus arteriosus or a branch of the pulmonary artery. Because these structures lie in close proximity, it can be difficult to place the pulsed Doppler cursor directly in the aortic arch. This is a very important distinction because fetuses will usually tolerate coarctations well in utero, but a constricted ductus can result in in utero death.

Color Doppler imaging is useful for assessing the arch in its entirety and for identifying areas of increased velocity or turbulence (Fig. 11–15). It may also be helpful in illuminating areas of narrowing within the arch or, in the case of an interrupted aortic arch, a blind ending. Once again, however, it should be stressed that the aortic arch may appear absolutely normal, even when a coarctation is present.

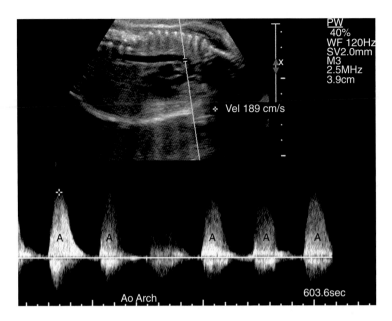

Figure 11-14 Pulsed Doppler tracing in a fetus with coarctation. The Doppler cursor is placed in the aorta, just distal to the left subclavian artery. An increased peak systolic velocity of 189 cm/second is appreciated.

A conservative approach would be to recommend a postnatal echo for any fetus with cardiac asymmetry in the second trimester. Many of these fetuses will not have a coarctation at follow-up, which should be emphasized to expectant parents. However, it should also be borne in mind that clinical or echographic signs of coarctation may not be evident until after closure of the ductus arteriosus.[30] Some centers have advocated following neonates in whom cardiac asymmetry was present in utero until they are 1 year of age.[13]

Treatment

The first line of treatment with coarctation is usually digoxin and diuretics to control congestive heart failure. Prostaglandin E may be initially used to maintain ductus arteriosus patency.[12] If medical therapy is ineffective, particularly in infants with an associated lesion such as a ventricular septal defect, immediate surgery is indicated.[4] Patients with mild coarctations may not require surgical repair.[33] Coarctation repair delayed beyond infancy has a reported correlation with increased chronic hypertension.[28,39]

Surgical management varies depending of the age of the patient, the severity of the coarctation, and the presence of associated abnormalities. Repair may be accomplished with one procedure or two depending on the extent of surgery required.[40]

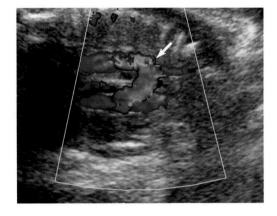

Figure 11-15 Sagittal view of the aortic arch in a fetus with a coarctation with color Doppler imaging showing an area of increased velocity *(arrow)* distal to the left subclavian artery.

The preferred method of surgical repair of coarctation has been to resect the aorta at the site of the coarctation, to remove the narrowed portion through a left lateral thoracotomy.[25,39] The two open ends are then reconnected in an end-to-end anastomosis of the vessel. End-to-side anastomoses are also used (Fig. 11–16). If the coarctation involves a long segment of the aorta, a patch

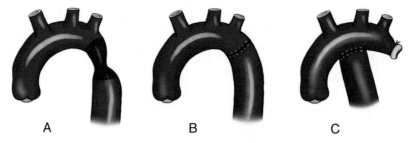

A   B   C

Figure 11–16 Diagram showing end-to-end and end-to-side repair of coarctation of the aorta. The narrowed area of the aorta **(A)** is resected and the ends of the normal caliber aorta are sewn together **(B)**. If an end-to-side repair is performed **(C)**, the narrowed portion of the aorta is resected and tied off. The aortic arch is then sewn to the descending aorta.

augmentation may be performed. This technique involves cutting across the obstruction and augmenting the area with a patch of prosthetic material.[41] A median sternotomy with use of cardiopulmonary bypass may be necessary for more extensive repair.[13,25]

Balloon angioplasty with or without stent placement is also gaining acceptance as an alternative to surgery in discrete membranous obstruction.[39,42]

Recurrent coarctation has been reported as a complication because of stricture formation at the anastomosis site.[43] This sequela usually occurs after repair of coarctation in young infants and usually within 1 year of operation.[44]

Surgical treatment for an interrupted aortic arch usually is an end-to-end anastomosis to bridge the gap.[44] Other surgical treatments include a turn up or turn down of one of the arch vessels to the aorta across the gap or bypassing the interruption with a prosthetic graft.[43]

Prognosis

Coarctation of the aorta is easily correctable when the diagnosis is made early but can be devastating if it goes undetected.[14] Neonates with severe coarctation or interrupted aortic arch frequently develop irreversible heart failure and acidosis.[1] Without surgery, 50% of these infants die during the first month of life, and greater than 80% die by 3 months of age.[13,41,44–46] Restenosis of the aorta at the site of repair may occur in up to 50% of cases. Survival after coarctation of the aorta depends on the presence of other cardiac malformations.[12] However, morbidity and mortality rates associated with coarctation repair are usually minimal.[45]

Affected children who progress to adulthood before symptoms appear have an average life expectancy of 35 years, with 60% to 70% dying by age 40 years. The cause of death in these individuals is most often rupture of the ascending aorta, intracranial hemorrhage, bacterial endocarditis, or congestive heart failure.[16,43] The mortality rate was higher in patients with preductal coarctations (32%) compared with postductal or juxtaductal locations (3%).[32]

Associated Anomalies

In most cases, coarctation is associated with other cardiac malformations (see Table 11–2). The most frequently associated lesion is a bicuspid aortic valve, occurring in 70% to 80% of cases. This often results in aortic stenosis.[15] As stated previously, ventricular septal defects are commonly found in conjunction with preductal coarctations as well as an interrupted aortic arch.[40,44] An association with persistent left superior vena cava (PLSVC) has also been reported. However, this may be a coincidental finding in that PLSVC can result in increased right heart size, which is also seen in the setting of coarctation. A direct relationship between the two has not been established.[13] Other associated cardiac anomalies include atrial septal defects, atrioventricular septal defects, hypoplastic left heart syndrome, and Shone complex.[27]

Coarctations occur in a variety of syndromes and chromosomal defects. The most common is Turner syndrome (XO), occurring in about 12% of patients.[47] An interesting theory regarding this association suggests that the distended lymphatics seen with Turner syndrome compress the developing aortic root, resulting in decreased blood flow.

This in turn leads to left-sided defects, including coarctation.[29] Trisomies 13, 18, and 21 and numerous syndromes also have a reported association. Therefore, genetic counseling and amniocentesis are warranted when a coarctation is detected in utero.

Several noncardiac anomalies have also been reported, including short umbilical cord, renal agenesis, polycystic kidney disease, horseshoe kidney, circle of Willis aneurysms, and tracheoesophageal fistula.[15,23,24] Coarctation of the aorta has also been associated with maternal ingestion of phenytoin and valproic acid and with maternal phenylketonuria and diabetes mellitus.

References

1. Waldhausen JA, Pae WE Jr: Thoracic great vessels. In: Welch KJ, Randolph JF, Ravitch MM, et al (eds): Pediatric Surgery. Chicago, Year Book Medical, 1986, pp 1399–1419.
2. Allan LD, Chita SK, Anderson RH, et al: Coarctation of the aorta in prenatal life: An echocardiographic, anatomical, and functional study. Br Heart J 1988; 59:356–360.
3. Hornberger LK: Aortic arch anomalies. In: Lindsey A, Lisa H, Gurleen S (eds): Textbook of Fetal Cardiology. London, Greenwich Medial Media, 2000, pp 307–331.
4. Amato JJ, Galdieri RJ, Cotroneo JV: Role of extended aortoplasty related to the definition of coarctation of the aorta. Ann Thorac Surg 1991; 52:615–620.
5. Salcedo E: Congenital Heart Disease: Atlas of Echocardiography, 2nd ed. Philadelphia, WB Saunders, 1985, pp 316–317.
6. Van Praagh R, Bernhard WF, Rosenthal A, et al: Interrupted aortic arch: Surgical treatment. Am J Cardiol 1971; 27:200–211.
7. Higgins CB, Silverman NH, Kersting-Sommerhoff BA, et al: Thoracic aortic abnormalities. In: Higgins CB, Silverman NH, Kersting-Sommerhoff BA (eds): Congenital Heart Disease. Echocardiography and Magnetic Resonance Imaging. New York, Raven Press, 1990, pp 292–293.
8. Wigglesworth JS, Singer DB: The Cardiovascular System: Textbook of Fetal and Perinatal Pathology. Boston, Blackwell Scientific, 1991, pp 725–729.
9. Menahem S, Rahayoe AU, Brawn WJ, et al: Interrupted aortic arch in infancy: A 10 year experience. Pediatr Cardiol 1992; 13:214–221.
10. Sell JE, Jonas RA, Mayer JE, et al: The results of a surgical program for interrupted aortic arch. J Thorac Cardiovasc Surg 1988; 96:864–877.
11. Beekman RH, Riemanschneider TA, Emmanouilides GC: Coarctation of the aorta. In: Moss and Adams' Heart Disease in Infants, Children and Adolescents, ed 5. Baltimore, Lippincott Williams & Wilkins, 1995, pp 1111–1133.
12. Bianchi DW, Crombleholme TM, D'Alton ME: Coarctation of the aorta. Fetology 2000; 46:365–369
13. Head CEG, Jowett VC, Sharland GK, et al: Timing of presentation and postnatal outcome of infants suspected of having coarctation of the aorta during fetal life. Heart 2005; 91:1070–1074.
14. Benacerraf BR, Saltzman DH, Sanders SP: Sonographic signs suggesting the prenatal diagnosis of coarctation of the aorta. J Ultrasound Med 1989; 8:65–69.
15. Hutchins GM: Coarctation of the aorta explained as a branch point of the ductus arteriosus. Am J Pathol 1971; 63:203–214.
16. Bankl H: Particular malformations: Congenital malformations of the heart and great vessels. In: Synopsis of Pathology, Embryology and Natural History. Baltimore, Urban and Schwarzenberg, 1977, pp 155–159.
17. Elkayam U, Gleicher N: Cardiac problems in pregnancy. In: Elkayam U, Gleicher N (eds): Diagnosis and Management of Maternal and Fetal Disease, 2nd ed. New York, Alan R Liss, 1990, pp 83–85.
18. Rosenthal E: Coarctation of the aorta from the fetus to adult: Curable condition or life long disease process? Heart Online: http://heart.bmj.com/cgi/content/full/91/11/1495. Accessed October 10, 2007.
19. Homberger LK, Sahn DJ, Kleinman CS, et al: Antenatal diagnosis of coarctation of the aorta: A multicenter experience. J Am Coll Cardiol 1994; 23:417–423.
20. Allan LD, Crawford DC, Handerson RH, et al: Spectrum of congenital heart disease detected echocardiographically in prenatal life. Br Heart J 1985; 54:523–526.
21. Ferencz C, Rubin JD, McCarte RJ, et al: Cardiac and noncardiac malformations: Observations in a population based study. Teratology 1987; 35:367–378.
22. Coleman EN: Serious congestive heart disease in infancy. Br Heart J 1965; 27:42–45.
23. Hodes HL, Steinfeld L, Blumenthal S: Congenital cerebral aneurysms and coarctation of the aorta. Arch Pediatr 1959; 76:28–30.
24. Blackburn W: Aorta, coarctation, infantile type. In: Buyse ML (ed): Birth Defects Encyclopedia. Dover, Blackwell Scientific, 1990, pp 157–158.
25. Simpson J: Fetal aortic arch measurements between 14 and 38 weeks' gestation: In-utero

ultrasonographic study. Ultrasound Obstet Gynecol 2006; 16:203.

26. Stos B, Le Bidois J, Fermont L, et al: Is antenatal diagnosis of coarctation of the aorta possible? Arch Mal Coeur Vaiss 2007; 100:428–432.

27. Pasquini L, Mellander M, Seale A, et al: Z-scores of the fetal aortic isthmus and duct: An aid to assessing arch hypoplasia. Ultrasound Obstet Gynecol 2007; 29:628–633.

28. Bharti S, Lev M: Coarctation of the aorta: Fetal or preductal coarctation-tubular hypoplasia of the transverse arch. In: Bharti S, Lev M (eds): The Pathology of Congenital Heart Disease. A Personal Experience with More Than 6300 Congenitally Malformed Hearts, vol 1. Armonk NY, Futura Publishing, 1996, pp 697–710.

29. Loscalzo ML, Van PL, Ho VB: Association between fetal lymphedema and congenital cardiovascular defects in Turner Syndrome. Pediatrics 2005; 115:732–735.

30. Jung E, Hye-Sung W, Lee PR, et al: Clinical implication of isolated right dominant heart in the fetus. Prenat Diagn 2007; 27:695–698.

31. Hornberger LK, Weintraub RG, Pesonen E, et al: Echocardiographic study of the morphology and growth of the aortic arch in the human fetus: Observations related to the prenatal diagnosis of coarctation. Circulation 1988; 86:741–745.

32. Goldberg SJ, Allen HD, Sahn DJ: Coarctation of the aorta. In: Goldberg SJ, Allen HD, Sahn DJ (eds): Pediatric and Adolescent Echocardiography, 2nd ed. Chicago, Year Book Medical, 1980, pp 419–425.

33. Shipp TD, Bromley B, Hornberger LK, et al: Levorotation of the fetal cardiac axis: A clue for the presence of congenital heart disease. Obstet Gynecol 1995; 85:97–102.

34. Riggs TW, Berry TE, Aziz KV, et al: Two-dimensional echocardiographic features of interruption of the aortic arch. Am J Cardiol 1982; 50:1385–1386.

35. Anderson RH, Lenox CC: Morphology of ventricular septal defect associated with coarctation of the aorta. Br Heart J 1983; 50:176–180.

36. Freedom RM, Bain HH, Esplugas E, et al: Ventricular septal defect in interruption of aortic arch. Am J Cardiol 1977; 39:572–575.

37. Higgins CB, French JW, Silverman JF, et al: Interruption of the aortic arch: Preoperative and postoperative clinical, hemodynamic, and angiographic features. Am J Cardiol 1977; 39:563–571.

38. Moene RJ, Oppenheimer-Dekker A, Wenink ACG: Relation between aortic arch hypoplasia of variable severity and central muscular ventricular septal defects. Am J Cardiol 1981; 48:111–116.

39. Giordano U, Giannico S, Turchetta A, et al: The influence of different surgical procedures on hypertension after repair of coarctation. Cardiol Young 2005; 15:477–480.

40. Kanter KR: Management of infants with coarctation and ventricular septal defect. Semin Thorac Cardiovasc Surg 2007; 19:264–268.

41. Shah S, Calderon DM: Aortic coarctation. eMedicine online: www.emedicine.com/med/topic154.htm. Accessed April 2, 2008.

42. Massoud Iel S, Farghly HE, Abdul-Monem A, et al: Balloon angioplasty for native aortic coarctation in different anatomic variants. Pediatr Cardiol 2008; 29:521–529.

43. Hallman GL, Cooley DA, Gutgesell HP: Coarctation of thoracic aorta. In: Hallman GL, Cooley DA (eds): Surgical Treatment of Congenital Heart Disease, 3rd ed. Philadelphia, Lea & Febiger, 1987, pp 33–50.

44. Van Son JAM, Falk V, Schneider P, et al: Repair of coarctation of the aorta in neonates and young infants. J Card Surg 1997; 12:139–146.

45. Alsoufi B, Cal S, Coles JG: Outcomes of different surgical strategies in the treatment of neonates with aortic coarctation and associated ventricular septal defects. Ann Thorac Surg 2007; 84:1331–1336.

46. Hager A, Kanz S, Kaemmerer H, et al: Coarctation long-term assessment (COALA): Significance of arterial hypertension in a cohort of 404 patients up to 27 years after surgical repair of isolated coarctation of the aorta, even in the absence of restenosis and prosthetic material. J Thorac Cardiovasc Surg 2007; 134:738–745.

47. Ho VB, Bakalov VK, Cooley M, et al: Major vascular anomalies in Turner syndrome: Prevalence and magnetic resonance angiographic features. Circulation 2004; 110:1694–1700.

CHAPTER 12

Ebstein Anomaly

Elizabeth R. Stamm

OUTLINE

Definition
Embryology
Occurrence Rate
Sonographic Criteria
Treatment
Prognosis
Associated Anomalies

Definition

Ebstein anomaly is defined as the displacement of the tricuspid valve leaflets from their normal location at the atrioventricular junction into the right ventricle. This results in a reduction in the size of the functional right ventricle caused by "atrialization" of the right ventricular inlet.

Ebstein anomaly is characterized by apical displacement of the septal, and usually the posterior, leaflet of the tricuspid valve into the right ventricle.[1] The degree of this displacement is inconsistent.[2] In addition, the septal and posterior leaflets of the tricuspid valve are adherent to the ventricular wall to a variable degree so that the relatively small, mobile portions of the leaflets may reside deep within the right ventricle. If there is substantial adherence of the leaflets to the right ventricular wall, only a small part of the valve cusps will be free to move. This contributes to tricuspid insufficiency.

The anterior leaflet is not displaced and may be relatively normal, although it is generally enlarged and redundant and has been described as sail-like in appearance.

The maximal amount of valve displacement occurs at the crux cordis, the commissure between the septal and posterior leaflets (Fig. 12–1). This inferior displacement of the tricuspid valve results in "atrialization" of the inflow portion of the right ventricle so that it behaves functionally like part of the right atrium. This atrialized portion of the right ventricle may have little or no residual myocardium and may closely resemble the right atrium associated with Uhl malformation. Frequently the right atrium is severely dilated. The nonatrialized apical portion of the right ventricle generally demonstrates a normal wall thickness but may be dilated.

In addition to the displacement, some degree of tricuspid dysplasia is virtually always present in the neonatal expression of Ebstein anomaly. This dysplasia may range from mild to severe.[2,3]

Last, the distal attachments of the anterior and septal leaflets of the tricuspid valve may be abnormal with thickened chordae and abnormal linear attachments between the valve cusps and the trabecula of the right ventricle, tethering the leaflet to the ventricular wall.[1] When there are numerous linear attachments, functional tricuspid stenosis can result. In its most severe form, this can mimic tricuspid atresia and has been termed the imperforate type of Ebstein anomaly.[4-6] In most cases of Ebstein anomaly, however, the displacement, dysplasia, and abnormal distal attachments of the tricuspid valve result in tricuspid insufficiency, which causes further enlargement of the right atrium and the right ventricle.

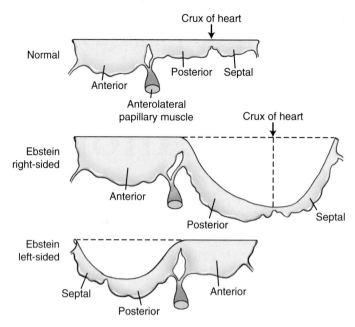

Figure 12–1 Diagram of the tricuspid valve opened out to show leaflets in a single plane. In both right-sided and left-sided Ebstein anomaly, the point of maximal displacement is at the commissure between the septal and posterior leaflets. This commissure is normally situated at the crux of the heart.

Ebstein anomaly is one of the few congenital heart defects to cause significant cardiac dysfunction in utero, frequently with resultant severe cardiomegaly, hydrops fetalis, and tachyarrhythmias.[7]

Embryology

The tricuspid valve leaflets and chordae tendineae are believed to be formed by undermining of the inner layers of the right ventricular inlet, a process called delamination (Fig. 12–2).[8] The valve leaflets and chordae tendineae are initially muscular structures but later develop fibrous components. The posterior and septal leaflets are formed at 12 to 16 weeks' gestation. In Ebstein anomaly, the delamination process is faulty, resulting in the abnormal apical insertion of the septal and posterior tricuspid valve leaflets at the junction of the inlet and trabecular portions of the right ventricle. The anterior leaflet is formed much earlier in embryological development and also has a muscular origin. It may contain various amounts of muscle and can even consist of a complete muscular diaphragm between the inlet and apical portions of the right ventricle. Zuberbuhler et al[4]

suggested that the anterosuperior leaflet arises from the trabecula septomarginalis.

Occurrence Rate

Ebstein anomaly is one of the less common congenital heart defects, accounting for 3% to 7% of cases of congenital heart disease in the fetal population.[9,10] It occurs in approximately 1 in 20,000 live births[11] and makes up 0.5% of congenital cardiac disease cases.[12] Males and females are affected equally.[13] Although the anomaly generally appears sporadically, there have been reports of familial Ebstein anomaly.[14–18] The risk of occurrence when one sibling is affected is approximately 1%.[19]

Ebstein anomaly has been associated with maternal ingestion of lithium carbonate, a first-line drug used to treat manic-depressive psychosis, suggesting that lithium is a specific teratogen.[11,20–24] Most data supporting this view came from the Danish Registry, in which more than 200 "lithium babies" (normal or congenitally abnormal babies born to mothers who ingested lithium during the first trimester of pregnancy) were registered. In this group, there was a 10% incidence of congenital

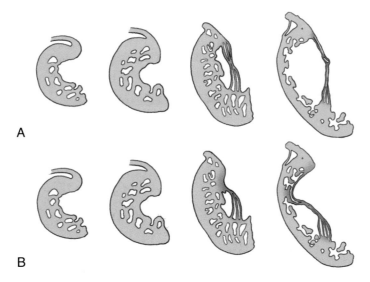

Figure 12–2 A, Diagram showing formation of a normal atrioventricular valve cusp. **B,** Diagram showing valve cusp formation in Ebstein anomaly.

heart disease compared with the 0.01% risk in the general population. Importantly, the Danish Registry recorded eight cases of Ebstein anomaly. Because Ebstein anomaly occurs sporadically in 1 in 20,000 live births, this suggested that maternal lithium ingestion increased the risk of Ebstein anomaly 500-fold over the incidence in the general population.

However, this conclusion was faulty because the data collection was biased in this study. Data were collected retrospectively by a voluntary reporting system. Notes were published periodically in general medical and psychiatric journals requesting physicians to report babies born to mothers who had ingested lithium. It would be expected that this design would lead to an over-representation of anomalies because the birth of an abnormal baby usually leads to a detailed history and workup, including inquiries regarding drugs ingested during pregnancy, whereas little attention may be paid to maternal drug use when a normal healthy baby is born. It is reasonable to expect that babies born to mothers who were treated with lithium were more likely to be recognized and reported when they had congenital anomalies.

The first major study that attempted to avoid this bias reported cardiac malformations in 7% of lithium-exposed fetuses but failed to link lithium with Ebstein anomaly.[24]

A case-control study on the association between first-trimester lithium exposure and Ebstein anomaly suggests that, if lithium increases the risk of Ebstein anomaly, the increased risk is not more than 28-fold—substantially less than the 500-fold increase estimated by the data from the lithium registries.[25] More recent retrospective, prospective, and meta-analysis studies failed to show a clear association between Ebstein anomaly and lithium.[26]

Sonographic Criteria

The diagnosis of Ebstein anomaly is readily made in utero.[7,27,28] Oberhoffer et al[28] retrospectively reviewed 19 postmortem cases of Ebstein malformation or tricuspid valvular dysplasia in fetuses who underwent echocardiography between 16 and 37 weeks' gestation. Death occurred between 20 and 40 weeks' gestation, and the time between fetal echocardiography and fetal death ranged from 1 to 12 weeks. This study clearly demonstrates that fetal echocardiography can not only detect but also can reliably differentiate various types of tricuspid valvular disease in utero.

Although an enlarged right atrium may be the first indication that congenital heart disease is present, apical displacement of the tricuspid septal leaflet is the most reliable sign of Ebstein anomaly. This displacement can be recognized by comparing the level of the insertion of the septal leaflet of the tricuspid valve with that of the mitral valve and determining the amount of offset between the two (Fig. 12–3). Several methods have been described to quantify the degree of tricuspid valve displacement. Ports et al[29] compared the mitral valve-to-apex and the tricuspid valve-to-apex distances (Fig. 12–4). This method becomes invalid when the size of either ventricle is abnormal. This group also measured the distance between the displaced tricuspid valve and the atrioventricular groove (Fig. 12–5). Because it is sometimes difficult to localize the atrioventricular groove reliably by ultrasonography, this method can be inaccurate.

Kambe et al[30] described the simplest and most reliable method of determining septal leaflet offset. They simply measured the distance between the septal leaflet of the tricuspid valve and the anterior leaflet of the mitral valve (Fig. 12–6). This can be accomplished in the subcostal or apical four-chamber view.

Because the insertion of the septal leaflet of the tricuspid valve is slightly more apical than that of the anterior mitral valve leaflet in the normal heart, the diagnosis of mild forms of Ebstein anomaly may be difficult. It is important to identify a cutoff value between normal and abnormal offsets. Gussenhover et al[31] determined the minimal and maximal offset of the septal leaflets of the mitral and tricuspid valves anatomically and with echocardiography in fetuses, infants, children, and adults with and without Ebstein anomaly. In the first trimester of pregnancy, it was impossible to detect any offset between the tricuspid and mitral valves in normal fetuses. Thereafter, the distance gradually increased in the normal heart; however, accurate measurements were not established for normal fetuses in the second and third trimesters of pregnancy. In normal infants, the offset was less than 8 mm, in normal children it was less than 15 mm, and in normal adults it was less than 20 mm.[31]

Oberhoffer et al[28] studied a group of fetuses with tricuspid valvular disease between 16 and 37 weeks' gestation. In two fetuses with pathologically proven Ebstein anomaly, the offset was only 5 mm. Displacement varied between 4 and 20 mm in 10 cases of fetal and neonatal Ebstein anomaly in the series of Lang et al.[32]

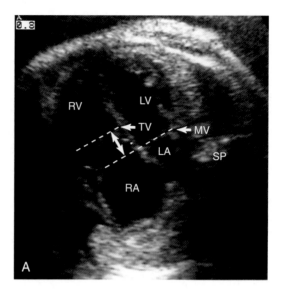

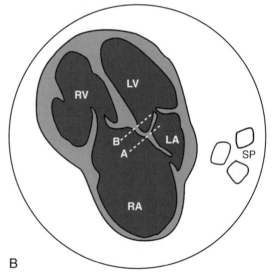

Figure 12–3 **A,** Apical four-chamber view showing inferior displacement of the tricuspid valve *(TV)* resulting in atrialization of the right ventricle *(RV)*. This displacement can be recognized by comparing the level of insertion of the septal leaflet of the tricuspid valve with that of the mitral valve *(MV)*. LA, Left atrium; *LV,* left ventricle; *RA,* right atrium; *SP,* spine. **B,** Diagram representing the same apical four-chamber view as seen in **A,** comparing the displaced level of insertion of the septal leaflet of the tricuspid valve *(B)* with the normal insertion site of the mitral valve leaflet *(A)*. LA, Left atrium; *LV,* left ventricle; *RA,* right atrium; *RV,* right ventricle; *SP,* spine.

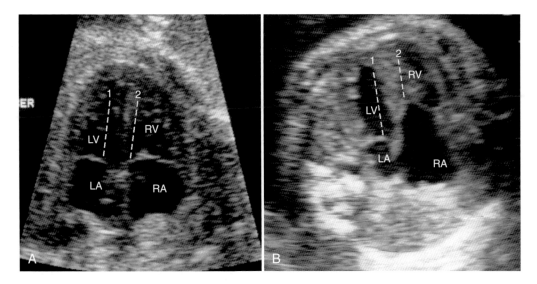

Figure 12–4 Apical four-chamber view, measuring the mitral valve-to-apex distance *(1)* and the tricuspid valve-to-apex distance *(2)* in a normal heart **(A)** and a heart with Ebstein anomaly **(B)**. *LA,* Left atrium; *LV,* left ventricle; *RA,* right atrium; *RV,* right ventricle.

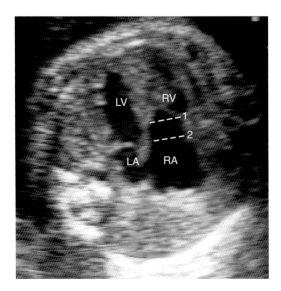

Figure 12–5 Apical four-chamber view showing the method of measuring the distance between the displaced tricuspid valve *(1)* and the atrioventricular groove *(2)*. *LA,* Left atrium; *LV,* left ventricle; *RA,* right atrium; *RV,* right ventricle.

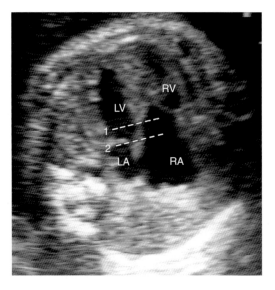

Figure 12–6 Apical four-chamber view measuring the distance between the displaced septal leaflet of the tricuspid valve *(1)* and the anterior leaflet of the mitral valve *(2)*. *LA,* Left atrium; *LV,* left ventricle; *RA,* right atrium; *RV,* right ventricle.

In the normal heart, the offset between the septal insertions of the mitral and tricuspid valves is maximized, with anterior angulation best visualized in the subcostal four-chamber view. In the heart with Ebstein anomaly, this relationship is reversed so that the offset of the atrioventricular valves is accentuated with posterior angulation of the subcostal four-chamber view.[31] This observation is important and can be particularly helpful in the diagnosis of milder forms of Ebstein anomaly (Fig. 12–7).

In some instances, a four-chamber view may appear normal in the setting of milder forms of Ebstein anomaly if the tricuspid valve orifice is mistaken for the valve itself (Fig. 12–8, *A*). This error is easily avoided by angling posteriorly in the four-chamber view and identifying the actual insertion site of the septal leaflet (Fig. 12–8, *B*).

Another common finding with Ebstein anomaly is severe levorotation of the fetal heart. The enlarged right atrium often associated with Ebstein anomaly causes the heart to rotate into an almost horizontal orientation within the fetal chest (Fig. 12–9).

Because some degree of tricuspid valve dysplasia is always present in Ebstein anomaly, the tricuspid valve must be carefully evaluated for signs of dysplasia, such as valvular thickening or nodularity (Fig. 12–10). The abnormal distal tricuspid valve attachments associated with Ebstein anomaly may be recognized on fetal echocardiogram by noting numerous accessory attachments, thickened chordae, or both. Frequently, tethering of the tricuspid valve is best visualized on the subcostal four-chamber view.

Right atrial enlargement is frequently severe in the setting of Ebstein anomaly. More subtle right atrial enlargement can be recognized by comparing the right and left atria. In the normal heart, the atria appear of equal size on ultrasonography. Any obvious size discrepancy should be considered abnormal (Figs. 12–11 and 12–12).

Careful evaluation of the right ventricle should always be performed when Ebstein anomaly is suspected. This may reveal some degree of right ventricular dysplasia manifested by right ventricular dilation, decreased wall thickness, dyskinesia, or a combination of these conditions (Fig. 12–13).

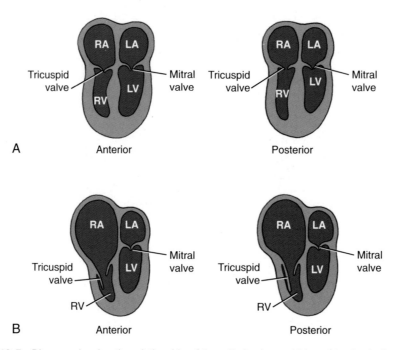

Figure 12–7 Diagram showing the relationship of the mitral valve and tricuspid valve in the normal heart **(A)** with anterior and posterior angulation of the transducer and in the heart with Ebstein anomaly **(B)**. *LA,* Left atrium; *LV,* left ventricle; *RA,* right atrium; *RV,* right ventricle.

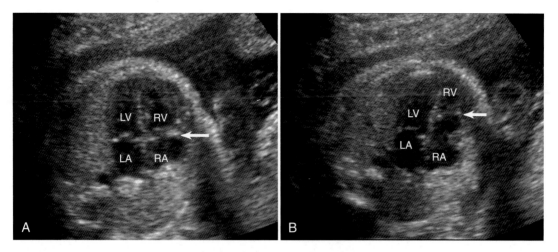

Figure 12–8 Apical four-chamber view of a fetal heart with Ebstein anomaly. **A,** An anterior angulation of the transducer gives the appearance of a normal four-chamber view, with the tricuspid valve annulus *(arrow)* mimicking the tricuspid valve. **B,** By angling the transducer more posteriorly, the actual tricuspid valve *(arrow)* is seen displaced apically, resulting in atrialization of the right ventricle *(RV)*. *LA,* Left atrium; *LV,* left ventricle; *RA,* right atrium.

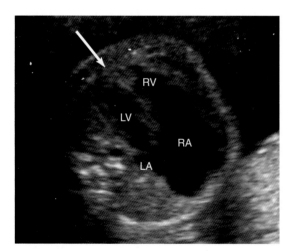

Figure 12–9 Severe levorotation of the fetal heart as a result of Ebstein anomaly. The heart is positioned horizontally in the chest, with the apex *(arrow)* pointing directly leftward. *LA,* Left atrium; *LV,* left ventricle; *RA,* right atrium; *RV,* right ventricle.

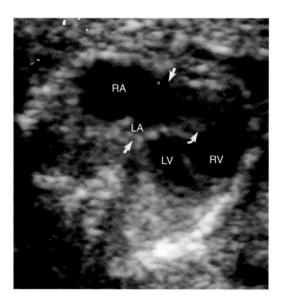

Figure 12–10 Subcostal four-chamber view in a fetus with Ebstein anomaly showing a thickened, displaced septal leaflet *(curved arrow)* of the tricuspid valve. *Straight arrows* mark the area of the atrioventricular groove. The right atrium *(RA)* is markedly enlarged and is compressing the left atrium *(LA)*. *LV,* Left ventricle; *RV,* right ventricle.

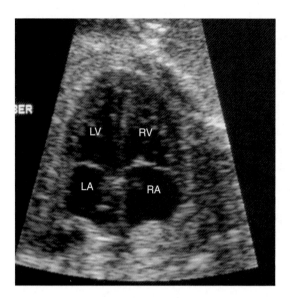

Figure 12–11 Comparison of the left atrium *(LA)* and the right atrium *(RA)* in an apical four-chamber view of a normal fetal heart. The atria appear to be of nearly equal size. *LV,* Left ventricle; *RV,* right ventricle.

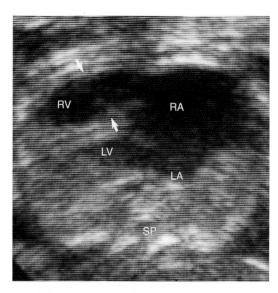

Figure 12–13 Subcostal four-chamber view of a fetal heart with Ebstein anomaly showing the decreased wall thickness of the right ventricle *(RV)* compared with that of the left ventricle *(LV).* Also noted is the dilated right atrium *(RA),* which is compressing the left atrium *(LA),* and the displaced leaflets *(arrows)* of the tricuspid valve. *SP,* Spine.

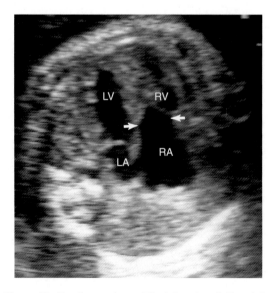

Figure 12–12 Comparison of the left atrium *(LA)* and the enlarged right atrium *(RA)* in an apical four-chamber view of a fetal heart with Ebstein anomaly. There is a discrepancy in the size of the atria resulting from displacement of the tricuspid valve *(arrows)* and compression of the left atrium by the enlarged right atrium. *LV,* Left ventricle; *RV,* right ventricle.

With right ventricular enlargement, paradoxical septal motion may result in alterations in left ventricular size and geometry because the interventricular septum compresses the left ventricle. This important finding can be associated with a poor outcome.

When the diagnosis of Ebstein anomaly is made, it is essential to search for complications. Arrhythmias, particularly supraventricular tachycardias, are common. Tricuspid insufficiency is almost always present (Fig. 12–14, *A* and *B*). Signs of hydrops fetalis such as pleural or pericardial effusions, ascites, and skin thickening may be present in severe cases, suggesting a poor outcome. As with any congenital heart defect, associated cardiac anomalies should be excluded. There is a high incidence of pulmonary atresia or stenosis in the setting of Ebstein anomaly.

Ebstein anomaly may be confused with several other entities, including Uhl anomaly, tricuspid valvular dysplasia or atresia, and idiopathic right atrial enlargement. Although all these anomalies are associated with an enlarged right atrium, the

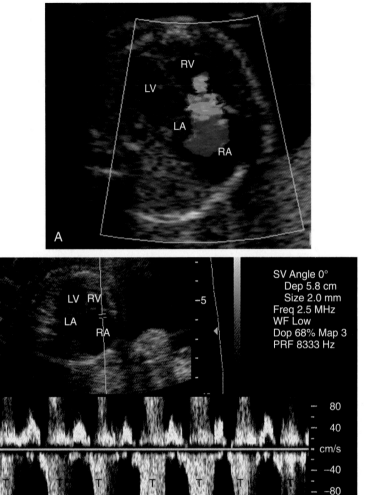

Figure 12–14 Massive tricuspid insufficiency associated with Ebstein anomaly. **A,** Color Doppler imaging of the regurgitant jet filling a significant portion of the dilated right atrium. **B,** Pulsed Doppler cursor placed in the dilated right atrium, showing tricuspid insufficiency below the baseline *(T)* occurring throughout systole. *LA,* Left atrium; *LV,* left ventricle; *RA,* right atrium; *RV,* right ventricle.

tricuspid valve is not inferiorly displaced in any of them.

Ebstein anomaly is one of the few congenital malformations that frequently causes in utero cardiac dysfunction, resulting in cardiomegaly, hydrops fetalis, and tachyarrhythmias. Because these abnormalities are easily identified by obstet-rical ultrasonography, Ebstein anomaly is frequently diagnosed in utero.

In summary, the following checklist can be used for the echocardiographic evaluation of suspected Ebstein anomaly:

- Is cardiomegaly present?
- Is the right atrium enlarged?

- Is severe levocardia present?
- Is the tricuspid valve abnormal?
  - Apical displacement of the septal leaflet?
  - Enlarged sail-like anterior leaflet?
  - Tricuspid valvular dysplasia?
  - Tethering of the tricuspid leaflets with abnormal distal attachments?
  - Tricuspid valvular insufficiency or regurgitation?
- Is the right ventricle abnormal?
  - Right ventricular dilation?
  - Right ventricular dyskinesia?
  - Decreased right ventricular wall thickness?
- Is there paradoxical septal motion?
- Is there left ventricular compression?
- Is there an arrhythmia?
- Are there signs of failure or hydrops fetalis?
- Are additional cardiac or noncardiac anomalies present?

Treatment

When the diagnosis of Ebstein anomaly is made in utero, the fetus should be monitored closely for progression of cardiac dysfunction with resultant cardiomegaly, hydrops fetalis, and tachyarrhythmia. The latter has been treated successfully in the fetus. Left untreated, these arrhythmias may result in new or worsening hydrops fetalis, which is an ominous sign associated with a poor prognosis.[33,34]

Delivery at an appropriate center with a neonatal intensive care unit, pediatric cardiologist, and pediatric anesthesiologist should be arranged. A treatment plan including resuscitation, medical therapy, and the options for surgical intervention should be discussed before delivery.

Even neonates with massive cardiomegaly, cyanosis, and congestive heart failure may improve dramatically with the decrease in pulmonary vascular resistance that occurs after birth, and they may remain stable for long periods. Alternatively, aggressive resuscitation including intubation with mechanical ventilation, administration of prostaglandins to maintain ductal patency and adequate pulmonary blood flow, bicarbonate infusion to reverse metabolic acidosis, and aggressive treatment of arrhythmias may be necessary in the neonate.

Although numerous reports in the literature have been devoted to the surgical correction of Ebstein anomaly, almost all patients were beyond the neonatal period at the time they underwent surgery. The youngest patient to be treated surgically in the extensive Mayo Clinic series was 11 months of age, and death resulted.[35]

Patients who survive the neonatal period may remain asymptomatic for a long time, requiring little or no treatment.[36,37]

When severe right ventricular outflow tract obstruction or atresia is present, palliative surgical procedures such as a Blalock-Taussig shunt or Glenn anastomosis may be useful in older infants or children.[38,39] In the past, many investigators favored tricuspid valve replacement with repair of the atrial septum and plication of a portion of the atrialized right ventricle.[40-42] Reports of tricuspid valvuloplasty alone have been encouraging.[43,44] Recently, catheterization techniques with radiofrequency ablation have been used to destroy the accessory pathways that predispose patients with Ebstein anomaly to supraventricular tachycardia.[45,46]

The overall surgical mortality rate in children and adults who have had surgical repair for Ebstein anomaly has dropped to less than 3%.[47]

For patients with severe forms of Ebstein anomaly that are not amenable to surgical correction or for individuals with numerous associated congenital cardiac anomalies, conventional surgical correction may be unrealistic and heart transplantation may be the only option.

Prognosis

The overall prognosis for fetuses diagnosed with Ebstein anomaly in utero is extremely poor. The majority of the literature has been devoted to the study of Ebstein anomaly in children and adults, in whom the prognosis is frequently excellent.[48] Only a few studies provide detailed information regarding the poor prognosis for fetuses diagnosed with Ebstein anomaly.

Hornberger et al[27] reviewed the fetal echocardiograms of 26 fetuses diagnosed in utero with tricuspid valvular disease and significant regurgitation in utero. Seventeen fetuses had Ebstein anomaly, and therapeutic abortion was performed in three of these cases. Of the remaining group with Ebstein anomaly, 44% died in utero, 36% of those who survived delivery died in the first 2 weeks of life, and only 3 of 14 infants survived beyond the neonatal period and were doing well at 3, 4, and 5 years of age. The overall mortality rate for fetuses diagnosed with Ebstein anomaly in utero in this study was approximately 80%. Hornberger et al[27] noted a high incidence of pulmonary hypoplasia in fetuses who died, with lung weights approximately half of that expected for body weight. This observation has been made with severe cardiomegaly, which presumably inhibits lung growth,[32,49] and in fetuses with right-sided abnormalities associated with reduced pulmonary flow or decreased pulmonary artery size.[50] It is well documented that Ebstein anomaly is frequently associated with pulmonary atresia with an intact ventricular septum[51,52] and with massive cardiomegaly. Therefore it is not surprising that the incidence of associated pulmonary hypoplasia is high in this fetal population. In their series, Lang et al[32] identified severe obstruction at the level of the pulmonary valve in 40% of the fetuses and neonates with Ebstein anomaly. This was associated with a high incidence of relatively small lungs.

In another study of 16 consecutive patients (five fetuses and 11 neonates) with Ebstein anomaly, Roberson and Silverman[7] identified four morphological features strongly associated with death by 3 months of age. These include the following:

- Tethered distal attachments of the anterior superior leaflet of the tricuspid valve, recognized by three or more accessory attachments between the valve and the right ventricular wall
- Marked right atrial enlargement, with the size of the right atrium being greater than that of the functional right ventricle, left ventricle, and left atrium together
- Dysplasia of the atrialized portion of the right ventricle manifested by decreased wall thickness (2 standard deviations below normal) and right ventricular dyskinesia
- Left ventricular compression with narrowing of the left ventricular outflow tract from leftward bulging of the intraventricular septum, best visualized on the long-axis view of the ventricular outflow tract

These findings are all potentially recognizable in the fetus with careful echocardiography. Roberson and Silverman's study[7] demonstrated an overall 3-month mortality rate of 80% for fetuses diagnosed with Ebstein anomaly in utero. Similar studies documented an equally grim prognosis, with mortality rates of approximately 90% in fetuses diagnosed with Ebstein anomaly in utero.

Because the most severe cases of Ebstein anomaly are often detected in utero and commonly progress during gestation with increasing tricuspid regurgitation, right atrial enlargement, generalized cardiomegaly, fetal hydrops, and lung hypoplasia, it has been suggested that management of the fetus with Ebstein anomaly should include frequent monitoring with fetal echocardiography and early delivery in the mid third trimester before decompensation occurs.[53]

Symptomatic neonates with Ebstein anomaly also have a poor prognosis. Marked cardiomegaly, cyanosis, and a high volume of tricuspid valve regurgitation are all indicative of neonatal death without surgery.[54]

As with other types of congenital heart disease, the prognosis becomes worse when additional cardiac, extracardiac, or chromosomal anomalies are present. This underscores the importance of a thorough obstetrical ultrasonographic examination and fetal karyotyping when the diagnosis of Ebstein anomaly is entertained.

In conclusion, the overall prognosis for fetuses with Ebstein anomaly diagnosed prenatally is extremely poor. Careful echocardiography can detect features associated with a particularly grim prognosis.

Associated Anomalies

Ebstein anomaly may be associated with a wide variety of cardiovascular abnormalities as well as noncardiac and some chromosomal abnormalities (Table 12–1). The association between Ebstein anomaly and pulmonary valvular stenosis or atresia is strong and widely recognized.[51,52,55] This association is almost certainly more common in utero because many of these fetuses do not survive to the neonatal period. In one large series of fetal tricuspid valvular disease, 10 of 16 (>60%) fetuses diagnosed with Ebstein anomaly in utero had an associated abnormality of the pulmonary valve.[9] Atrial septal defects and ventricular septal defects are common in fetuses with Ebstein anomaly.[7,32] Atrial septal defects have been documented in 42% to 60% of children and adolescents with Ebstein anomaly.[15] The prenatal diagnosis of atrial septal defect is difficult because of the normal patency of the foramen ovale in utero, and many will be missed by ultrasonography in this population.[28]

Corrected transposition of the great vessels may occur in the fetus with Ebstein anomaly.[7,9,32] Other

TABLE 12–1 Conditions Associated with Ebstein Anomaly

Maternal		Fetal	
Drug Use	Associated Cardiac Abnormalities	Chromosome Abnormalities	Syndromes
Lithium (?)	Atrial septal defect Coarctation Corrected transposition of the great arteries Pulmonary atresia Pulmonary stenosis Supraventricular tachycardia Tetralogy of Fallot Tricuspid insufficiency Ventricular septal defect	Trisomy 13 (Patau syndrome) Trisomy 21 (Down syndrome)	Craniofacial Digital

lesions, including tetralogy of Fallot, atrioventricular septal defect, and coarctation of the aorta, have been reported with Ebstein anomaly but are less common.

Extracardiac anomalies associated with Ebstein include craniofacial and digital abnormalities.[7] Although the incidence of associated chromosomal anomalies is much higher with some other forms of congenital heart disease, Ebstein anomaly may be associated with abnormal chromosomes, including trisomy 13,[27,32] trisomy 18,[56] and trisomy 21.[7] Obstetrical management must include not only a detailed fetal echocardiogram to rule out associated cardiac anomalies but also amniocentesis for chromosomal evaluation.

References

1. Zuberbuhler JR, Anderson RH: Ebstein's malformation of the tricuspid valve: Morphology and natural history. In: Anderson RH, Park SC, Nechs WH, et al (eds): Perspectives in Pediatric Cardiology, vol 1. Mount Kisco, NY, Futura, 1988, pp 99–112.
2. Anderson KR, Zuberbuhler JR, Anderson RG, et al: Morphologic spectrum of Ebstein's anomaly of the heart: A review. Mayo Clin Proc 1979; 54:174–180.
3. Becker AE, Becker MJ, Edwards JE: Pathologic spectrum of dysplasia of the tricuspid valve: Features in common with Ebstein's malformation. Arch Pathol 1971; 91:167–178.
4. Zuberbuhler JR, Becker KE, Anderson RH, et al: Ebstein's malformation and the embryological development of the tricuspid valve: With a role of the nature of "clefts" in the atrioventricular valves. Pediatr Cardiol 1984; 5:289–296.
5. Zuberbuhler JR, Allword SP, Anderson RH: The spectrum of Ebstein's anomaly of the tricuspid valve. J Thorac Cardiovasc Surg 1979; 77:202–211.
6. Rao PS, Jue KL, Isabel-Jones J, et al: Ebstein's malformation of the tricuspid valve with atresia: Differentiation from isolated tricuspid atresia. Am J Cardiol 1973; 32:1004–1009.
7. Roberson DA, Silverman NH: Ebstein's anomaly: Echocardiographic and clinical features in the fetus and neonate. J Am Coll Cardiol 1989; 14:1300–1307.
8. Van Mierop LHS, Gessner IH: Pathogenetic mechanisms in congenital cardiovascular malformations. Prog Cardiovasc 1972; 15:67–85.
9. Sharland GK, Chita SK, Allan LD: Tricuspid valve dysplasia or displacement in intrauterine life. J Am Coll Cardiol 1991; 117:944–949.
10. Copel JA, Pilo G, Green J, et al: Fetal echocardiographic screening for congenital heart disease: The importance of the four-chamber view. An J Obstet Gynecol 1987; 157:648–655.
11. Nora JJ, Nora AH, Tolcus WH: Lithium, Ebstein's anomaly and other congenital heart defects. Lancet 1974; 2:594–596.
12. Fyler DC, Buckley LP, Hellenbrand WE, et al: Report of the New England Regional Infant Cardiac Program. Pediatrics 1980; 65:375–461.
13. Genton E, Blount SG Jr: Spectrum of Ebstein's anomaly. Am Heart J 1967; 73:395–420.
14. Bialostosky D, Horitz S, Espino-Vela J: Ebstein's malformation of the tricuspid valve: A review of 65 cases. Am J Cardiol 1972; 29:826–830.
15. Watson H: Natural history of Ebstein's anomaly of tricuspid valve in childhood and adolescence: An international cooperative study of 505 cases. Br Heart J 1974; 36:417–427.
16. Emanuel R, O'Brien K, Ng R: Ebstein's anomaly: Genetic study of 26 families. Br Heart J 1976; 38:5–7.

17. Gueron M, Hirsch M, Otern J, et al: Familial Ebstein's anomaly with emphasis on surgical treatment. Am J Cardiol 1966; 18:105–111.
18. Lo KS, Loventhal JP, Walton JA: Familial Ebstein's anomaly. Cardiology 1979; 64:246–255.
19. Nora JJ, Frazer FC: Cardiovascular disease. In: Nora JJ, Frazer FC (eds): Medical Genetics: Principles and Practice. Philadelphia, Lea & Febiger, 1989, pp 321–337.
20. Nora JJ, Nora AH: The evolution of specific genetic and environmental counseling in congenital heart disease. Circulation 1978; 57:205–213.
21. Schou M, Goldfield MD, Weinstein MR, et al: Lithium and pregnancy, 1: Report from the Register of Lithium Babies. BMJ 1973; 2:135–136.
22. Weinstein MR, Goldfield MD: Cardiovascular malformations with lithium use during pregnancy. Am J Psychiatry 1975; 132:529–531.
23. Park JM, Sridaromont S, Ledbetter EO, et al: Ebstein's anomaly of the tricuspid valve associated with prenatal exposure to lithium carbonate. Arch Pediatr Adolesc Med 1980; 134:703–704.
24. Kallen B, Tandberg A: Lithium and pregnancy: A cohort study on manic-depressive women. Acta Psychiatr Scand 1983; 68:134–139.
25. Zalzstein E, Gideon K, Einarson T, et al: A case control study on the association between first trimester exposure to lithium and Ebstein's anomaly. Am J Cardiol 1990; 65:817–818.
26. Jenkins KJ, Correa A, Feinstein JA, et al: Noninherited risk factors and congenital cardiovascular defects: current knowledge: A scientific statement from the American Heart Association Council on Cardiovascular Disease in the Young. Circulation 2007; 115:2995–3014.
27. Hornberger LK, Sahn DJ, Kleinman CS, et al: Tricuspid valve disease with significant tricuspid insufficiency in the fetus: Diagnosis and outcome. J Am Coll Cardiol 1991; 17:167–173.
28. Oberhoffer R, Cook C, Lang D, et al: Correlation between echocardiographic and morphological investigations of lesions of the tricuspid valve diagnosed during fetal life. Br Heart J 1992; 68:580–585.
29. Ports TA, Silverman NH, Schiller NB: Two dimensional echocardiographic assessment of Ebstein's anomaly. Circulation 1978; 58:336–343.
30. Kambe T, Ichimiya S, Toguchi M, et al: Apex and subxiphoid approaches to Ebstein's anomaly using cross-sectional echocardiography. Am Heart J 1980; 100:53–57.
31. Gussenhover EJ, Steuart PA, Beckert A, et al: "Offsetting" of the septa tricuspid leaflet in normal hearts and in hearts with Ebstein's anomaly. Am J Cardiol 1984; 54:172–176.
32. Lang D, Oberhoffer R, Cook A, et al: Pathologic spectrum of malformations of the tricuspid valve in prenatal and neonatal life. J Am Coll Cardiol 1991; 17:1161–1167.
33. Allan LD, Crawford DC, Sheridan R, et al: Aetiology of non-immune hydrops: The value of echocardiography. Br J Obstet Gynaecol 1986; 93:223–225.
34. Kleinman CS, Donnerstein RL, DeVore GR, et al: Fetal echocardiography for evaluation of in utero congestive heart failure. N Engl J Med 1982; 306:568–575.
35. Mair DD, Seward JB, Driscoll DJ, et al: Surgical repair of Ebstein's anomaly: Selection of patients and early and late operative results. Circulation 1985; 72(2 Suppl):70–77.
36. Kumar AE, Flyer DC, Miettinen OS, et al: Ebstein's anomaly: Clinical profile and natural history. Am J Cardiol 1971; 28:84–95.
37. Seward JB, Tajik AJ, Feist DJ, et al: Ebstein's anomaly in an 85-year-old-man. Mayo Clin Proc 1979; 54:193–196.
38. Scott LP, Dempsey JJ, Timmis HH, et al: A surgical approach to Ebstein's disease. Circulation 1963; 27:574–577.
39. Weinberg M Jr, Bicoff JP, Agustsson MH, et al: Surgical palliation in patients with Ebstein's anomaly and congenital hypoplasia of the right ventricle. J Thorac Cardiovasc Surg 1960; 40:310–320.
40. Barbero-Marcial M, Verginelli G, Ward M, et al: Surgical treatment of Ebstein's anomaly. J Thorac Cardiovasc Surg 1979; 78:416–422.
41. Bove EL, Kirsh MM: Valve replacement for Ebstein's anomaly of the tricuspid valve. J Thorac Cardiovasc Surg 1979; 78:229–232.
42. Timmis HH, Harady JD, Watson DG: The surgical management of Ebstein's anomaly: The combined use of tricuspid valve replacement, atrioventricular placation and arterioplasty. J Thorac Cardiovasc Surg 1967; 53:385–391.
43. Danielson GK, Driscoll DJ, Mair DD, et al: Operative treatment of Ebstein's anomaly. J Thorac Cardiovasc Surg 1992;104:1195–1202.
44. Quaegebeur JM, Seeram N, Fraser AG, et al: Surgery for Ebstein's anomaly: The clinical and echocardiographic evaluation of a new technique. J Am Coll Cardiol 1991;17:722–728.
45. Cappato R, Hebe J, Weib C, et al: Radiofrequency current ablation of accessory pathways in Ebstein's anomaly [abstract]. J Am Coll Cardiol 1993; 21(A Suppl):172A.
46. Drago F, Brancaccio G, Grutter G, et al: Successful radiofrequency ablation of atrial tachycardias in surgically repaired Ebstein's anomaly using the Carto XP system and the QwikStar catheter. J Cardiovasc Med 2007; 8:459–462.

47. Stulak JM, Dearani JA, Danielson GK. Surgical management of Ebstein's anomaly. Semin Thorac Cardiovasc Surg Pediatr Card Surg Annu 2007; 10:105–111.

48. Kapusta L, Eveleigh RM, Poulino SE, et al: Ebstein's anomaly: Factors associated with death in childhood and adolescence: a multi-centre, long-term study. Eur Heart J 2007; 28:2661–2666.

49. Sahn DJ, Heldt GP, Roed KL, et al: Fetal heart disease with cardiomegaly may be associated with lung hypoplasia as a determinant of poor prognosis [abstract]. J Am Coll Cardiol 1988; 11:9A.

50. Allan LD, Crawford DC, Tynan MJ: Pulmonary atresia in prenatal life. J Am Coll Cardiol 1986; 8:1131–1136.

51. Freedom RM, Dische MR, Rowe RD: The tricuspid valve in pulmonary atresia and intact ventricular septum. Arch Pathol Lab Med 1978; 102:28–31.

52. Zuberbuhler JP, Anderson RH: Morphological variations in pulmonary atresia with intact ventricular septum. Br Heart J 1979; 41:281–288.

53. McElhinney DB, Salvin JW, Colan SD, et al. Improving outcomes in fetuses and neonates with congenital displacement (Ebstein's malromation) or dysplasia of the tricuspid valve. Am J Cardiol 2005; 96:582–586.

54. Attenhofer Jost CH, Connolly HM, Dearani JA, et al: Congenital heart disease for the adult cardiologist: Ebstein's anomaly. Circulation 2007; 115:277–285.

55. Roberson HA, Silverman NH, Zuberbuhler JR: Congenitally enlarged tricuspid orifice: Its differentiation from Ebstein's malformation in association with pulmonary atresia with an intact ventricular septum. Pediatr Cardiol 1990; 11:86–90.

56. Copel JA, Cullun M, Green JJ, et al: The frequency of aneuploidy in prenatally diagnosed congenital heart disease: An indication for fetal karyotyping. Am J Obstet Gynecol 1988; 158:409–413.

CHAPTER 13

Tetralogy of Fallot

Danielle M. Bolger

OUTLINE

Definition

Tetralogy of Fallot (TOF) is a common malformation in children born with congenital heart disease (CHD). It occurs in about 1 in 3600 live births and in roughly 3.5% to 7% of infants with CHD.[1] As the name implies, this condition consists of four classic features (Fig. 13–1). They include the following:

- A ventricular septal defect (VSD)
- Aortic override of the defect
- Pulmonary stenosis (PS) or atresia (PA)
- Right ventricular hypertrophy

Because of the various shunts that exist in the fetal circulation, right ventricular hypertrophy may not be present in utero. TOF is frequently associated with extracardiac anomalies, maternal conditions, and genetic syndromes, including DiGeorge syndrome, Down syndrome, Apert syndrome, thrombocytopenia, and phenylketonuria; it has also been associated with teratogens such as trimethadione and thalidomide.[2] Neonates with the classic form of TOF, which includes PS rather than PA, may be asymptomatic at birth and present with a murmur or increasing cyanosis over the first month of life.[1]

Ventricular Septal Defect

As with any malformation, there is a broad spectrum in the degree of severity of the anatomical defects. The VSD associated with TOF is typically subaortic. Less frequently, it is linked to absence or deficiency of the infundibular septum. This type of VSD is also referred to as a supracristal or doubly committed subarterial defect.[3] In about 1.5% of patients, the VSD is part of a complete atrioventricular septal defect.[4] The septal defect may be solely infundibular, but more commonly it extends into the membranous septum.[5] The margin of the VSD is composed of an anterior border delineated by muscular bundles that correlate with the malpositioned crista supraventricularis, whereas the crest of the muscular ventricular septum provides the inferior border. Posteriorly, the margin can be either fibrous (incomplete membranous septum and fibrous continuity of the aortic and tricuspid valves) or muscular (inferior portion of a divided parietal band). There is no distinct margin superiorly because the defect is continuous with the aortic ostium. The aorta is in

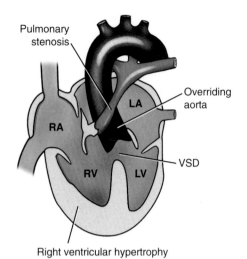

Figure 13-1 Diagram showing the four abnormalities associated with TOF: overriding aorta, VSD, pulmonary stenosis, and right ventricular hypertrophy (not usually apparent in utero). *LA*, Left atrium; *LV*, left ventricle; *RA*, right atrium; *RV*, right ventricle.

direct contact with the free wall of the right ventricle.[6]

Anderson et al[7] reviewed 53 specimens with TOF. They identified three different types of VSDs. In 41 hearts, the defect extended cephalad and anterior and was bordered by the infundibular septum. Caudally, the defects were marginated by the trabecula septomarginalis. These perimembranous septal defects were related to the malalignment of the infundibular muscles and trabecular components of the ventricular septum. Defects consisting of a complete muscular rim were found in 11 specimens. One case was classified as being subarterial because of its position under the aortic and pulmonary valve rings.[7]

Overriding Aorta

The overriding aorta in TOF occurs as a result of the subaortic location of the VSD in the majority of cases.[6] The amount of override can vary from a small degree to as much as 75%. This is a result of abnormal anterior extension of the aortic root in relation to the ventricular septum, a consequence of maldevelopment of the conotruncus.[2] Extreme aortic overriding can occur when there is severe stenosis or atresia of the pulmonary infundibulum. In these hearts, no direct fibrous continuity

exists between the anterior leaflet of the mitral valve and the noncoronary and left coronary leaflets of the aortic valve, as is present in the normal heart. Only the right aortic leaflet is in direct continuity, suggesting that the aortic ostium is abnormally positioned to the right. The sinuses of Valsalva are also abnormally located.[6] Instead of facing rightward and posteriorly, the noncoronary sinus is directed more rightward. The right coronary sinus faces anteriorly and leftward instead of completely anteriorly. The left coronary sinus is positioned less to the left than is normal and more posteriorly. This severe degree of override is important with respect to surgery because the anterior descending coronary artery can originate from the right coronary artery.[6]

Pulmonary Outflow Tract Obstruction

The degree of right ventricular outflow tract obstruction is thought to be the key factor in determining the type and amount of dysfunction that a patient with TOF displays. The severity of pulmonary obstruction ranges from mild PS to pulmonary atresia (PA). The pulmonary blood supply in TOF with PA is mediated through a patent ductus arteriosus in two thirds of patients and through major aortopulmonary collateral arteries in one third of patients. There are three clinically distinguishable types of TOF relating to the type of pulmonary obstruction: (1) TOF with PS, (2) TOF with PA with a patent ductus arteriosus, and (3) TOF with PA and major aortopulmonary collaterals.[8] Obstruction to pulmonary flow most commonly occurs in the right ventricular infundibulum or subvalvular area. The pulmonary valve and annulus are usually abnormal, and supravalvular narrowing of the pulmonary trunk occurs in 50% of patients. Infundibular stenosis usually occurs as the only major obstruction; however, a combination of obstruction sites may be present, the most common being infundibular in conjunction with valvular obstruction, which is found in 25% of patients.[6]

Although most patients have at least a minor pulmonary valve abnormality, the valve orifice is at least equal in size to or larger than the smallest diameter of the infundibular opening. As a result, the valves may be anomalous with respect to the number of cusps or the degree of stenosis.[2] Pulmonary infundibular stenosis is created when the outlet septum inserts anteriorly and the septal and parietal insertions are both toward the anterior ventricular wall. The parietal band is displaced superiorly and toward the septum, causing obstruction to blood flow.[2] Frequently, septoparietal trabeculations located anteriorly may form a muscular ring, which can be narrowed further by fibrous tissue.[9] This hypertrophy infringes on the outflow tract in both systole and diastole. If the hyperplasia is diffuse, there is overall narrowing of the infundibulum. In some cases, however, the tapering may be at the orifice of the infundibulum only, beyond which the infundibulum widens to create an "infundibular chamber." Malformed pulmonary valves can be tricuspid, bicuspid, unicuspid, or dome shaped. Each cusp is usually small and rigid and lacks mobility.[6] A narrowed and hypoplastic pulmonary annulus may be present as a single entity or may occur in conjunction with a deformed pulmonary valve. Severe hypoplasia or congenital absence of the pulmonary valve has also been reported.

In the normal heart, the diameter of the pulmonary orifice is greater than 80% of the diameter of the aortic orifice. If the pulmonary orifice is between 50% and 80% of the aortic orifice, mild to moderate stenosis is considered to exist. Severe stenosis is present when the diameter of the pulmonary orifice is less than 50% of the aortic orifice.[6]

Hypoplasia of the pulmonary trunk and its branches almost always occurs in conjunction with obstruction at the pulmonary valve or infundibulum, or both. A relationship exists between the pulmonary valve and the pulmonary trunk. The pulmonary trunk decreases in caliber as the number of pulmonary cusps decreases and as the degree of pulmonary valvular stenosis increases. The most extreme form of pulmonary outflow obstruction is PA. When this occurs, there is no communication between the right ventricle and the pulmonary trunk, and the ventricular infundibulum can end blindly against an atretic valve, muscle, or vestigial valvular tissue.[6]

Right Ventricular Hypertrophy

Because of pulmonary outflow tract obstruction, the right ventricle can demonstrate pressure-induced hypertrophy. The left ventricle is often of normal size or rarely smaller than the right ventricle. Right ventricular hypertrophy usually is not present in the fetus because of the foramen ovale and ductus arteriosus, which act as shunts that allow the blood to bypass the right ventricle and fetal lungs. These shunts offer little resistance to blood flow and thus help to prevent pressure overload in the right ventricle. Even in cases of severe PS or PA, right ventricular output can be diverted into the aorta, and pulmonary blood flow can be supplied by retrograde flow through the ductus arteriosus. After birth, however, hemodynamic problems occur as a result of ductal closing, and right ventricular hypertrophy develops.

Embryology

From a developmental standpoint, TOF is caused by a single embryonic error. There is an unequal division of the conus resulting from an anterior displacement of the truncoconal septum.[9] This anterior displacement occurs primarily in the lower portion of the conus septum, dividing the conus into a smaller anterior right ventricular section and a larger posterior portion.[10] This results in narrowing of the right ventricular outflow region or pulmonary infundibular stenosis.[9] This displacement also prohibits the crista supraventricularis from forming, thus preventing the closure of the interventricular septum (IVS). The resulting large interventricular septal defect, in turn, inhibits the aortic valve from residing in its normal position. Because the aortic valve's free edge is so far removed from the tricuspid valve, it is unable to participate in the formation of that valve. Subsequently, this explains the absence of the medial papillary muscle and the abnormally formed tricuspid valve, which may also be present in TOF. The truncal septum is usually anteriorly displaced, which partially attributes to the small pulmonary trunk and the disproportionately large aorta.[9] The aorta arises directly above the septal defect overriding both ventricles. Dilation of the aorta appears to be related to the increased aortic flow, which varies inversely with the caliber of the pulmonary outflow tract. This aortic dilation can increase the degree to which the aorta overrides the ventricular septum.[6]

Occurrence Rate

TOF is reported to occur in 3.5% to 7% of children with CHD. In the pediatric population, TOF is estimated to occur in 1 in 3600 live births.[1] The risk of occurrence in a sibling is approximately 2.5%. The empirical risk of occurrence is 2.6% in the child of an affected mother. If the father is affected, the empirical risk is 1.4%. The incidence in males versus females is approximately 3:2.[11]

As with most congenital cardiac diseases, the occurrence rate in the fetus is thought to be higher before spontaneous or elective termination.

Sonographic Criteria

To diagnose TOF in utero, an aortic root overriding the IVS must be identified. It must be borne in mind that the right ventricular hypertrophy associated with TOF does not usually manifest itself in utero. Additionally, infundibular PS may not be apparent in early pregnancy. The prenatal diagnosis of a VSD with an overriding aorta has been reported as early as 14 weeks' gestation.[12]

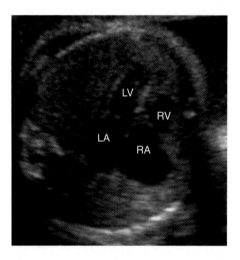

Figure 13–2 Normal-appearing subcostal four-chamber view in a fetus with TOF. All four cardiac chambers appear normal in size. *LA,* Left atrium; *LV,* left ventricle; *RA,* right atrium; *RV,* right ventricle.

Recently, an association between an increased nuchal translucency measurement in the first trimester and the diagnosis of TOF, even in the absence of a chromosomal anomaly, has been reported.[1]

It can be difficult to make the diagnosis of TOF on either the subcostal or apical four-chamber view alone. Because of the inherent shunts in the fetal heart, all four heart chambers will usually appear of equal size (Fig. 13–2). Severe levocardia may be appreciated in some cases (Fig. 13–3). The perimembranous VSD may be seen on the subcostal four-chamber view; however, color Doppler imaging may be necessary to confirm the defect.[13]

A slight cephalad angulation of the transducer from a four-chamber view should allow a five-chamber view including the aorta to be obtained. From this projection, an overriding aorta is often apparent (Fig. 13–4).

Angling toward the fetus' right shoulder from a subcostal four-chamber view into a long-axis view of the aorta will allow evaluation of discontinuity between the anterior wall of the aorta and the IVS, also confirming the presence of an overriding aorta (Fig. 13–5). However, the artifactual appearance of septoaortic discontinuity is possible (Fig. 13–6). Again, color Doppler imaging may be helpful in confirming that a defect is present.

If the override is extreme, the aortic root may appear to originate exclusively from the right ventricle and resemble a double-outlet right ventricle. Many investigators use the "50% rule" to assist in the diagnosis. If more than 50% of the aorta overlies the left ventricle, TOF is present. Conversely,

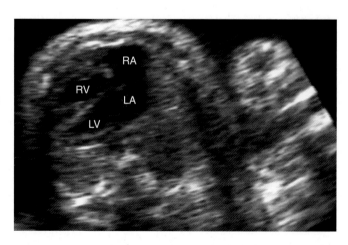

Figure 13–3 Four-chamber view in a fetus with TOF. All four chambers appear normal in size; however, severe levocardia is present. *LA,* Left atrium; *LV,* left ventricle; *RA,* right atrium; *RV,* right ventricle.

if more than 50% of the aorta overlies the right ventricle, double-outlet right ventricle is more likely.[14]

The size of the aortic root should also be assessed. In one study, the aortic root diameter in seven fetuses with TOF and 45 unaffected control fetuses between 18 and 34 weeks' gestation was measured. These measurements were compared with a biventricular outer dimension of the heart (epicardium to epicardium) and with noncardiac growth parameters, such as biparietal diameter, head circumference, abdominal circumference, and femur length. All fetuses with TOF demonstrated dilation of the aortic root compared with any of the parameters used.[15] Dilation appeared to progress throughout pregnancy. This dilation is thought to result from blood being received from both the right and left ventricles as a result of the septal defect.[14] In contrast, Hornberger et al[16] found that 87% of fetuses studied with TOF had normal aortic diameters at initial the ultrasonographic examination, suggesting that aortic dilation may not be apparent in midgestation.

The five-chamber view may also be helpful when pulsed Doppler or color Doppler imaging is used to evaluate the aortic valve for insufficiency that may result from root dilation. If a regurgitant jet is present, it can be quantitated with pulsed Doppler imaging to follow the progression of the anomaly throughout pregnancy.

Once an overriding aorta has been identified, the next step in diagnosing TOF relies on the eval-uation of the right ventricular outflow tract. It is best evaluated in either a long-axis view of the pulmonary artery (Fig. 13–7), which is obtained by acquiring a subcostal four-chamber view and then angling the transducer toward the fetal right shoulder, or turning into a sagittal view of the fetus and acquiring a short-axis view of the great vessels (Fig. 13–8). If the pulmonary artery is present but abnormally small (which can make it difficult to identify), TOF should be suspected. The

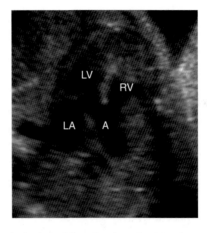

Figure 13–4 Apical five-chamber view showing the aorta overriding a VSD in a fetus with TOF. *A,* Aorta; *LV,* left ventricle; *LA,* left atrium; *RV,* right ventricle.

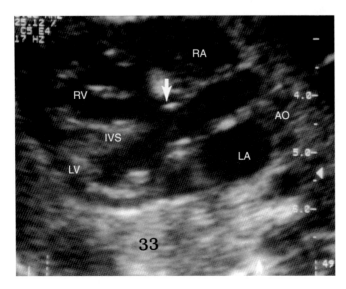

Figure 13–5 Long-axis view of the aorta in a fetus with TOF showing the aorta *(arrow)* overriding a VSD. *AO,* Aorta; *IVS,* interventricular septum; *LA,* left atrium; *LV,* left ventricle; *RA,* right atrium; *RV,* right ventricle.

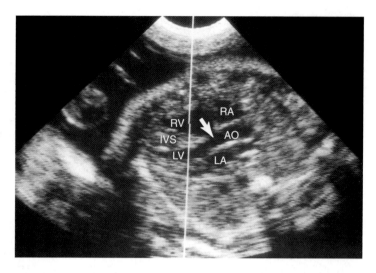

Figure 13–6 Long-axis view of the aorta in a fetus with a normal heart showing artifactual septoaortic discontinuity *(arrow).* *AO,* Aorta; *IVS,* interventricular septum; *LA,* left atrium; *LV,* left ventricle; *RA,* right atrium; *RV,* right ventricle.

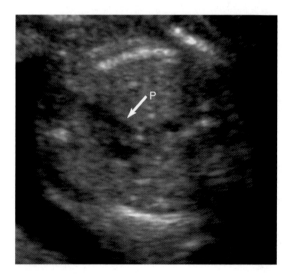

Figure 13–7 Long-axis view of the pulmonary artery *(P)* in a fetus with TOF. The size of the pulmonary artery is markedly decreased.

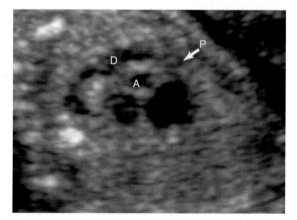

Figure 13–8 Short-axis view of the great vessels in a fetus with TOF. The small pulmonary artery *(P)* is very difficult to visualize. *D,* Ductus arteriosus; *A,* aorta.

differential diagnosis includes PA with a VSD or truncus arteriosus. If a connection between the overriding artery and pulmonary arteries can be demonstrated, the diagnosis of truncus arteriosus can be made.

If a pulmonary artery can be identified, the outer diameter should be measured. One study followed the progression of PS associated with TOF in utero. Both the aorta and pulmonary arteries were measured serially. All measurements were taken 0.5 cm above the valve so that the valve sinuses were not included in the measurement. In the normal heart, the pulmonary artery is larger than the aorta in utero because of the larger contribution of the right ventricle to the combined cardiac output. Also, pulsed Doppler velocities are usually slightly lower in the pulmonary artery than in the aorta in the fetus. This study of fetuses with TOF found that by 29 weeks' gestation the pulmonary artery diameter was approximately 40% smaller than that of the aorta. By 37 weeks' gestation, this discrepancy had increased to ap-

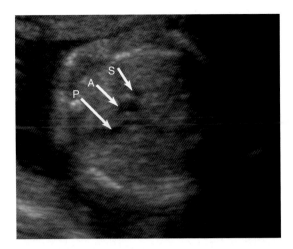

Figure 13–9 Three-vessel view in a fetus with TOF. The caliber of the pulmonary artery *(P)* is very small compared with the aorta *(A)*. *S,* Superior vena cava.

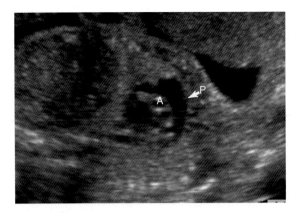

Figure 13–10 Short-axis view of the great vessels in a fetus with TOF showing a dilated pulmonary artery *(P)* resulting from absence of the pulmonic valve. *A,* Aorta.

proximately 55%. In addition, the pulmonary artery velocities were increased over aortic velocities by approximately 14%.[17]

The three-vessel view is useful for allowing a side-by-side comparison of the size of the aorta and the pulmonary artery (Fig. 13–9).

The study by Hornberger et al[16] reported similar findings and studied postnatal outcomes. They found that main pulmonary artery hypoplasia on initial examination was consistent in fetuses with more severe disease postnatally. However, branch pulmonary artery size was normal in most fetuses during mid gestation, even those with severe disease at birth. During the second half of gestation, the growth of the pulmonary branches remained within normal limits or was reduced. Pulmonary valve atresia may also be present in fetuses with TOF. On postmortem examinations, 3% to 6% of fetuses with TOF had absence of the pulmonic valve.[18]

Aneurysmal dilation of the pulmonary artery should prompt the diagnosis of absence of the pulmonic valve (Fig. 13–10). Doppler imaging of the pulmonary artery demonstrates severe pulmonic insufficiency in these cases. Also, a relationship between severe dilation of the pulmonary arteries and an absent ductus arteriosus has been reported.[17] Severely dilated pulmonary arteries were also associated with tracheobronchial compression, resulting in respiratory distress and cardiac failure at birth. Therefore an absent pul-

monic valve can be an important indicator of a poor prognosis after delivery.[19]

Pulsed Doppler interrogation of the pulmonary artery is extremely useful in evaluation of fetuses with TOF. Doppler echocardiography can identify pulmonary outflow tract obstruction by demonstrating flow disturbances in the pulmonary artery.[20] Doppler velocities are usually increased in the pulmonary artery compared with those of the aorta in fetuses with TOF. Usually, the higher the peak systolic velocity, the more severe the pulmonary stenosis (Fig. 13–11). In extreme cases, retrograde flow in the main pulmonary artery from the ductus arteriosus, with no detectable antegrade right ventricular flow, is seen.[16] Color Doppler imaging may also be useful in detecting retrograde flow from the descending aorta through the ductus arteriosus into the main pulmonary artery. This reversal of flow can occur along with a high-velocity turbulent jet in the pulmonary artery. Thus, in severe obstruction of the right ventricular outflow tract, it may be possible to visualize two opposite jets in the main pulmonary artery.[21]

Finally, laterality of the aortic arch should be assessed because approximately 25% of patients with TOF have a right-sided aortic arch.[14] An ideal view for evaluating this relationship is usually the three-vessel trachea view. In the normal heart, both the aorta and pulmonary artery will be located to the left of the trachea. If a right-sided aortic arch is present, it will lie to the right of the trachea. A transverse view through the fetal chest showing the descending aorta to the right of

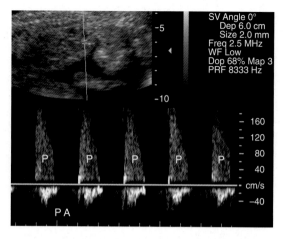

Figure 13–11   Increased pulsed Doppler velocity *(P)* through the pulmonic valve in a fetus with TOF. The peak systolic velocity of 160 cm/second is indicative of PS.

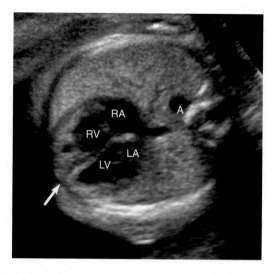

Figure 13–12   Transverse image of the fetal chest in a fetus with TOF showing the descending aorta *(A)* abnormally positioned on the right side of the spine. The apex of the heart *(arrow)* is correctly pointing toward the fetal left chest. *LA,* Left atrium; *LV,* left ventricle; *RA,* right atrium; *RV,* right ventricle.

the fetal spine will also confirm this diagnosis (Fig. 13–12).

Fetuses with an enlarged ascending aorta and also dilated pulmonary arteries may have tracheal and esophageal compression, which can result in polyhydramnios and further respiratory distress and swallowing difficulties.[22] Extreme cases of in utero TOF have also been associated with nonimmune hydrops fetalis.

Treatment

Once the diagnosis of TOF is confirmed by postnatal echocardiography, the infant usually undergoes cardiac catheterization to identify collateral vessels and to assess the pulmonary and coronary artery anatomy.[2] Although the definitive treatment of this heart lesion is surgical, medical management both before and after surgery is important. Indications for surgical intervention include hypercyanotic episodes (tet spells), hypotension, excessively high hemoglobin and hematocrit readings, altered consciousness, and a diminished exercise tolerance.[21,23]

In the past, various systemic-to-pulmonary shunts have been used to increase pulmonary blood flow. This is commonly referred to as a palliative procedure that temporarily restores blood flow to the lungs, therefore diminishing hypoxia. These procedures include subclavian artery–

to–pulmonary artery (Blalock-Taussig), descending aorta–to–left pulmonary artery (Potts), and ascending aorta–to–right pulmonary (Waterson) anastomoses.[19] In neonates with severe hypoxic spells, prostaglandins may be used to re-establish ductal patency.[23]

Controversy continues to surround the role of palliative surgery for TOF. It was previously thought that is was best to initially place a systemic-to-pulmonary shunt to stabilize the patient until further surgical intervention was necessary. A second surgery could then be performed later in life, once the infant was strong enough, to completely correct the deficiencies. Recent publications suggest that traditional early palliative surgery followed by complete repair at a later time can cause secondary damage to the heart and other organ systems, primarily the brain, resulting from chronic hypoxia.[24] Currently, most institutions have elected to treat TOF with one-stage primary complete repair because of the benefits of early intervention (<90 days of age) and the desire to avoid the risks and inconvenience of a palliative procedure.[25] Benefits include promotion of normal growth and development of organs, elimination of hypoxemia, the ability to minimize or avoid right ventricular muscle excision, and decreased late arrhythmias. Early resolution of right ventricular hypertrophy and fibrosis are thought to be important in decreasing the incidence of late right ventricular dysfunction and ventricular arrhythmias, which remains the most common cause of death (35%–45%) after repair of TOF.[26,27] Intraventricular scarring and fibrosis are thought to provide anatomical substrates of abnormal depolarization and repolarization causing re-entrant ventricular arrhythmias.[27]

Exceptions to complete primary repair of TOF include infants with hypoplastic pulmonary arteries, small left ventricle, anomalous origin of the left coronary artery, and multiple VSDs.[25]

The goals of the intracardiac repair are to close the VSD (or VSDs) completely and permanently, to relieve the right ventricular outflow tract obstruction, discontinue preexisting shunts, and correct any other associated heart defects.[2] In most institutions, the surgical mortality rate is low. One study reported a hospital mortality rate that ranged from 1.6% with surgery at 5 years of age to 4.1% with surgery at 1 year of age (7.7% if a transannular patch was used).[19] Eighty-seven percent of patients surviving complete correction of TOF have an excellent late clinical and hemodynamic result without functional disability, need for medication, or significant residual cardiac abnormalities.[2] However, postsurgical cardiovascular events, including congestive heart failure, arrhythmias, and death, do occur. Most commonly, late congestive heart failure is a result of the residual VSD. Reoperation is recommended in such cases and in those cases involving pulmonary valve insufficiency and residual ventricular outflow tract obstruction. Conduction abnormalities, namely, right bundle branch block, are also common after surgical repair. Rarely, a risk of sudden unexpected death long after surgical repair, thought to be caused by ventricular ectopy, has been reported.[19]

Prognosis

The prognosis for patients with TOF is variable and is primarily dependent on the severity of the pulmonary stenosis.[6] Pooled data from 2001 reported a 97% survival rate at 1 year with surgical repair. Of the survivors, 98% would be expected to be alive at 20 years.[1] Recent statistics have shown a survival rate 30 years after total correction of TOF close to 90%, and a perioperative death rate of less than 1%.[27] The prognosis for TOF with PA or absence of the pulmonic valve is not as good. This severe form of TOF may cause congestive heart failure in the fetus or neonate.[28] The mortality rates for patients with TOF left untreated are 25% at 1 year of age, 40% at 3 years, and 70% at 10 years.[22]

Tracheobronchial compression resulting from dilated pulmonary arteries and an enlarged ascending aorta are likely to contribute to bronchial and pulmonary hypoplasia, resulting in respiratory distress in the neonate. It has also been speculated that the hemodynamic changes caused by the back-and-forth blood flow between the right ventricle and the dilated pulmonary arteries produce elevated right ventricular end-diastolic pressure that can lead to congestive heart failure.[29] Polyhydramnios indicates a poor prognosis.

Clinically, the spectrum of TOF ranges from the distressed, cyanotic, hypoxemic neonate to the young adult with no cyanosis and few symptoms.[19] Again, this range in sequelae is related to the severity of the right-sided outflow obstruction. Cyanosis may be present at birth or may appear later in life. Occasionally, an older infant may present with TOF. These infants have a net left-to-right shunt and are considered to have "pink" tetralogy. As they mature and more infundibular narrowing develops, they exhibit cyanosis at rest and become prone to hypercyanotic episodes.[2] These children can also have clubbing of the fingers and toes.[10]

In severe cases of TOF, such as those accompanied by severe PS or PA, sudden death usually occurs early in infancy. This may be the consequence of acute hypoxia or cerebral venous thrombosis. The average life expectancy of a severely affected child does not extend beyond the first decade of life. Approximately 20% of patients live to the age of 20 years or beyond.[6] Death is most commonly the result of hypoxia or complications such as cerebral venous thrombosis, cerebral embolism from venous thrombosis, pneumonia, cerebral abscess, subacute bacterial endocarditis, or pneumonia. In general, the life expectancy of a patient with TOF who does not undergo surgery is around 12 years.

Fortunately, advances in cardiac surgery over the past few decades have greatly improved the prognosis of this anomaly. A study performed on a large group of TOF survivors found that 91% had not had any late events (congestive heart failure,

TABLE 13–1   Conditions Associated with Tetralogy of Fallot

Maternal		Fetal		
Condition	Drug Use	Associated Cardiac Abnormalities	Chromosome Abnormalities	Syndromes
Diabetes Phenylketonuria Thrombocytopenia	Alcohol Thalidomide Trimethadione	Absent ductus arteriosus Absent pulmonic valve Atrial septal defect Atrioventricular septal defect Cor triatriatum Hypoplastic left heart syndrome Interrupted inferior vena cava Isolated subclavian artery Left superior vena cava Mitral stenosis Partial anomalous pulmonary venous connection Pulmonary atresia Right-sided aortic arch Supravalvular aortic stenosis Total anomalous pulmonary venous connection	Partial monosomy 11P Trisomy 14 mosaic Trisomy 16P Trisomy 21 (Down syndrome)	Absent radius Apert syndrome Arthrochalasis multiplex congenita Cardiofacial syndrome Cat-eye syndrome Cayler syndrome CHARGE (coloboma, heart disease, atresia choanae, retarded growth and development or central nervous system anomalies, genital hypoplasia, and ear anomalies or deafness) syndrome CHIME (coloboma, heart anomaly, ichthyosis, mental retardation, ear anomaly) syndrome DiGeorge syndrome Duodenal atresia Ehlers-Danlos syndrome Elfin facies Fetal alcohol syndrome Goldenhar syndrome Halarz syndrome Hydrocephaly Intestinal lymphangiectasia Johanson-Blizzard Noonan syndrome Oculoauriculo-vertebral anomaly Omphalocele Pentalogy of Cantrell Renal tubular dysgenesis Scimitar syndrome Situs inversus Venolobar syndrome Williams-Beuren syndrome

need for reoperation, arrhythmias, or death) by 8 years after surgery.[19]

Associated Anomalies

Approximately 57% of patients with TOF have associated cardiac anomalies (Table 13–1).[1,6] A right-sided aortic arch occurs in roughly 25% of patients with TOF. Of these patients, 90% have mirror-image branching, and 10% have an aberrant left subclavian artery.[22] In some cases of right-sided aortic arch, a complete or incomplete double arch may be discovered.[14]

There is also a high incidence of interatrial communication associated with TOF. In an autopsy study of 85 cases, Rao et al[30] found that 47 patients had a patent foramen ovale and 23 had an atrial septal defect. Thus only 17% had an atrial septum that was intact. This complex has been referred to as pentalogy of Fallot.

Absence of the pulmonary valve may accompany TOF. The left pulmonary artery has been reported to be absent or hypoplastic in 14% of patients. Absence of the ductus arteriosus is also possible.[31,32]

Atrioventricular septal defects can accompany TOF. This is caused by an anterior deviation of the infundibular septum. The aortic valve is contiguous with a large VSD, and, most commonly, there is a continuation between the leaflets of a common atrioventricular valve.[4] This combination of malformations has a higher association with Down syndrome than with isolated TOF.

Various venous anomalies have also been reported. A left superior vena cava draining into the coronary sinus has been reported, as has intrahepatic interruption of the vena cava with azygos continuation. Partial and total anomalous pulmonary venous connections have been associated with TOF in a few cases.[33]

Other rare cardiac findings include a small or hypoplastic left ventricle, aortic valve abnormalities, aortic stenosis, aortic regurgitation, cor triatriatum, and anastomosis between the pulmonary and subclavian arteries.[6]

Associated extracardiac abnormalities are found in up to 50% of cases.[1,33] The defects vary in type and severity, including tracheoesophageal fistula, cleft lip/palate, hypertelorism, abdominal wall defects, single umbilical artery, renal anomalies, and talipes.[1,8] Extracardiac defects occur even in cases in which a chromosomal anomaly has been ruled out.[1] Chromosome abnormalities are present in 12% of live-born infants with TOF and in 50% of fetuses.[34] Most frequent are DiGeorge syndrome (22q11.2 deletion) in 8% to 17% of cases, Down syndrome in 8%, and Noonan syndrome in approximately 1%.[19] Therefore obstetrical management should include amniocentesis for chromosomal evaluation and a detailed anatomical survey.

References

1. Poon LCY, Huggon IC, Zidere V, et al: Tetralogy of Fallot in the fetus in the current era. Ultrasound Obstet Gynecol 2007; 29:625–627.
2. Pinsky AE: Tetralogy of Fallot. Pediatr Clin North Am 1990; 37:179–180.
3. Higgins C, Kersting-Sommerhoff B, Silverman N, et al: Right heart obstructive lesions, congenital heart disease. In: Higgins C, Kersting-Sommerhoff B, Silverman N (eds): Echocardiography and Magnetic Resonance Imaging. New York, Raven Press, 1990, pp 220–221.
4. Uretzky G, Puga FJ, Danielson GK, et al: Complete atrioventricular canal associated with tetralogy of Fallot. J Thorac Cardiovasc Surg 1984; 87:756–780.
5. Snider R, Serwer G: Defects in cardiac septation. In: Lampert R (ed): Echocardiography in Pediatric Heart Disease. Chicago, Year Book Medical, 1990, pp 150–153.
6. Bankl H: Particular malformations. In: Bankl H (ed): Congenital Malformations of the Heart and Great Vessels. Baltimore, Urban & Schwarzenberg, 1977, pp 46–52.
7. Anderson RH, Allwork SP, Ho SY, et al: Surgical anatomy of tetralogy of Fallot. J Thorac Cardiovasc Surg 1981; 81:887–891.
8. Maeda J, Yamagishi H, Matsuoka R, et al: Frequent association of 22q11.2 deletion with tetralogy of Fallot. Am J Med Genet 2000; 92:269–272.
9. Sadler TW: Cardiovascular system. In: Sadler TW (ed): Langman's Medical Embryology. Baltimore, Williams & Wilkins, 1990, pp 199–202.
10. Netter FH: Congenital anomalies. The Ciba Collection of Medical Illustrations—The Heart, vol 5. Summit, NJ, Ciba-Geigy Corp, 1978, pp 148–150.
11. Buyse M: Heart, tetralogy of Fallot. In: Buyse M (ed): Heart, Birth Defects Encyclopedia. Cambridge, Blackwell Scientific, 1990, pp 846–848.
12. Bronshtein M, Siegler E, Yoffe N, et al: Prenatal diagnosis of ventricular septal defect and

overriding aorta at 14 weeks' gestation, using transvaginal sonography. Prenat Diagn 1990; 10:697–702.

13. Anderson C, McCurdy C, McNamara M, et al: Case of the day. 8. Diagnosis: Color Doppler aided diagnosis of tetralogy of Fallot. J Ultrasound Med 1994; 13:341–342.

14. Silverman N, Sinder A: Conditions with override of the ventricular septum by the systemic artery. In: Hachtel G (ed): Two-Dimensional Echocardiography in Congenital Heart Disease. Norwalk, CT, Appleton-Century-Crofts, 1982, pp 149–155.

15. DeVore G, Siassi B, Platt L: Aortic route dilatation: A marker for tetralogy of Fallot. Am J Obstet Gynecol 1988; 8:129–136.

16. Hornberger L, Sanders S, Sahn D: In utero pulmonary artery and aortic growth and potential for progression of pulmonary outflow tract obstruction in tetralogy of Fallot. J Am Coll Cardiol 1995; 25:739–745.

17. Rice M, McDonald R, Reller M: Progressive pulmonary stenosis in the fetus: Two case reports. Am J Perinatol 1993; 10:424–426.

18. Rein AJJT, Singer R, Simcha A: Prenatal diagnosis of tetralogy of Fallot with absence of the leaflets of the pulmonic valve. Int J Cardiol 1992; 34:211–213.

19. Zuberbuhler J: Tetralogy of Fallot. In: Emmanouilides G, Riemenschneider T, Allen H, et al (eds): Moss and Adams' Heart Disease in Infants, Children and Adolescents: Including the Fetus and Young Adult, 5th ed, vol 2. Baltimore, Williams & Wilkins, 1995, pp 998–1016.

20. Goldberg S, Alan H, Sahn D: Conotruncal abnormalities. In: Goldberg S, Alan H, Sahn D (eds): Pediatric and Adolescent Echocardiography, 2nd ed. Chicago, Year Book Medical, 1980, pp 350–360.

21. Gembruch U, Weinraud Z, Bald R, et al: Flow analysis in the pulmonary trunk in fetuses with tetralogy of Fallot by colour Doppler flow mapping: Two case reports. Eur J Obstet Gynaecol Reprod Biol 1990; 35:259–265.

22. Greenberg SB: Tetralogy of Fallot. E Medicine. Accessed September 8, 2007. http://www.emedicine.com/radio/TOPIC685.HTM.

23. Jacobs JP, Singh VN: Tetralogy of Fallot: Surgical perspective. E Medicine. Accessed October 24, 2007. http://www.emedicine.com/ped/TOPIC2832.HTM.

24. Pigula FA, Khalil PN, Mayer JE, et al: Repair of Tetralogy of Fallot in neonates and young infants. Circulation 1999; 100(2 Suppl):157–161.

25. Alexiou C, Mahmoud H, Al-Khaddour A, et al: Outcome after repair of tetralogy of Fallot in the first year of life. Ann Thorac Surg 2001; 71:494–500.

26. Hirsch JC, Mosca RS, Bove EL: Complete repair of tetralogy of Fallot in the neonate: Results in the modern era. Ann Surg 2000; 232:508–514.

27. Folino AF, Daliento L: Arrhythmias after tetralogy of Fallot repair. Ind Pacing Electrophysiol J 2005; 5:312–324.

28. Callan N, Kan J: Prenatal diagnosis of tetralogy of Fallot with absent pulmonary valve. Am J Perinatol 1991; 8(1):15–17.

29. Sameshima H, Nishibatake M, Ninomiya Y, et al: Antenatal diagnosis of tetralogy of Fallot with absent pulmonary valve accompanied by hydrops fetalis and polyhydramnios. Fetal Diagn Ther 1993; 8:305–308.

30. Rao BNS, Anderson RC, Edwards JE: Anatomic variations in tetralogy of Fallot. Am Heart J 1971; 81:361–365.

31. Rao PS, Lawrie GM: Absent pulmonary valve syndrome. Br Heart J 1983; 50:586–590.

32. Ohba T, Matsui K, Nakamura S, et al: Tetralogy of Fallot with absent pulmonary valve detected by fetal echocardiography. Int J Gynecol Obstet 1990; 32:71–74.

33. Nyberg D, Emerson D: Cardiac malformations. In: Nyberg D, Mahoney B, Pretorius D (eds): Diagnostic Ultrasound of Fetal Anomalies. St Louis, Mosby–Year Book, 1990, pp 323–330.

34. Crawford DC, Chita SK, Allan LD: Prenatal detection of congenital heart disease: Factors affecting obstetric management and survival. Am J Obstet Gynecol 1988; 159:352–356.

CHAPTER 14

Persistent Truncus Arteriosus

Cynthia L. Rapp
Julia A. Drose

OUTLINE

Definition

Truncus arteriosus is a rare cardiac anomaly first described in 1864.[1] It is one of several truncoconal defects accounting for approximately 0.4% to 2.8% of all congenital heart defects among live births.[2] In the fetus it accounts for 1% of cardiac lesions.[3] Truncus arteriosus results from failure of the truncoconal ridges to fuse.[4] These ridges normally divide the truncus arteriosus into separate aortic and pulmonary arterial trunks. The result is a single great vessel arising from the heart that overrides the interventricular septum. The systemic, pulmonary, and coronary circulations are all supplied with blood by this one great vessel. This failure of fusion of the truncoconal ridges also results in a ventricular septal defect (VSD). The single semilunar valve, or truncal valve, lies directly above the VSD in 42% of patients. In another 42%, it is dominantly positioned over the right ventricle, and in the remaining 16% of patients, it is positioned predominantly over the left ventricle.[4] This single great vessel receives blood from both the right and left ventricles.[5,6] With truncus arteriosus, the pulmonary arteries arises from the undivided truncus (Fig. 14–1).[7] The single semilunar valve usually has three cusps but can have between one and six cusps.[3–5,8,9] In one large multicenter study involving pathological evaluation of 536 cases of truncus arteriosus, 66% were tricuspid, 22% had four leaflets, and 11% were unicuspid. Fewer than 1% had five or six cusps.[10] Truncus arteriosus is frequently associated with valve dysplasia, leading to insufficiency or stenosis. Valvular insufficiency occurs more frequently than stenosis.[11] The mitral and tricuspid valves are usually normal. In approximately 50% to 75% of cases the ductus arteriosus is absent, and a right-sided aortic arch is associated 30% of the time.[12,13]

Truncus arteriosus has been variously referred to as aorticopulmonary trunk, truncus arteriosus communis, and persistent truncus arteriosus.[1] Generally, it is abbreviated truncus arteriosus for simplicity and clarity. However, the truncus arteriosus is actually a normal embryological heart structure that becomes anomalous only when it persists throughout cardiac development; therefore persistent truncus arteriosus would be the most appropriate term to describe this abnormality.

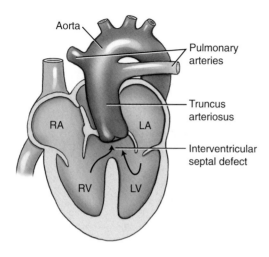

Figure 14–1 Diagram of truncus arteriosus showing the common trunk that overrides the interventricular septal defect. The pulmonary arteries originate from the common trunk. *LA,* Left atrium; *LV,* left ventricle; *RA,* right atrium; *RV,* right ventricle.

Collett and Edwards[5] described an anatomical classification for persistent truncus arteriosus on the basis of the location of the pulmonary artery origins from the truncus:

- Type I: a short main pulmonary artery arising from the left lateral aspect of the truncus, then dividing into right and left branches
- Type II: separate but closely positioned right and left pulmonary arteries arising from the posterior-lateral aspect of the truncus
- Type III: widely separated pulmonary arteries arising laterally from the truncus
- Type IV: pulmonary arteries arising from the descending aorta

These divisions represent different stages of failure in the embryological development of the heart.

In 1965, Van Praagh and Van Praagh[8] modified these classifications (Fig. 14–2). They proposed the following classifications:

- Type 1A: similar to the type I described by Collett and Edwards
- Type 2A: combination of type II and type III
- Type A3: a single pulmonary artery originating from the truncus, usually the right, with either a ductus arteriosus or collateral vessels supplying the contralateral side
- Type A4: truncus arteriosus with an interrupted aortic arch

The type IV classification originally described by Collett and Edwards was eliminated because it was thought to more accurately describe pulmonary atresia with a VSD. Types A1 and A2 are the most common forms of persistent truncus arteriosus, with occurrence rates of 49% and 43%, respectively. Type A3 is found in only 6% of cases and type A4 is found in 2%.[8]

In the fetus, the hemodynamic concern is the presence or absence of truncal valve insufficiency. Both ventricles in the fetus function as a single chamber; mixing of blood occurs by way of the VSD. If the truncal valve is competent, no significant problems are evident in utero. However, an incompetent or insufficient truncal valve can result in regurgitation of blood back into the ventricles and subsequent congestive heart failure (CHF). Soon after birth, the foramen ovale and ductus arteriosus (if present) close, resulting in a large left-to-right shunt that increases as the pulmonary vascular resistance falls. This, along with the truncal valve regurgitation that is present in about 50% of patients, results in a pressure overload to the already volume-overloaded ventricles.[12,14,15] Pulmonary vascular obstructive disease usually develops by 6 months of age. Cyanosis and progressive CHF are common.[16]

Embryology

Persistent truncus arteriosus results from a failure of septation of the embryonic truncus arteriosus and the conal septum.[17,18] In the normally developing heart, a single heart tube elongates and divides into ventricular and atrial components, with a small, narrow mid portion becoming the bulbus cordis.[17,18] The mid portion of the bulbus cordis forms the outflow tracts of the right and left ventricles and is referred to as the cornus cordis. The inferior portion of the bulbus cordis gives rise to a short arterial trunk, the truncus arteriosus.[17,18] Beginning at approximately 27 days' gestation, spiral ridges of endocardial tissue form within the lumen of the truncus arteriosus. These ridges fuse together, resulting in the aorticopulmonary or spiral septum. It is this septum that divides the truncus into an anterior pulmonary artery and a posterior aorta (Fig. 14–3).[18] Concurrently, the conal septum forms to divide the bulbus cordis. The spiral and conal septa merge, resulting in right ventricular-to-pulmonary artery continuity.[18] The aortic and pulmonary valves form at the level of fusion of these septa.

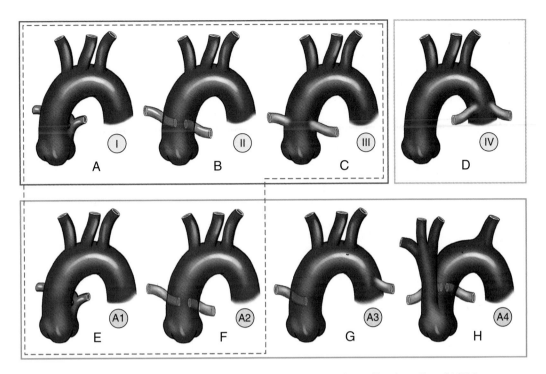

Figure 14–2   A through **D,** Collett-Edwards types I, II, III, and IV classifications. Type IV **(D)** is now considered pulmonary atresia with a VSD. **E** through **H,** Van Praagh modifications of Collett-Edwards classifications. Collett-Edwards types I, II, and III (**A** to **C**) and Van Praagh types A1 and A2 (**E** and **F**) are similar, differing only in the number and location of the pulmonary arteries originating from the truncus. Van Praagh type A3 **(G)** has a single pulmonary artery arising from the truncus and the second pulmonary artery from the descending aorta. In Van Praagh type A4 **(H),** a hypoplastic aortic arch and a patent ductus arteriosus arise from the truncus arteriosus. Pulmonary arteries originate from the posterior aspect of the truncus arteriosus.

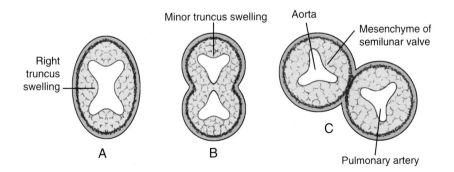

Figure 14–3   Transverse sections through the truncus arteriosus at the level of the semilunar valves at 5 **(A),** 6 **(B),** and 7 **(C)** weeks of development, showing fusion of the truncoconal ridges that results in formation of an anterior pulmonary artery and a posterior aorta.

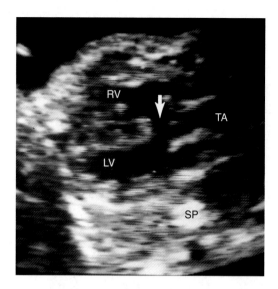

Figure 14–4 Subcostal five-chamber view in a fetus with truncus arteriosus. The single trunk *(TA)* can be seen overriding the VSD *(arrow)*. *LV,* Left ventricle; *RV,* right ventricle; *SP,* spine.

Failure of the spiral septum to form results in a single great vessel and a single outflow tract. This developmental failure also produces a large defect in the infundibular septum. The size and position of the concurrent VSD is determined by the degree of deficiency of the conal septum.[19] Failure of fusion usually occurs in the sixth or seventh week of gestation. This developmental failure also results in a variety of malformations of the truncal valve leaflets because two semilunar valves are normally formed from embryological tubercles on the truncal wall.[17,18] The truncal valve may have thickened or poorly formed cusps. The cusps may prolapse, resulting in regurgitation. The truncal valve is anatomically continuous with the mitral valve but frequently not with the tricuspid valve.

The truncal root may be dilated as a result of receiving both the right and left ventricular components of the circulation. The ductus arteriosus may be absent, or if present it can be large in association with a hypoplastic or interrupted aorta. One of the pulmonary arteries may be absent, most commonly ipsilateral to the aortic arch. Also, the coronary arteries may vary in their origins. Failure of septation of the truncus arteriosus is thought to result from failure of neural crest cell migration.[20] The fact that maternal diabetes is associated with an increased risk of persistent truncus arteriosus supports this theory.[21]

Occurrence Rate

Persistent truncus arteriosus is a rare anomaly, accounting for 0.4% to 2.8% of all congenital heart defects.[2,5,14,22,23]

As is true of most congenital heart defects, the occurrence risk in siblings of an affected infant is slightly higher than in the general population. With truncus arteriosus, the occurrence risk in a sibling is approximately 1.2%.[24]

In general, males have a higher incidence of cardiac anomalies and a higher incidence of lethal anomalies. However, truncus arteriosus appears to occur equally in males and females.[25]

Sonographic Criteria

The in utero diagnosis of persistent truncus arteriosus can be challenging.[26-28] However, increased equipment resolution and improved operator expertise have contributed to improved prenatal identification. The predominant finding is a single large truncal vessel overriding a VSD (Fig. 14–4). When this is present, the differential diagnosis includes tetralogy of Fallot or pulmonary atresia with a VSD. The definitive diagnosis can be made only if more than three leaflets are identified within the truncal valve or if the origin of the pulmonary arteries can be identified arising from the trunk.[25]

The apical four-chamber view of the heart usually appears normal in fetuses with truncus arteriosus (Fig. 14–5). Anterior angulation of the transducer from the apical four-chamber view will result in a five-chamber view, which should allow visualization of the single trunk overriding the accompanying VSD (Fig. 14–6).

The subcostal four-chamber view can also appear unremarkable; however, because the incident beam is perpendicular to the ventricular septum in this projection, the VSD may be easier to visualize. Angling toward the fetal right shoulder from the subcostal four-chamber view allows visualization of a long-axis view of the aorta. From this projection, the single vessel overriding the VSD should be seen (Fig. 14–7).

The truncal valve orifice is commonly dilated. The long-axis view of the aorta may also allow visualization of the multileaflet truncal valve doming into the left ventricular outflow tract, if valvular insufficiency is present (Fig. 14–8).[28] A

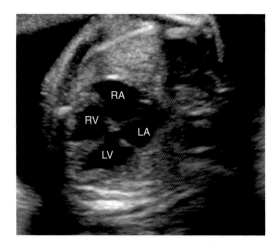

Figure 14–5   Normal-appearing four-chamber view of the heart in a fetus with truncus arteriosus. *LA,* Left atrium; *LV,* left ventricle; *RA,* right atrium; *RV,* right ventricle.

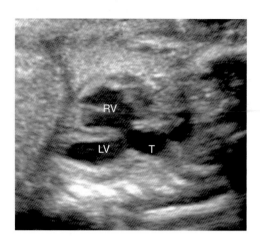

Figure 14–7   Long-axis view showing the large truncal artery *(T)* overriding a VSD. *LV,* Left ventricle; *RV,* right ventricle.

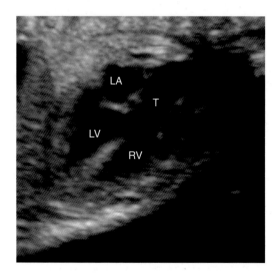

Figure 14–6   Angulation of the transducer into an apical five-chamber view reveals the large truncal artery *(T)* overriding a large VSD. *LA,* Left atrium; *LV,* left ventricle; *RV,* right ventricle.

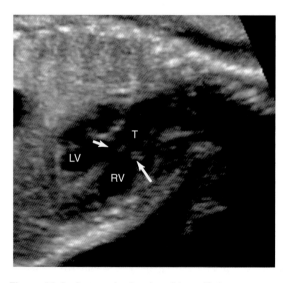

Figure 14–8   Long-axis view in a fetus with truncus arteriosus showing the valve leaflets *(arrows)* of the single truncal valve *(T)* doming into the ventricles. *LV,* Left ventricle; *RV,* right ventricle.

continuation of this rotation, into a long-axis view of the pulmonary artery, should result in an inability to identify a normal right ventricular outflow tract.

A short-axis view of the great vessels should show the single large truncal valve. In this view the number of leaflets present in the vessel may be appreciated. The truncal valve leaflets can also appear thickened. Again, the absence of a normally positioned pulmonary artery should be apparent. By sliding superiorly on the vessel, from either a long or short axis, it may be possible to

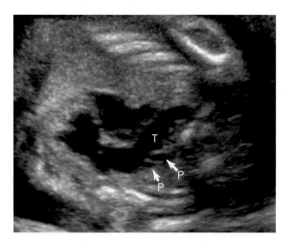

Figure 14–9 Anomalous pulmonary arteries *(P)* arising from the large truncal artery *(T)* in persistent truncus arteriosus.

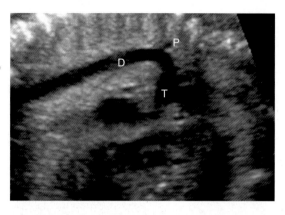

Figure 14–10 Truncal arch *(T)* in a fetus with persistent truncus arteriosus. An anomalous pulmonary artery *(P)* is seen originating from the descending aorta *(D)*.

identify the pulmonary arteries as they arise from the trunk (Fig. 14–9). Because the ductus arteriosus is absent in 50% to 75% of cases, a thorough attempt should be made to identify it in either a short-axis or ductal arch view.[14,26,27] Evaluating the fetal aortic arch is important for several reasons. A right-sided aortic arch has been reported in 15% to 30% of patients.[8,14,22,28,29] Interruption of the aortic arch has also been associated with persistent truncus arteriosus.[9] Additionally, as described previously, the aberrant pulmonary arteries may arise from the descending aorta (Fig. 14–10). The three-vessel view in this setting should look abnormal with only one great vessel present.

Pulsed-wave and color flow Doppler imaging are also important in making the diagnosis of persistent truncus arteriosus. Once the single trunk has been identified, Doppler imaging should be used to identify the presence of valvular insufficiency or stenosis (Fig. 14–11). Mild to moderate valvular regurgitation is present in 40% to 50% of cases.[3] Although the VSD is usually readily apparent on two-dimensional imaging alone, color or pulsed Doppler imaging can be used for confirmation. A lack of a Doppler signal in the ductus arteriosus or in the aortic arch may indicate agenesis or interruption. Color Doppler imaging is also helpful in identifying the small pulmonary artery branches arising from the common trunk.

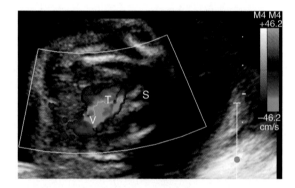

Figure 14–11 Color Doppler imaging showing regurgitant blood flow *(blue)* returning into the ventricle *(V)* from the truncal artery *(T)*. S, Spine.

Once the diagnosis of truncus arteriosus has been established in utero, serial sonographic examinations should be performed to monitor for signs of CHF. Nonimmune hydrops fetalis suggests a dismal outcome and may alter obstetrical management. Genetic counseling is warranted because of the association of chromosomal defects and other anomalies.

Treatment

Pulmonary artery size and pulmonary vascular resistance determine the clinical sequelae in patients with persistent truncus arteriosus. Normal pulmonary vasculature and low resistance result in increased blood flow and mild or no cyanosis in the infant; cyanosis may become worse, however, on exertion. Conversely, poorly developed pulmonary arteries, a single pulmonary artery, or high pulmonary vascular resistance result in severe cyanosis.[9] Symptoms may also include polycythemia, dyspnea, and respiratory infections.

Physical examination often reveals normal blood pressure and increased liver size resulting from CHF. The first heart sound, which represents closure of the atrioventricular valves, is normal. The second heart sound, representing truncal valve closure, is loud and may be followed by a murmur, indicating the presence of valvular insufficiency.[6,9] An electrocardiogram usually exhibits normal sinus rhythm.

On a chest film, the heart may or may not appear enlarged, depending on the amount of left-to-right shunting. As this shunting decreases with increasing pulmonary vascular resistance, the heart size will decrease. Cardiac catheterization provides information regarding the oxygen saturation in the trunk and in the pulmonary arteries and pressure measurements of the right ventricle. This pressure is equal to the systemic pressure. The degree of truncal valve regurgitation and pulmonary artery size can also be evaluated.[6]

Persistent truncus arteriosus invariably requires operative repair. The onset of symptoms may occur in the first day or so if severe truncal valve regurgitation is present.[25,30] Early corrective surgery is usually necessary to prevent pulmonary vascular disease and CHF. Fluid restriction, diuretic therapy, or digitalis administration may all be used initially to improve the sequelae associated with CHF and to allow the infant to stabilize and grow.[31] These measures are only temporary, however, with surgery usually recommended within the first 2 months of life.[31,32] If severe CHF is not present, surgery can be delayed until after neonatal pulmonary vascular resistance has fallen. Persistent, severe CHF requires that surgical repair be undertaken immediately.

Surgical management of persistent truncus arteriosus has undergone significant evolution.[33] Until successful surgical repair was achieved in the late 1960s, treatment in infants with truncus arteriosus was mostly palliative. Pioneering work in the surgical correction of truncus arteriosus was carried out by Rastelli et al,[34] followed by early procedures performed by McGoon.[35] In 1984 Ebert et al[36] reported an overall mortality rate of 19% in 106 infants who had surgery before 6 months of age. Truncal valve insufficiency contributed to a higher postoperative mortality rate. The surgical mortality increases significantly for repairs performed after 6 months of age because of the possibility of ventricular dysfunction and the high probability that pulmonary vascular disease has already developed. One-stage surgical repair in the early neonatal period has now become the gold standard.[37]

A Rastelli procedure is often the surgery of choice in the repair of persistent truncus arteriosus (Fig. 14–12). It involves excising the pulmonary artery from the trunk and closing the resulting defect. The VSD is also closed with a synthetic patch, resulting in blood being ejected into the common trunk from the left ventricle only, thereby establishing it as the systemic artery. Valved conduits are then used to reconstruct the right ventricular outflow tract, providing a connection between the right ventricle and the origin of the main pulmonary artery. These conduits consist of a homograft aorta or pulmonary artery,

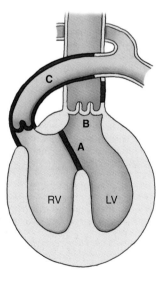

Figure 14–12 Diagram of the Rastelli procedure showing the VSD repair *(A)*, the repair to the defect in the truncal valve *(B)*, and the placement of a conduit *(C)* between the right ventricle and the pulmonary artery. *LV,* Left ventricle; *RV,* right ventricle.

including the valve, or they can be made of polyester and contain a porcine valve.[34,35] A disadvantage of the homografts has been a tendency toward wall calcification creating an obstruction to outflow. However, newer cryopreservation techniques have led to improved results. Pearl et al[37] reported a 14% incidence of homograft obstruction over the first 3 postoperative years compared with a 71% incidence of obstruction in the polyester-porcine grafts over 6 years. Very young patients must have the conduit replaced with a larger one once they are older, but this seems to be a low-risk procedure.

Truncal valve regurgitation increases the surgical risk significantly and determines the type of surgical correction, depending on the patient's age.[38] In infants, valve repair is preferred over replacement whenever possible. In older patients, the valve can be replaced at the same time as the surgical repair if the regurgitation is severe enough to warrant it.

Interrupted aortic arch occurs in 15% of patients. The operative mortality in patients with associated interrupted aortic arch is 37% compared with 20% in patients without an interrupted aortic arch.[37,39]

Postoperative complications include tamponade and bronchial and coronary artery compression. These specific problems are thought to result from the limited space in the thorax secondary to conduit placement.[39,40] Conduction system injury may occur, depending on the position of the atrioventricular bundle in relation to the VSD.[41] Cardiac pacing may be required in some cases. Pulmonary

TABLE 14–1   Conditions Associated with Truncus Arteriosus

| Maternal | Fetal | | |
Condition	Associated Cardiac Abnormalities	Chromosome Abnormalities	Syndromes
Diabetes	Aberrant origin of right subclavian artery	Monosomy lq4	CHARGE (coloboma, heart disease, atresia choanae, retarded growth and development or central nervous system anomalies, genital hypoplasia, and ear anomalies or deafness) syndrome
	Aberrant origin of brachiocephalic trunk	Monosomy 11q	
	Aberrant origin of left subclavian artery	Trisomy lq32-qter	Cryptophthalmus-syndactyly syndrome
	Aneurysm of fossa ovalis		DiGeorge syndrome
	Atrial septal defect		Distichiasis-lymphedema
	Atrioventricular septal defect		Femoral-facial syndrome
	Common brachiocephalic artery		Fraser syndrome
	Complete heart block		Hydrolethalus syndrome
	Dextrocardia		Johanson-Blizzard syndrome
	Dextroversion		Tracheal agenesis–multiple anomaly association
	Diverticulum of right ventricle		
	Interrupted aortic arch		
	Incomplete cor triatriatum		
	Left superior vena cava		
	Mitral atresia		
	Narrowing of right pulmonary artery and subclavian artery, forming collateral anastomosis to pulmonary artery		
	Partial anomalous pulmonary venous connection		
	Single ventricle		
	Supraventricular tachycardia		
	Total anomalous pulmonary venous connection		
	Tricuspid insufficiency		
	Wolfe-Parkinson-White syndrome		

hypertension and right heart failure have also been reported.[42,43]

Prognosis

Persistent truncus arteriosus is well tolerated in utero.[44] However, survival beyond infancy is uncommon. Left untreated, patients have a dismal prognosis, with a 65% 6-month and a 75% 1-year mortality rate.[5,33] Death is usually the result of CHF or pulmonary vascular disease.[31] In some patients, heart failure may occur because of truncal valve insufficiency. Sudden death has been reported in neonates who have a stenotic truncal valve.[33] Prenatal pulsed Doppler velocities above 2 meters/second are associated with adverse neonatal outcome.[33]

Reported surgical mortality rates after persistent truncus arteriosus repair are variable, ranging from 13% to 50%.[35,37,38,43] Long-term survival after surgical correction has been reported to range from 30% to 83% at 15 years of age.[37,43]

Children with a 22q11 microdeletion and congenital heart disease are at a higher risk for morbidity and death as determined by both the severity of the cardiac lesions and the extracardiac anomalies associated with the microdeletion.[45]

Associated Anomalies

Approximately 43% to 48% of infants affected with persistent truncus arteriosus have associated extracardiac abnormalities, including holoprosencephaly, agenesis of the corpus callosum, ventriculomegaly, cleft lip and palate, renal abnormalities and duodenal atresia.[3] Persistent truncus arteriosus has been reported with a variety of syndromes and chromosome abnormalities (Table 14–1), the most significant being the 22q11 microdeletion associated with DiGeorge syndrome, which has been reported in 33% of patients.[46–49] Conversely, a 21% incidence of truncus arteriosus has been reported in infants affected with DiGeorge syndrome.[7] Persistent truncus arteriosus and double-outlet right ventricle are the primary cardiac lesions found in infants of diabetic mothers, with a risk factor of approximately 13%.[2]

Persistent truncus arteriosus is also associated with other cardiac abnormalities in 35% of cases, including atrial septal defect, truncal valve abnormalities, partial anomalous pulmonary venous connection, and rarely mitral valve or tricuspid valve atresia.[3,23] Abnormalities of the aorta—namely, right-sided aortic arch—have been reported in approximately 15% to 30% of patients.[8,22,28,29] The presence of the VSD in truncus arteriosus may account for associated arrhythmias, such as supraventricular tachycardia and complete heart block.[35]

References

1. Langford Kidd BS: Persistent truncus arteriosus. In: Keith JD, Rowe RD, Vlad P (eds): Heart Disease in Infancy and Childhood, 3rd ed. New York, Macmillan, 1978, pp 457–469.
2. Ferencz C: A case-control study of cardiovascular malformations in liveborn infants: The morphogenetic relevance of epidemiologic findings. In: Clark EB, Takao A (eds): Developmental Cardiology; Morphogenesis and Function. Mount Kisco, NY, Futura, 1990, pp 526–551.
3. Volpe P, Paladini D, Marasini M, et al: Common arterial trunk in the fetus: characteristics, associations, and outcome in a multicentre series of 23 cases. Heart 2003; 89:1437–1441.
4. Mavroudis C, Backer CL: Truncus arteriosus. In: Mavroudis C (ed): Pediatric Cardiac Surgery. St Louis, Mosby–Year Book, 1994, pp 237–245.
5. Collett RW, Edwards JE: Persistent truncus arteriosus: A classification according to anatomic types. Surg Clin North Am 1949; 29:1245–1270.
6. Hillis LD, Firth BG, Willerson JT: Truncus arteriosus. In: Manual of Clinical Problems in Cardiology, 2nd ed. New York, Little, Brown, 1984, pp 187–189.
7. Nyberg DH, Emerson DS: Cardiac malformations. In: Nyberg DA, Mahoney BS, Pretorius DS (eds): Diagnostic Ultrasound of Fetal Anomalies. Text and Atlas. Chicago, Year Book Medical, 1990, pp 324–328.
8. Van Praagh R, Van Praagh S: The anatomy of common aorticopulmonary trunk (truncus arteriosus communis) and its embryologic implications: A study of 57 necropsy cases. Am J Cardiol 1965; 16:406–423.
9. Nadas AS, Fyler DC: Communications between systemic and pulmonary circuits with predominantly left to right shunts. Pediatric Cardiology, 3rd ed. Philadelphia, WB Saunders, 1972, pp 438–443.
10. Elami A, Laks H, Pearl J: Truncal valve repair: Initial experiences with infants and children. Ann Thorac Surg 1994; 57:397–402.
11. Chawki E, Michel I, Sulekha K, et al: Severe truncal valve stenosis: Diagnosis and management. J Card Surg 2005; 20:589–593.
12. Allan LD, Crawford DC, Anderson RH: Spectrum of congenital heart disease detected

echocardiographically in prenatal life. Br Heart J 1984; 54:523–526.

13. Perloff JK: Truncus arteriosus communis. In: Bharati S, Lev M (eds): The Pathology of Congenital Heart Disease; A Personal Experience with More Than 6,300 Congenitally Malformed Hearts, vol I. Armonk, NY, Futura, 1996, pp 353–380.

14. Calder L, Van Praagh R, Van Praagh S, et al: Truncus arteriosus communis. Clinical, angiocardiographic, and pathologic findings in 100 patients. Am Heart J 1976; 92:23–38.

15. Romero R, Pilu G, Jeanty P, et al: The heart. In: Romero R, Pilu G, Jeanty P, et al (eds): Prenatal Diagnosis of Congenital Anomalies. Norwalk, CT, Appleton & Lange, 1987, pp 168–171.

16. Cheng W, Nichols DG, Cameron DE: Truncus arteriosus. In: Nichols DG, Cameron DE, Greeley WJ, et al (eds): Critical Heart Disease in Infants and Children. St Louis, Mosby–Year Book, 1995, pp 797–807.

17. Sadler TW: Cardiovascular system. In: Sadler TW (ed): Langman's Medical Embryology, 6th ed. Baltimore, Williams & Wilkins, 1990, pp 179–227.

18. Moore KL: In: The Circulatory System. The Developing Human, 4th ed. Philadelphia, WB Saunders, 1988, pp 286–333.

19. Verrier ED, Hanley FL, Turley H: Truncus arteriosus. In: Congiel LD (ed): Cardiac Surgery; State of the Art Reviews. Philadelphia, Hanley & Belfus, 1989, pp 201–215.

20. Leatherbury L, Connock DM, Gauldin HE, et al: Hemodynamic changes and compensatory mechanisms during early cardiogenesis after neural crest ablation in chick embryos. Pediatr Res 1990; 30:509–512.

21. Ferencz C, Rubin JD, McCarter RJ, et al: Maternal diabetes and cardiovascular malformations: Predominance of double outlet right ventricle and truncus arteriosus. Teratology 1990; 41:319–326.

22. Crupi GM, McCartney FJ, Anderson RH: Persistent truncus arteriosus: A study of 66 autopsy cases with special reference to definition and morphogenesis. Am J Cardiol 1977; 40:569–578.

23. Fyler DC, Buckley LP, Hellenbrand WE, et al: Report of the New England Regional Infant Cardiac Program. Pediatrics 1980; 65:374–461.

24. Keith JD: Prevalence, incidence, and epidemiology. In: Keith JD, Rowe RD, Vlad P (eds): Heart Disease in Infancy and Childhood, 3rd ed. New York, Macmillan, 1978, pp 3–13.

25. Tometzki AJ, Suda K, Kohl T, et al: Accuracy of prenatal echocardiographic diagnosis and prognosis of fetuses with conotruncal anomalies. J Am Coll Cardiol 1999; 33:1696–1701.

26. deAraujo LML, Schmidt KG, Silverman WH, et al: Prenatal diagnosis of truncus arteriosus by ultrasound. Pediatr Cardiol 1987; 8:261–263.

27. Allan LD, Crawford DC, Chita SK, et al: Prenatal screening for congenital heart disease. BMJ 1986; 292:1717–1719.

28. Kleinman CS, Santulli TV: Ultrasonic evaluation of the fetal human heart. Semin Perinatol 1983; 7:90–101.

29. Hastreiter AR, D'Cruz IA, Cantez T: Right-sided aorta. Br Heart J 1966; 28:722–725.

30. Lev M, Shaphiro O: Truncus arteriosus in the first six months of life. Ann Surg 1984; 200:451–456.

31. Castaneda AR, Mayer JE Jr, Jonas RA, et al: The neonate with critical congenital heart disease: Repair—A surgical challenge. J Thorac Cardiovasc Surg 1989; 98:869–875.

32. Mair DD, Edwards WD, Julsrud PR, et al: Truncus arteriosus. In: Emmanouilides GC, Riemenschnieder TA, Allen HD, et al (eds): Moss & Adams' Heart Disease in Infants and Children and Adolescents: Including the Fetus and Young Adult, 5th ed, vols 1 and 2. Baltimore, Williams & Wilkins, 1995, pp 1026–1041.

33. Turley K: Current method of repair of truncus arteriosus. J Cardiovasc Surg 1992; 7:1–4.

34. Rastelli GC, Titus JL, McGoon DC: Homograft of ascending aorta and aortic valve as a right ventricular outflow: An experimental approach to the repair of truncus arteriosus. Arch Surg 1967; 95:698–708.

35. McGoon DC, Rastelli GC, Ongley PA: An operation for the correction of truncus arteriosus. JAMA 1968; 205:59–62.

36. Ebert PA, Turley K, Stanger P, et al: Surgical treatment of truncus arteriosus in the first six months of life. Ann Surg 1984; 200:451–456.

37. Pearl JM, Laks H, Drinkwater DC Jr, et al: Repair of conotruncal abnormalities with the use of the valved conduit: Improved early and mid-term results with the cryopreserved homograft. J Am Coll Cardiol 1992; 20:191–196.

38. Hanley FL, Heinemann MK, Jonas RA, et al: Repair of truncus arteriosus in the neonate. J Thorac Cardiovasc Surg 1993;105:1047–1056.

39. Sano S, Brawn WJ, Mee RB: Repair of truncus arteriosus and interrupted aortic arch. J Cardiovasc Surg 1990; 5:157–162.

40. Harris JP, Stewart S, Anderson V, et al: Coronary artery injury by a valved external conduit. Ann Thorac Surg 1981; 31:271–273.

41. Bharati S, Karp R, Lev M: The conduction system in truncus arteriosus and its surgical significance: A study of five cases. J Thorac Cardiovasc Surg 1992; 104:954–960.

42. Davis DA, Russo P: Successful treatment of acute postoperative pulmonary hypertension with nifedipine. Ann Thorac Surg 1992; 53:148–150.

43. Miyamoto T, Sinzobahamvya N, Kumpikaite D, et al: Repair of truncus arteriosus and aortic arch interruption: outcome analysis. Ann Thorac Surg 2005; 79:2077–2082.

44. Duke C, Sharland GK, Jones AMR, et al: Echocardiographic features and outcome of truncus arteriosus diagnosed during fetal life. Am J Cardiol 2001; 88:1379–1384.

45. Kyburz A, Bauersfeld U, Schinzel A, et al: The fate of children with microdeletion 22q11.2 syndrome and congenital heart defect: Clinical course and cardiac outcome. Pediatr Cardiol 2008; 29:76–83.

46. Van Mierop LH, Kutsche LM: Cardiovascular anomalies in DiGeorge syndrome and importance of neural crest as a possible pathogenetic factor. Am J Cardiol 1986; 58:133–137.

47. Radford DJ, Perkins L, Lachman R, et al: Spectrum of DiGeorge syndrome in patients with truncus arteriosus: Expanded DiGeorge syndrome. Pediatr Cardiol 1988; 9:95–101.

48. Goldmuntz E, Clark BJ, Mitchell LE, et al: Frequency of 22q11 deletions in patients with conotruncal defects. J Am Coll Cardiol 1998; 32:492–498.

49. Volpe P, Marasini M, Caruso G, et al: 22q11 deletions in fetuses with malformations of the outflow tracts or interruption of the aortic arch: impact of additional ultrasound signs. Prenat Diagn 2003; 23:752–757.

CHAPTER 15

Complete and Congenitally Corrected Transposition of the Great Arteries

Elizabeth M. Shaffer

Transposition of the great arteries (TGA) occurs in many complex forms of congenital heart disease. Two types of TGA are described: complete transposition and congenitally corrected transposition.[1] These two types of TGA are entirely different entities in embryology, anatomy, physiology, and treatment. The term "d-transposition" is sometimes used when referring to complete transposition of the great arteries and "l-transposition" when referring to congenitally corrected transposition of the great arteries. The d- and l- refer to the position of the aorta in relationship to the pulmonary artery with d- meaning to the right of (dextro) and l- to the left of (levo) the pulmonary artery. In both cases, the pulmonary artery is connected to the left ventricle and the aorta is connected to the right ventricle. There are major differences between complete transposition and corrected transposition that warrant discussing the two syndromes individually.

Complete Transposition of the Great Arteries

Definition

TGA is defined as the aorta arising from the right ventricle and the pulmonary artery arising from the left ventricle. The majority of fetuses with TGA have complete or d-transposition. In patients with complete transposition, the connections between the atria and the ventricles are normal or concordant, meaning that the right atrium connects through the tricuspid valve to the morphological right ventricle and the left atrium connects through the mitral valve to the morphological left ventricle. However, the aorta arises from the right ventricle and the pulmonary artery arises from the left ventricle (Fig. 15–1). In the normal heart, the pulmonary and systemic circulations function in series. In complete transposition, the pulmonary and systemic circulations function in parallel, resulting in cyanosis after birth (Fig. 15–2). Therefore the only possible mixing of venous and arterial blood with complete transposition occurs through atrial, ventricular, or great artery connections.

Before surgical correction, at least one avenue of mixing between the pulmonic and systemic circulations must be present to support life. The right ventricle serves as the systemic ventricle in complete transposition, leading to potential right ventricular hypertrophy and dysfunction. This fact has important consequences for the management of complete transposition.

Embryology

By the end of the fourth week after conception, the truncus arteriosus divides into the aorta and the pulmonary artery. This is accomplished by the caudal spiral growth of the conotruncal ridges so that, in the normal heart, the aorta rises from the left ventricle and the pulmonary artery arises from the right ventricle. If the septum grows downward in a straight manner instead of spiraling manner, the expected relationship between the ventricles and the great vessels is disrupted. As a result, not only do the aorta and pulmonary arteries originate from the ventricles opposite those in the normal heart, but they are also oriented parallel to each other and do not cross.

The heart and abdominal organs are positioned in the normal fashion (situs solitus) in 95% of patients with complete transposition.[2]

Occurrence Rate

Complete transposition of the great arteries occurs in 5% to 8% of infants born with congenital heart disease, or 0.206 per 1000 live births.[1] It makes up 5.5% of all heart disease in the fetal population.[3]

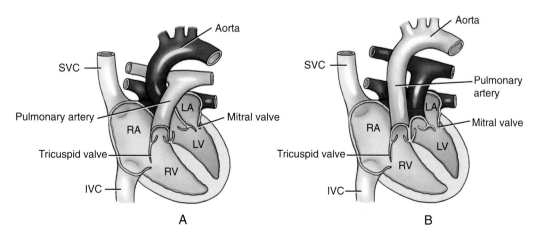

Figure 15–1 Diagram of the anatomical findings associated with complete TGA **(B)** compared with a normal heart **(A)**. The right-sided aorta arises from the right ventricle, and the left-sided pulmonary artery arises from the left ventricle. *IVC,* Inferior vena cava; *LA,* left atrium; *LV,* left ventricle; *RA,* right atrium; *RV,* right ventricle; *SVC,* superior vena cava.

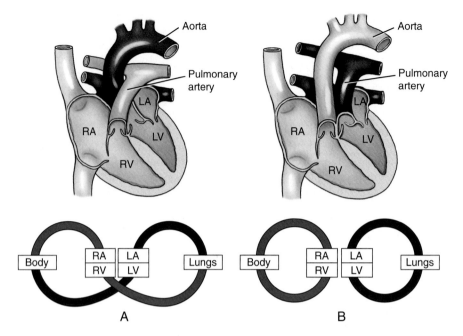

Figure 15–2 Diagram of the parallel circulation that occurs in complete transposition **(B)** compared with the series circulation of a normal heart **(A).** *LA,* Left atrium; *LV,* left ventricle; *RA,* right atrium; *RV,* right ventricle.

There is a male predominance in complete transposition.

Sonographic Criteria

To evaluate the transposition complexes, chamber identification must be reviewed. The cardiac chambers and great vessels are identified by morphological characteristics rather than by location or position in the chest. The atria are identified by their atrial appendages and the foraminal flap. The left atrial appendage is long and fingerlike, whereas the right atrial appendage is broad based and has pectinate muscles. The atrial appendages may be difficult to identify by fetal echocardiography, but the foraminal flap, which will be seen opening into the left atrium in the normal heart, is usually well seen and is a morphological marker of the left atrium. The ventricles are identified by their atrioventricular valve and musculature. The tricuspid valve is associated with the right ventricle and is slightly more apically positioned than is the mitral valve. The tricuspid valve has attachments to the ventricular septum, whereas the mitral valve does not. The right ventricle also has a prominent moderator band near the apex that

is easily appreciated on fetal echocardiography. The left ventricle is smooth walled with no muscle bundles. The pulmonary artery is distinguished from the aorta because it branches into left and right pulmonary arteries, whereas the head and neck vessels and the coronary arteries arise from the aorta.

The prenatal detection of complete transposition by fetal echocardiography has been reported by numerous authors but remains a challenge.[4–6] In a recent study, only 7% (25 of 346) of patients with TGA were diagnosed prenatally.[7] The prenatal diagnosis of complete transposition has been shown to improve the outcome of patients.[8] The apical and subcostal four-chamber views are usually completely normal with complete transposition of the great arteries.[9] The ventricular outflow tracts must be imaged if complete transposition is to be diagnosed in the fetus. From the subcostal four-chamber view, the transducer should be angled toward the fetal right shoulder to appreciate the outflow tracts. In complete transposition, the great vessels are parallel, not crossing, at the level of the semilunar valves (Fig. 15–3). The ascending aorta is seen arising from the right

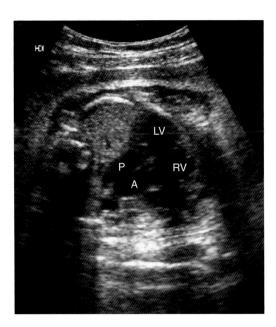

Figure 15–3 Parallel outflow tracts in a fetus with complete TGA. *A,* Aorta; *LV,* left ventricle; *P,* pulmonary artery; *RV,* right ventricle.

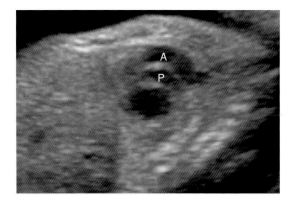

Figure 15–4 Short-axis view of the great vessels in a fetus with complete transposition, showing the aorta *(A)* and pulmonary artery *(P)* arising in a parallel fashion.

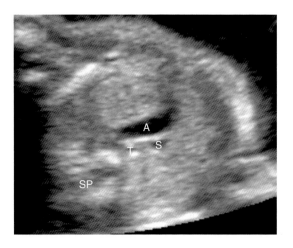

Figure 15–5 Three-vessel tracheal view in a fetus with complete TGA showing only the aorta *(A)* and superior vena cava *(S)*. *SP,* Spine; *T,* trachea.

ventricle and continuing as the aortic arch and the descending aorta. The pulmonary artery arises from the left ventricle, branches into the left and right pulmonary arteries, and continues as the ductal arch.

The short-axis view at the level of the great vessels is also useful in diagnosing complete transposition of the great arteries. In this view, the great vessels lose their normal orientation of the right ventricular outflow tract and pulmonary artery wrapping around the circular aorta. Instead, they will appear as two side-by-side circular structures or as parallel vessels arising in an oblique fashion (Fig. 15–4).

A three-vessel view (3VV) is also useful in diagnosing complete transposition. This view is obtained by sliding the transducer cephalad from an apical four-chamber view. In the normal heart, the aorta and pulmonary artery will form a "V" from the fetal spine. In the setting of complete transposition, the vessels may assume a more parallel orientation.

In a study by Vinals et al,[10] the examination of the fetal heart by a series of transverse short-axis views from the fetal abdomen to the trachea proved helpful in the diagnosis of TGA. The trans-verse cardiac sweeps obtained were four-chamber, five-chamber, 3VV, and three-vessel trachea (3VVT) views. The most reliable characteristics of complete transposition were a branching great artery arising from the left ventricle seen in the five-chamber view, and two vessels (aortic arch and superior vena cava) rather than three seen at the level of the 3VVT view (Fig. 15–5).

Associated Anomalies

Other cardiac defects that are commonly present with complete transposition include ventricular

TABLE 15–1 Conditions Associated with Complete and Corrected Transposition of the Great Arteries

Maternal		Fetal		
Condition	Drug Use	Associated Cardiac Abnormalities	Chromosome Abnormality	Syndromes
Diabetes	Accutane	Arrhythmia	Monosomy 22q	Carpenter syndrome
	Amphetamine	Atrial septal defect		CHIME (coloboma, heart anomaly, ichthyosis, mental retardation, ear abnormality) syndrome
	Retinoic acid	Coarctation		
	Thalidomide	Dextrocardia		
	Trifluoperazine	Double-outlet right ventricle		
	Trimethadione	Ebstein anomaly		Cryptophthalmos syndrome
		Hypoplastic left heart syndrome		DiGeorge syndrome
				Fraser syndrome
		Hypoplastic right ventricle		Johanson-Blizzard syndrome
		Mesocardia		Klippel-Feil syndrome
		Pulmonary atresia		Pena-Shokeir syndrome
		Pulmonary stenosis		Polydactyly-chondrodystrophy types 1 and 2
		Tricuspid insufficiency		
		Ventricular septal defect		Short rib polydactyly

septal defects in 20% of patients and left ventricular outflow tract obstruction in 5% to 40% of patients.[2,3] Extracardiac anomalies are seen in association with complete transposition of the great arteries in approximately 8% of patients. Chromosomal anomalies are rarely associated with this condition (Table 15–1).

Treatment and Prognosis

Two major surgical techniques have been applied to complete transposition: the atrial switch procedure and the arterial switch procedure. Aside from palliative procedures targeted toward maintaining an interatrial communication, the first successful surgical treatment for complete transposition was an atrial switch.[11] This procedure involves interatrial baffles that direct the pulmonary venous flow to the right ventricle (systemic ventricle) and the systemic venous flow to the left ventricle (pulmonary ventricle).[12] The Senning and Mustard procedures produced a remarkable improvement in the survival rates of infants with transposition of the great arteries, from 10% at 1 year to 89% at 10 years.[13,14] Atrial switch procedures have been performed for three decades or more, allowing for significant follow-up data. Progressive late death occurs after the Mustard procedure at a rate of 0.5% per year. Sinus rhythm persists in only 57% of the patients 8 years after the procedure.[15]

Tachyarrhythmias and bradyarrhythmias are common, but tachyarrhythmias are of particular concern because they are associated with sudden death.[14,16] The cause of the increased incidence of arrhythmias is not known precisely but may be related to damage to the sinus node and interruption of the atrial internodal tracts at the time of surgery.[17] About 20% of patients require pacing and additional medication to suppress supraventricular arrhythmias.[18]

Eventual right ventricular dysfunction occurs in many patients after the atrial switch procedure and is related to approximately 20% of the late deaths.[1] With right ventricular dysfunction comes an increased risk of arrhythmias and tricuspid insufficiency.

Repair or replacement of the tricuspid valve is rarely successful in the long term. With complete transposition of the great vessels and no other associated complex lesions, survival of patients who have undergone an atrial switch procedure is 78% at 20 years after surgery.[13] The majority of survivors are classified as having New York Heart Association class I or II disease and report having a relatively normal lifestyle. Careful analysis, including exercise tolerance testing, actually reveals diminished ventricular function in most patients, which is not evident at rest.[19-21]

In contrast to the atrial switch procedure, the arterial switch operation, which was first performed successfully by Jatene et al[6] in 1974, has become the procedure of choice for complete transposition. The procedure involves surgically correcting the ventricular-arterial connections so that a neoaorta and a neopulmonary artery are created to provide outflow to the left and right ventricles, respectively.

The long-term patient follow-up period is significantly shorter for the arterial switch than for the atrial switch; however, it is hoped that fewer complications relating to arrhythmias and ventricular dysfunction will occur.

Initial reports suggest an excellent postsurgical course for most patients. Ventricular function is good and the majority of patients are asymptomatic.[22,23] The arterial switch procedure requires that the coronary arteries be implanted into the neoaorta. Coronary arterial lesions are present in 5% of long-term survivors of the neonatal arterial switch procedure.[24] The long-term complications of the coronary artery disease seen in this group of patients is unknown and warrants further study. Issues with the neoaortic valve and root have also surfaced, but overall the long-term results have been extremely promising.[25]

Congenitally Corrected Transposition of the Great Arteries

Definition

Congenitally corrected or l-transposition of the great arteries is a rare form of congenital heart disease with a prevalence of ≈0.5%.[26] Congenitally corrected transposition of the great arteries (CCTGA) has both atrioventricular and ventriculoarterial discordant connections (double discordance). Double discordance results in normal physiological features. In contrast to patients with complete TGA, patients with CCTGA are acyanotic after birth; however, the right ventricle is the systemic ventricle. In CCTGA, the right atrium connects to the left ventricle and the left ventricle connects to the pulmonary artery. The left atrium connects to the right ventricle and the right ventricle connects to the aorta.[27] In most cases, the right and left atria remain in their usual right and left positions; however, in 20% to 25% of CCTGA in postnatal life, dextrocardia is present.[28] Dextrocardia was present in 17% of fetuses diagnosed with CCTGA.[29]

Figure 15–6 illustrates the anatomy of CCTGA and compares it with that of the normal heart. Blood circulation in CCTGA is in series, so the individuals are acyanotic (Fig. 15–7). In the absence of other abnormalities, surgery may not be necessary; however, the majority of individuals do have associated abnormalities.

Embryology

Complete TGA is a defect associated with abnormal division of the truncus arteriosus. In contrast, CCTGA is a defect associated with abnormal looping of the heart tube. By the third week after conception, the primitive heart tube begins to fold

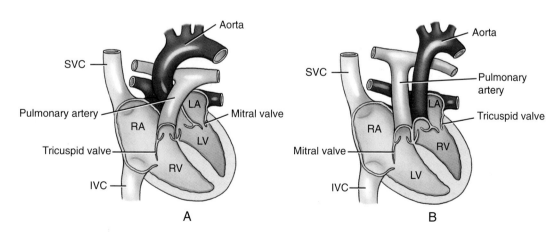

Figure 15–6 Diagram of the anatomical characteristics of corrected TGA **(B)** compared with the normal heart **(A)**. The pulmonary artery arises from the incorrectly located left ventricle *(LV)*, and the aorta arises from the incorrectly located right ventricle *(RV)*. *IVC*, Inferior vena cava; *LA*, left atrium; *RA*, right atrium; *SVC*, superior vena cava.

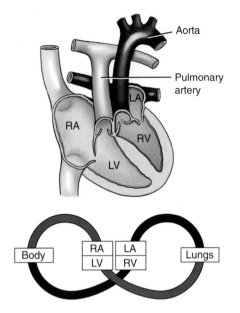

Figure 15–7 Diagram showing circulation in corrected TGA, which remains in series, similar to a normal heart. *LA,* Left atrium; *LV,* left ventricle; *RA,* right atrium; *RV,* right ventricle.

or loop. This is the beginning of the development of the four-chambered heart. Normally, the rapid growth of the heart tube around fixed proximal and distal attachments results in looping of the tube to the right (d loop). This is why the right ventricle comes to lie anterior and to the right of the left ventricle.

The atrioventricular valves passively follow the looping process so that the three-leaflet tricuspid valve sits between the right atrium and the right ventricle and the two-leaflet mitral valve lies between the left atrium and the left ventricle.

Within days of ventricular looping, the truncus arteriosus is divided by the caudal, spiral growth of the conotruncal ridges so that the aorta becomes the leftward and posterior outflow tract for the left ventricle, whereas the pulmonary artery lies anterior and to the right, forming the outflow tract for the right ventricle.

If looping occurs to the left instead of the right (l loop), the ventricle with right ventricular morphological features is displaced to the left, whereas the ventricle with left ventricular morphological features develops to the right. The truncus arteriosus develops by spiral, downward growth of the conotruncal ridges, leading to the pulmonary

artery connecting to the ventricle occupying the rightward position, which has left ventricular morphological features.

The outflow tract for the ventricle on the left, which has right ventricular morphological features, is the aorta. The origin of the aorta is displaced anteriorly and more leftward than is normal.

The conduction system is abnormal in CCTGA. The atrioventricular node and penetrating bundle of His are positioned more anteriorly than is normal and are subject to fibrosis, leading to heart block as a complicating factor in some patients.[1] The incidence of complete heart block is 2% each year, and pacemaker implantation is required in many of these patients.[30]

Occurrence Rate

CCTGA is a rare cardiac anomaly accounting for fewer than 1% of congenital cardiac lesions. As is the case in complete transposition, congenitally corrected transposition is more common in males than in females.

Sonographic Criteria

Correct identification of the cardiac chambers is crucial to the diagnosis of CCTGA. The most obvious finding in the four-chamber view is the position of the right ventricle, which is to the left instead of anterior and rightward. The right ventricle is identified by the apically positioned tricuspid valve and the prominent moderator band (Fig. 15–8). The great vessels are abnormally oriented and exit the heart in parallel (Fig. 15–9). The posterior and rightward great vessel is the pulmonary artery (Fig. 15–10). The pulmonary valve is tucked between the atrioventricular valves. The aorta exits from the left-sided morphological right ventricle in an anterior and leftward course.[1] Two large series of CCTGA in the fetal population have recently been reported.[29,31] In the study by Sharland et al,[31] parallel or abnormal orientation of the great arteries was seen in all 34 fetuses diagnosed with CCTGA; the moderator band identifying the right ventricle in an abnormal position was appreciated in 88%; reversed differential insertion of the tricuspid valve was identified in 76%. All these features were identified in 71%. Isolated CCTGA was present in only 5 of 34 fetuses (15%). The associated cardiac defects included ventricular septal defect (62%), pulmonary stenosis (35%), Ebstein anomaly (23%), and coarctation of the

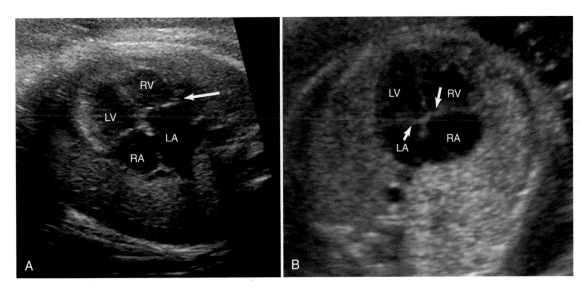

Figure 15–8 A, Apical four-chamber view in a fetus with CCTGA, showing the atrioventricular valve on the anatomic left side abnormally displaced apically *(arrow)*. This is due to the right and left ventricles being "switched." **B,** A normal fetal heart showing the normal position of the sepal leaflet of the tricuspid valve *(long arrow)*, which inserts slightly more apically than the mitral valve *(short arrow). LA,* Left atrium; *LV,* left ventricle; *RA,* right atrium; *RV,* right ventricle.

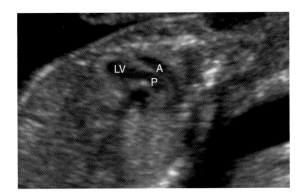

Figure 15–9 Short-axis view of the great vessels in a fetus with CCTGA. The aorta *(A)* and pulmonary artery *(P)* are arising abnormally in a parallel fashion. *LV,* Left ventricle.

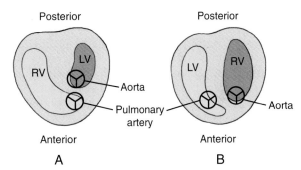

Figure 15–10 Cross-sectional diagrams of the heart showing the great vessel relationship to the ventricles in a normal heart **(A)** and in a heart with CCTGA **(B).** In **B** the great vessels are malpositioned, with the pulmonary artery arising from the right-sided left ventricle and the aorta arising from the left-sided right ventricle. *LV,* Left ventricle; *RV,* right ventricle.

aorta (18%). CCTGA may also be present in fetal hearts with mesocardia, the apex pointing directly midline. The intra-atrial septum can also be positioned more toward the left atrium in this setting.

In addition to structural abnormalities, fetuses with CCTGA may have heart block.[32,33] Jaeggi et al[32] reported 59 consecutive fetal cases of complete atrioventricular block. In this population, 41% had underlying major congenital heart disease. The majority of these fetuses had left atrial isomerism; however, three patients had CCTGA.

Associated Anomalies

Coexisting intracardiac defects are the rule rather than the exception[34] (see Table 15–1). As noted previously, ventricular septal defect, pulmonary stenosis, tricuspid valve abnormalities, coarctation of the aorta, and heart block are the most frequent cardiac abnormalities.

Abnormal cardiac axis (dextrocardia or mesocardia) is present in 20% to 25% of patients with CCTGA.[26,28] Situs inversus may accompany CCTGA; however, the most common situation is situs solitus. With situs inversus, the abdominal viscera are located in positions that are the mirror images of normal, and the atria are also reversed. The morphological left atrium, which is right sided, empties into the right ventricle, which is connected to the aorta; the morphological right atrium, which is left sided, empties into the left ventricle, which is connected to the pulmonary artery. In either situs solitus or situs inversus, the circulation is in series, and the pulmonary and systemic blood flow is normal.[27] As with complete transposition, chromosomal abnormalities are rarely associated.

Treatment and Prognosis

The management of CCTGA is controversial. CCTGA in isolation may not require surgery, but there are concerns about the long-term function of a systemic right ventricle. Some congenital heart disease centers advocate a double switch procedure to have the morphological left ventricle act as the systemic ventricle. Surgical intervention to repair associated lesions is less controversial, but there are many surgical approaches.

If an isolated ventricular septal defect is present, the indications for closure are the same as those for patients without transposition of the great arteries. In the most common situation, a ventricular septal defect is associated with pulmonary stenosis that causes outflow obstruction of the left ventricle (pulmonary ventricle).

When significant obstruction to pulmonary blood flow is present, cyanosis results from right-to-left shunting across the ventricular septal defect. If a simple transannular patch is used, complete heart block is likely to occur as a result of the abnormal course of the conduction system.[27] Extracardiac conduits are required to bypass the narrowed pulmonic tract while preserving normal conduction. It is uncommon for pulmonic obstruction to be significant enough to require correction

in infancy, and procedures are usually delayed until the patient is 2 years of age. If necessary, a palliative systemic-to-pulmonary shunt can be performed early in life, with the definitive procedure performed later. In the setting of CCTGA with an isolated large ventricular septal defect, an alternative to simple closure of the ventricular septal defect has recently been suggested: an atrial and arterial switch in addition to closure of the ventricular septal defect.[35,36] This double-switch procedure is relatively new, and the long-term outlook is not known. The double switch is commonly reserved for patients in whom right ventricular dysfunction or tricuspid (systemic) valve incompetence exists. With a double-switch procedure, the ventricle with left ventricular morphological features becomes the systemic ventricle when the proximal main pulmonary artery is anastomosed to the distal ascending aorta. The ventricle with right ventricular morphological features and the aortic valve are connected to the pulmonary artery bifurcation in the same manner as described for the standard arterial switch procedure in hearts with atrioventricular concordance.[6] The atrioventricular discordance is corrected by a Senning[11] or Mustard[12] procedure, potentially leaving these patients vulnerable to conduction defects and arrhythmias similar to those described in the section on complete transposition of the great arteries.[37]

For patients with pulmonary stenosis, an arterial switch procedure cannot be performed because of left ventricular outflow obstruction; therefore an atrial switch with a Rastelli procedure is an option.[38,39]

A patch is placed through the ventricular septal defect to channel left ventricular blood through the ventricular septal defect to the aortic valve. Right ventricle–to–pulmonary artery continuity is established by placing a conduit from a right ventricle to the pulmonary artery.

The prognosis for patients with CCTGA depends on the nature of the associated lesions. The early postsurgical mortality rate varies from 5% for simple closure of a ventricular septal defect[40] to 15% for closure of the ventricular septal defect in addition to a double-switch procedure.[35,36] Late mortality rates for all patients with surgical repair of lesions in the presence of CCTGA show a moderate but steady increase over time. Although improvement in survival has occurred progressively over the last decade because of improved surgical techniques, survival rates for patients operated on before 1983 were 76% at 5 years, 68% at 10 years, and 46% at 20 years in one large study.[40] The factors that most commonly result in death are systemic ventricular failure, tricuspid valve regurgitation, and complete heart block.[41] Whether the double-switch procedure results in an improvement in survival rates is not known. The answer to this question must await a longer follow-up period.

References

1. Webb GD, McLaughlin PR, Gow RM, et al: Transposition complexes. Cardiol Clin 1993; 11:651–664.
2. Heimansohn DA, Turrentine MW, Kesler KA, et al: New trends in the management of congenital heart disease. World J Surg 1993; 17:356–362.
3. Allan LD, Crawford DC, Anderson RH, et al: The spectrum of congenital heart disease detected echocardiographically in prenatal life. Br Heart J 1985; 54:523–526.
4. Kirklin JW, Colvin EV, McConnell ME, et al: Complete transposition of the great arteries: Treatment in the current era. Pediatr Clin North Am 1990; 37:171–176.
5. Romero R, Pilu G, Jeanty P, et al: Prenatal Diagnosis of Congenital Anomalies. Norwalk, CT, Appleton & Lange, 1988, pp 160–164.
6. Jatene AD, Fontes VF, Paulista PP, et al: Anatomic correction of transposition of the great vessels. J Thorac Cardiovasc Surg 1976; 72:364–370.
7. Bartlett JM, Wypij D, Bellinger DC, et al: Effect of prenatal diagnosis on outcomes in D-transposition of the great arteries. Pediatrics 2004;e335–e340.
8. Bonnet D, Coltri A, Butera G, et al: Detection of transposition of the great arteries in the fetuses reduces neonatal morbidity and mortality. Circulation 1999; 99:916–918.
9. Chaoui R: The four-chamber view: four reasons why it seems to fail in screening for cardiac abnormalities and suggestions to improve detection rate. Ultrasound Obstet Gynecol 2003; 22:3–10.
10. Vinals F, Ascenzo R, Poblete P, et al: Simple approach to prenatal diagnosis of transposition of the great arteries. Ultrasound Obstet Gynecol 2006; 28:22–25.
11. Senning A: Surgical correction of transposition of the great vessels. Surgery 1959; 45:966–980.
12. Mustard WT: Successful two-stage correction of transposition of the great arteries. Surgery 1964; 55:469–472.
13. Liebman J, Cullum L, Belloc NB: Natural history of transposition of the great arteries: Anatomy and birth and death characteristics. Circulation 1969; 40:237–262.
14. Williams WG, Trusler GA, Kirklin JW, et al: Early and late results of a protocol for simple transposition leading to an atrial switch (Mustard) repair. J Thorac Cardiovasc Surg 1988; 95:717–726.
15. Flinn CF, Wolff GS, Dick M, et al: Cardiac rhythm after the Mustard operation for complete transposition of the great arteries. N Engl J Med 1984; 310:1635–1638.
16. Fukushige J, Porter CJ, Hayes DL, et al: Antitachycardia pacemaker treatment of postoperative arrhythmias in pediatric patients. Pacing Clin Electrophysiol 1991; 14:546–556.
17. El-Said G, Rosenberg HS, Mullins CE, et al: Dysrhythmias after Mustard's operation for transposition of the great arteries. Am J Cardiol 1972; 30:526–532.
18. Akiba T, Neirotti R, Becker AE: Is there an anatomic basis for subvalvular right ventricular outflow tract obstruction after an arterial switch repair for complete transposition? J Thorac Cardiovasc Surg 1993; 105:142–146.
19. Musewe NN, Reisman J, Benson LN, et al: Cardiopulmonary adaptation at rest and during exercise 10 years after Mustard atrial repair for transposition of the great arteries. Circulation 1988; 77:1055–1061.
20. Ensing GJ, Heise CT, Driscoll DJ: Cardiovascular response to exercise after the Mustard operation for simple and complex transposition of the great vessels. Am J Cardiol 1988; 62:617–622.
21. Bowyer JJ, Busst CM, Till JA, et al: Exercise ability after Mustard's operation. Arch Dis Child 1990; 65:865–870.
22. Quaegebeur JM, Rohmer J, Ottenkamp J, et al: The arterial switch operation: An eight-year experience. J Thorac Cardiovasc Surg 1986; 92:361–365.
23. Jex RK, Puga FJ, Julsrud PR, et al: Repair of transposition of the great arteries with intact ventricular septum and left ventricular outflow tract obstruction. J Thorac Cardiovasc Surg 1990; 100:682–686.
24. Raisky O, Bergoend E, Agnoletti G, et al: Late coronary artery lesions after neonatal arterial switch operation: Results of surgical coronary revascularization. Eur J Cardiothorac Surg 2007; 31:894–898.
25. Cohen MS, Wernovsky G: Is the arterial switch operation as good over the long term as we thought it would be? Cardiol Young 2006; 16:117–124.

26. Freedom RM, Yoo S, Mikailian HJ, et al: Conditions with double discordance (congenitally corrected transposition of the great arteries). In: The Natural and Modified History of Congenital Heart Disease. New York, Blackwell Publishing, 2004, pp356–365.

27. Bove EL: Congenitally corrected transposition of the great arteries: Ventricle to pulmonary artery connection. Semin Thorac Cardiovasc Surg 1995; 7:139–144.

28. Rutledge JM, Nihill MR, Fraser CD, et al. Outcome of 121 patients with congenitally corrected transposition of the great arteries. Pediatr Cardiol 2002; 23:137–145.

29. Paladini D, Volpe P, Marasini M, et al. Diagnosis, characterization and outcome of congenitally corrected transposition of the great arteries in the fetus: a multicenter series of 30 cases. Ultrasound Obstet Gynecol 2006; 27:281–285.

30. Huhta JC, Maloney JD, Ritter DG, et al: Complete atrioventricular block in patients with atrioventricular discordance. Circulation 1983; 67:1374–1377.

31. Sharland G, Tingay R, Jones A, et al: Atrioventricular and ventriculoarterial discordance (congenitally corrected transposition of the great arteries): Echocardiographic features, associations, and outcome in 34 fetuses. Heart 2005;91:1453–1458.

32. Jaeggi ET, Hornberger LK, Smallhorn JF, et al: Prenatal diagnosis of complete atrioventricular block associated with structural heart disease: Combined experience of two tertiary care centers and review of the literature. Ultrasound Obstet Gynecol 2005; 26:16–21.

33. Berg C, Geipel A, Kohl T, et al: Atrioventricular block detected in fetal life: associated anomalies and potential prognostic markers. Ultrasound Obstet Gynecol 2005; 26:4–15.

34. Fink BW: Congenital Heart Disease: A Deductive Approach to Its Diagnosis. Chicago, Year Book Medical, 1985, pp 147–150.

35. Yagihara T, Kishimoto H, Isobe F, et al: Double switch operation in cardiac anomalies with atrioventricular and ventriculoarterial discordance. J Thorac Cardiovasc Surg 1994; 107:351–358.

36. Yamagishi M, Imai Y, Hoshino S, et al: Anatomic correction of atrioventricular discordance. J Thorac Cardiovasc Surg 1993; 105:1067–1076.

37. Imai Y, Sawatari K, Hoshino S, et al: Ventricular function after anatomic repair in patients with atrioventricular discordance. J Thorac Cardiovasc Surg 1994; 107:1272–1283.

38. DiDonato RM, Troconis CJ, Marino B, et al: Combined Mustard and Rastelli operations. J Thorac Cardiovasc Surg 1992;104:1246–1248.

39. Ilbawi MN, DeLeon SY, Backer CL, et al: An alternative approach to the surgical management of physiologically corrected transposition with ventricular septal defect and pulmonary stenosis or atresia. J Thorac Cardiovasc Surg 1990; 100:410–415.

40. Kirklin JW, Barratt-Boyes BG: Congenitally corrected transposition of the great arteries. In: Cardiac Surgery, 2nd ed. New York, Churchill Livingstone, 1993, pp 1511–1533.

41. Graham TP, Parrish MD, Boucek RJ, et al: Assessment of ventricular size and function in congenitally corrected transposition of the great arteries. Am J Cardiol 1983; 51:244–251.

CHAPTER 16

Anomalous Pulmonary Venous Connection

Elizabeth R. Stamm

Definition

Total anomalous pulmonary venous connection (TAPVC) is a condition in which all the pulmonary venous return drains either directly into the right atrium or into channels that ultimately terminate in the right atrium. In all cases, a right-to-left shunt (atrial septal defect [ASD]) is present, allowing return of blood to the left heart and systemic circulation. TAPVC is also referred to as total anomalous pulmonary venous return.

Although several different classification systems have been proposed for TAPVC, the most widely used is that of Craig et al,[1] which is based on the anatomical location of the anomalous connection.[1] With this system, TAPVC is divided into four categories (Fig. 16–1), listed here in order of frequency:

- Type I: supracardiac
- Type II: cardiac
- Type III: infracardiac
- Type IV: mixed anomalous connections

There is some variation in the reported frequencies for these four types of TAPVC; however, in most large series, the order of frequency is as listed, with supracardiac anomalous connection comprising the majority of cases.[2] A large retrospective study reviewed the medical records of 377 children with TAPVC between 1946 and 2005. In this study the anomalous venous connection was supracardiac in 44%, infracardiac in 26%, cardiac in 21%, and mixed in 9%.[3]

Obstruction to pulmonary venous return can occur at any level between the pulmonary veins (or the common pulmonary venous confluence characteristic of TAPVC) and the right atrium. Obstruction may occur at a discrete level because

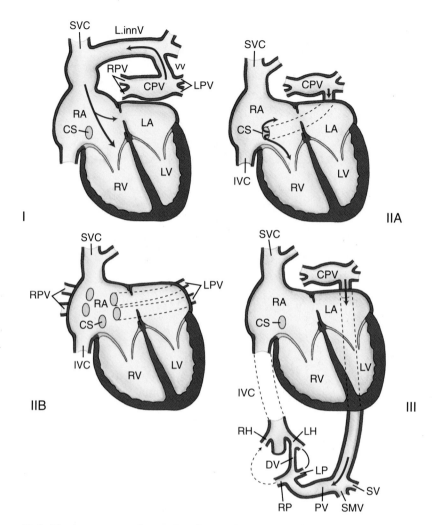

Figure 16–1 The four common forms of total anomalous venous connection. **I,** Supracardiac. Confluence of four pulmonary veins posterior to the left atrium connect via a vertical vein to the left innominate vein, which in turn, enters the right superior vena cava. **IIA,** Cardiac. Pulmonary vein confluence enters the right atrium via the coronary sinus, or **IIIB,** Cardiac. All four pulmonary veins enter the right atrium directly. **III,** Infracardiac. Pulmonary vein confluence connects via an anomalous channel to the portal vein. This in turn communicates with the inferior vena cava (*IVC*). Type IV, mixed, may consist of any of the above connections. *CPV,* Common pulmonary vein; *CS,* coronary sinus; *DV,* ductus venosus; *LA,* left atrium; *LH,* left hepatic vein; *L.innV,* left innominate vein; *LP,* left portal vein; *LPV,* left pulmonary vein; *LV,* left ventricle; *PV,* portal vein; *RA,* right atrium; *RH,* right hepatic vein; *RP,* right portal vein; *RPV,* right pulmonary vein; *RV,* right ventricle; *SMV,* superior mesenteric vein; *SV,* splenic vein; *SVC,* superior vena cava; *vv,* vertical vein.

of intrinsic narrowing of a vessel or compression from external structures, or it may be more generalized as when a large volume of pulmonary venous blood is forced through the liver in the setting of TAPVC of the infracardiac type. Karamlou et al[3] found that at the time of presenta-

tion 48% of children with TAPVC had some degree of obstruction.

Type I (Supracardiac)

Most cases of TAPVC fall into the supracardiac category. Most commonly, the four pulmonary veins (two from each lung) form a confluence posterior to the left atrium. An anomalous vertical vein originates from the left aspect of the confluence and courses cephalad and anterior to the left main bronchus and left pulmonary artery, to join the left innominate vein, which, in turn, enters the right superior vena cava (SVC). A second, less common type of anomalous supracardiac connection consists of a connection between an anomalous trunk arising from the right side of the pulmonary venous confluence and the right SVC.

Obstruction is rare with both types of supracardiac connection; however, it may occur when the left vertical vein is compressed between the left main stem bronchus and pulmonary artery or when there is a restrictive connection to the SVC. Complex cardiac malformations are common with anomalous connection to the right SVC.[4]

Type II (Cardiac)

In the cardiac type of TAPVC, the anomalous veins empty into the coronary sinus (more common) or into the posterior right atrium directly (less common) or through a short common trunk. Although several studies have suggested that obstruction is rare with direct cardiac connection,[5,6] a subsequent series found obstruction in 22% of patients with TAPVC to the coronary sinus.[7]

Type III (Infracardiac)

In infracardiac TAPVC, the four pulmonary veins generally join to form a confluence posterior to the left atrium. An anomalous descending vein extends from the confluence downward just anterior to the esophagus and accompanies the esophagus through the diaphragm by way of esophageal hiatus. In approximately 80% of cases, the anomalous vein drains into the portal venous system (usually at the portal confluence or splenic vein).[1,8] Rarely, this anomalous descending vein empties into one of the hepatic veins, the ductus venosus, or the inferior vena cava (IVC).[8]

Infracardiac TAPVC, unlike supracardiac TAPVC, is almost always associated with some degree of obstruction. This obstruction to venous return is frequently severe and may occur at any level, including the esophageal hiatus, the portal vein–to–anomalous vessel connection, or the ductus venosus (particularly after the normal obliteration of this vessel). In all cases, some degree of generalized obstruction occurs at the hepatic sinusoidal level when the large volume of pulmonary venous blood entering the portal venous system is forced through the liver.

Type IV (Mixed Anomalous Connections)

Mixed anomalous connection is the least common type of TAPVC. A large variety of pulmonary venous drainage patterns may occur in this subgroup. Most commonly, the left pulmonary veins drain into the left innominate vein through an anomalous vertical vein and the right pulmonary veins drain into the coronary sinus or directly into the right atrium. Obstruction can occur at one or more levels.

With partial anomalous pulmonary venous connection (PAPVC), one or more, but not all four, pulmonary veins connect directly to the right atrium or to a tributary that terminates in the right atrium. PAPVC is also commonly referred to as partial anomalous pulmonary venous return (PAPVR).

Similar to TAPVC, four common forms of PAPVC are usually described (Fig. 16–2)[9,10]:

- The right pulmonary veins enter the right atrium via the SVC. The left pulmonary veins enter the left atrium. A sinus venosus ASD is usually present.
- The right pulmonary veins enter the right atrium via the IVC. The left pulmonary veins enter the left atrium. In this form, the atrial septum is usually intact (excluding the normal foramen ovale). This type of PAPVC has been associated with hypoplasia of the right lung, hypoplasia of the right pulmonary artery, dextroposition, and other cardiac anomalies.[10]
- The left pulmonary veins enter the left innominate vein, which then connects with the SVC and drains into the right atrium. The right pulmonary veins may enter the left atrium, the coronary sinus, the IVC, the SVC, or the left subclavian vein. An ostium secundum ASD is often present. This form of PAPVC has been associated with a variety of cardiac anomalies and syndromes, including polysplenia, asplenia, Turner syndrome, and Noonan syndrome.
- The least common form of PAPVC involves the left pulmonary veins draining into the coronary sinus, the IVC, the SVC, the right atrium, or the left subclavian vein. The right

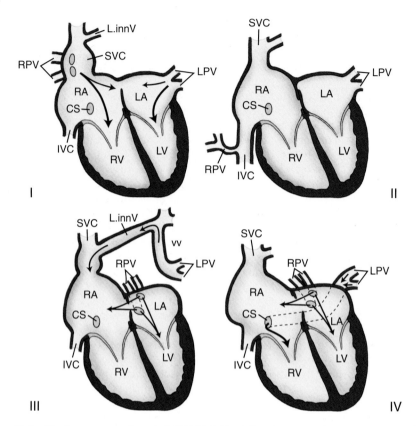

Figure 16–2   The four common forms of PAPVC. **I,** The left pulmonary veins connect correctly to the left atrium, and the anomalous right pulmonary veins connect to the right superior vena cava *(SVC)*. **II,** The left pulmonary veins connect correctly to the left atrium, and the anomalous right pulmonary veins connect to the inferior vena cava *(IVC)*. **III,** The right pulmonary veins connect correctly to the left atrium, and the anomalous left pulmonary veins connect to the left innominate vein by a vertical vein. This in turn connects to the right SVC. **IV,** The right pulmonary veins connect correctly to the left atrium, and the anomalous left pulmonary veins connect to the right atrium via the coronary sinus. *CS,* Coronary sinus; *LA,* left atrium; *L.innV,* left innominate vein; *LPV,* left pulmonary veins; *LV,* left ventricle; *RA,* right atrium; *RPV,* right pulmonary veins; *RV,* right ventricle; *vv,* vertical vein.

pulmonary veins usually maintain their normal connection to the left atrium.

Embryology

A brief review of the embryology of the pulmonary venous system is helpful to fully understand the complicated anatomy of TAPVC.

The embryonic lungs, larynx, and tracheobronchial tree are derived from the foregut. The primitive lungs are in close contact with the vascular plexus of the foregut (the splanchnic plexus), a portion of which later forms the pulmonary vascular bed. Initially, there is no direct venous connection between the heart and the lungs, and the pulmonary vascular bed drains with the splanchnic system into the cardinal and umbilico-vitelline venous systems. Between 27 and 29 days' gestation, the common pulmonary vein begins to form from an outpouching located to the left of the septum primum on the roof of the common atrium (Fig. 16–3, *A*). By gestational day 30, the atrial outpouching (common pulmonary vein) and the pulmonary venous portion of the splanchnic system have joined, forming a direct connection between the heart and the pulmonary veins (Fig. 16–3, *B*). When this occurs, the more

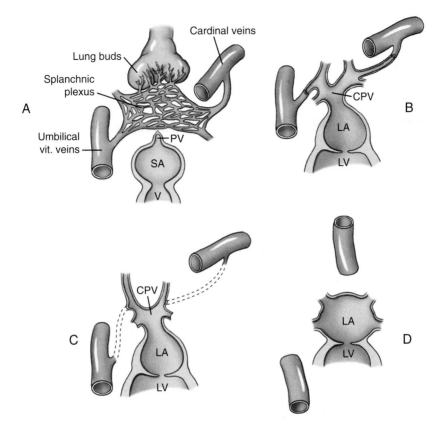

Figure 16–3 Embryological development of the pulmonary veins. **A,** The common pulmonary vein begins to form between 27 and 29 days' gestation. **B,** By gestational day 30, the common pulmonary vein and the splanchnic system have joined, forming a direct connection between the heart and the pulmonary veins. **C,** The primitive pulmonary venous drainage system begins to involute and eventually disappears, leaving the pulmonary vascular bed to drain through four major pulmonary veins into the left atrium by way of the common pulmonary vein. **D,** The individual pulmonary veins are incorporated into the left atrium, and the common pulmonary vein no longer exists as an anatomical structure. *CPV,* Common pulmonary vein; *LA,* left atrium; *LV,* left ventricle; *SA,* sinoatrial system; *V,* ventricle.

primitive system of pulmonary venous drainage through the umbilicovitelline and cardinal veins begins to involute and eventually disappears, leaving the pulmonary vascular bed to drain through four distinct major pulmonary veins into the left atrium by way of the common pulmonary vein (Fig. 16–3, *C*). The common pulmonary vein becomes incorporated into the left atrium, resulting in the familiar adult anatomical arrangement in which the four pulmonary veins drain separately into the left atrium (Fig. 16–3, *D*).

If normal development of the common pulmonary vein is interrupted early in gestation, flow is redirected into the collateral pathways between the splanchnic plexus and the cardinal or umbilicovitelline system, or both. Either of these pathways may then persist and enlarge, resulting in PAPVC or TAPVC as blood flow is redirected through these anomalous pathways.

Occurrence Rate

The exact incidence of TAPVC in the general population is difficult to determine because the defect is rare. It occurs in approximately 0.087 in 1000, or 8.7 in 100,000, live births.[11] TAPVC made up

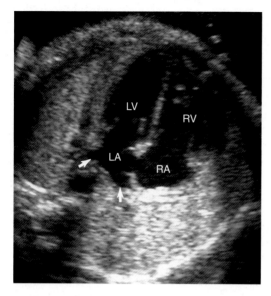

Figure 16–4 Apical four-chamber view showing the two superior pulmonary veins *(arrows)* draining into the left atrium *(LA)*. *LV,* Left ventricle; *RA,* right atrium; *RV,* right ventricle.

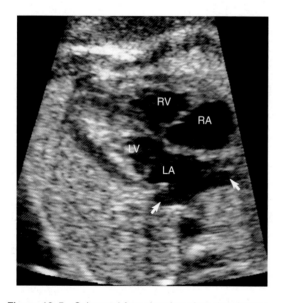

Figure 16–5 Subcostal four-chamber view showing the two superior pulmonary veins *(arrows)* draining into the left atrium *(LA)*. *LV,* Left ventricle; *RA,* right atrium; *RV,* right ventricle.

2.6% of all congenital heart disease in the New England Regional Infant Cardiac Program.[12]

Although the male-to-female distribution is equal in most types of TAPVC, TAPVC to the portal vein is twice as common in males as in females.[13]

No association between the occurrence of TAPVC and environmental toxins was identified in the New England Regional Infant Cardiac Registry.[12] In other studies, however, it has been suggested that there may be an association between TAPVC and paint, paint remover chemicals, lead, and pesticides.[14]

Although the genetics of TAPVC remain unclear, a monogenetic pattern of inheritance has been suggested by studies of siblings with the defect.[15–17]

Sonographic Criteria

Although echocardiography with pulsed and color Doppler imaging has been instrumental in making the diagnosis of PAPVC or TAPVC in neonates and older patients, the diagnosis is much more difficult in the fetal population. However, technical improvements in equipment and increased operator experience has made it feasible.[15]

In the normal fetus, at least the two superior pulmonary veins can generally be identified entering the left atrium on an apical four-chamber view (Fig. 16–4) or a subcostal four-chamber view (Fig. 16–5). The two inferior pulmonary veins are usually more difficult to appreciate on ultrasonography. This usually requires meticulous attention in defining individual veins. Pulsed Doppler (Fig. 16–6) and color flow Doppler imaging (Fig. 16–7) may help to identify the pulmonary veins and confirm the direction of blood flow. The diagnosis of TAPVC can be excluded if one or more of the four pulmonary veins terminate normally in the left atrium. Unless all four normal connections are identified entering the left atrium, the diagnosis of PAPVC cannot be excluded.

Commonly, ultrasonography affords a detailed evaluation of the anomalous pulmonary venous connections of TAPVC after birth (Fig. 16–8). Unfortunately, it can be difficult to identify these anomalous confluences in the fetal population because pulmonary blood flow in utero is minimal compared with that after birth. In addition, these anomalous vessels are frequently small in caliber and often follow a complex and variable course (Fig. 16–9). Making this diagnosis in utero more difficult because the right-to-left atrial shunt seen in all neonates with TAPVC is a normal finding in the fetus. Many cases of anomalous pulmonary venous connections are still routinely missed prenatally.[16,17] Limited reports of prenatal diagnosis of TAPVC have been published. Allan[18] diagnosed

fetal TAPVC to the coronary sinus. DiSessa et al[19] detected infracardiac TAPVC in a fetus with asplenia syndrome. More recently, Volpe et al[20] reported seven cases of TAPVC diagnosed in utero. These included three cases of anomalous supracardiac drainage to the innominate vein, cardiac to the

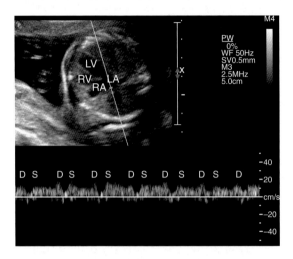

Figure 16–6 Pulsed Doppler tracing of a normal pulmonary vein draining into the left atrium *(LA)*. *D*, Diastole; *LV*, left ventricle; *RA*, right atrium; *RV*, right ventricle; *S*, systole.

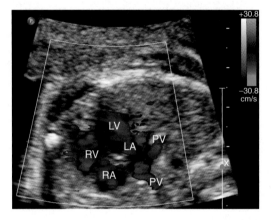

Figure 16–7 Apical four-chamber view using color Doppler imaging to identify the pulmonary veins *(PV)* draining into the left atrium *(LA)*. *LV*, Left ventricle; *RA*, right atrium; *RV*, right ventricle.

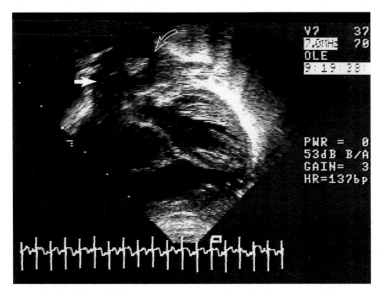

Figure 16–8 Subcostal four-chamber view in a neonate showing anomalous connection of the pulmonary veins *(open arrow)* into the SVC *(solid arrow)*.

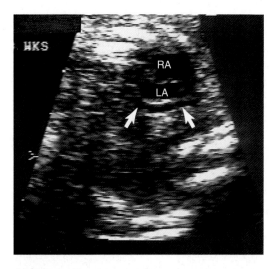

Figure 16–9 Short-axis view through the atria in a 23-week-old fetus showing anomalous pulmonary veins *(arrows)* coursing behind but not entering the left atrium *(LA)*. *RA*, Right atrium.

coronary sinus in two, and infracardiac to the portal vein in the remaining two cases. Patel et al[21] reviewed 13 cases of TAPVC diagnosed prenatally over a 13-year period. In their cohort, seven fetuses with supracardiac, two with cardiac, and four with infracardiac TAPVC were identified.

In the normal fetus, the right and left ventricles are similar in size, and the two superior pulmonary veins can almost always be identified draining into the left atrium. A subtle clue that TAPVC is present is enlargement of the right atrium and ventricle, with bowing of the interatrial septum toward the left atrium. Volpe et al[20] found this asymmetry present in four of seven cases of TAPVC; however, it was usually not apparent until later in pregnancy. This finding may be subtle in the fetus because of the presence of the foramen ovale. Identification of an abnormal confluence of vessels eventually draining into the right atrium or an abnormal number of venous vessels on a three-chamber view (due to visualization of a persistent left SVC or a vertical vein) are more reliable criteria. Color and pulsed Doppler imaging should be used to aid in identification of the vertical vein, which usually runs from the confluence to the innominate vein, which in turn terminates at the right SVC. The SVC may also appear enlarged compared with the aorta on the three-vessel view.

The most reliable sonographic criteria for making the diagnosis of PAPVC is identifying pulmonary veins entering both the right and left atria. Some component of pulmonary veins will always remain connected to the left atrium in this setting. The anomalous vessels will connect directly to the right atrium or terminate in the right atrium through the coronary sinus or the IVC or SVC.

Treatment

The definitive treatment in all cases of TAPVC is surgery, and most surgeons advocate immediate repair as soon as the diagnosis of TAPVC is made. When possible, the diagnosis should be confirmed and the anatomy defined with echocardiography as opposed to angiography. The exact anatomy of the anomalous connections is frequently well demonstrated with echocardiography alone, and this type of examination has served as the sole diagnostic procedure before surgery.

In complex (particularly mixed) cases of TAPVC, cardiac catheterization may be necessary to delineate the anatomy of the anomalous connections adequately. Omitting the cardiac catheterization when possible not only spares the patient an invasive procedure with a large contrast (osmotic) load but also shortens the delay to surgery and may reduce mortality rates.[22]

Medical management in the setting of TAPVC is limited, consisting of intubation with mechanical ventilation and correction of metabolic imbalances such as acidosis. Nonetheless, this type of management may be vital in stabilizing the neonate in the first few hours of life. Preliminary evidence suggests that prostaglandin E_1 may be beneficial in maintaining patency of the ductus venosus and thus decreasing pulmonary venous obstruction in patients with infracardiac TAPVC to the portal venous system.[23-25]

Prognosis

The prognosis for the neonate with PAPVC or TAPVC is directly related to the degree of pulmonary venous obstruction and the volume of intracardiac (right-to-left) shunting. Because the pulmonary and systemic circulations both return to the right heart, survival is impossible without a right-to-left shunt. This almost always occurs at the atrial level through a patent foramen ovale. If the right-to-left connection is small or restrictive, symptoms are more pronounced. The presence and severity of additional cardiac or extracardiac abnormalities also contributes to survival.

The degree of cyanosis is determined by the ratio of pulmonary to systemic blood exiting the left atrium toward the systemic circulation. This ratio is largely determined by the resistance in the systemic versus the pulmonary vascular beds and, importantly, by the presence and degree of pulmonary venous obstruction and the amount of restriction of blood flow at the atrial level.

Cyanosis is a prominent feature in neonates with TAPVC and severe pulmonary venous obstruction. These infants commonly experience severe respiratory distress in the first few hours of life and rarely survive more than several weeks without surgery.[13] Feeding may acutely exacerbate symptoms in babies with anomalous connection below the diaphragm, presumably because the distended esophagus compresses and further obstructs the anomalous vein at the esophageal hiatus.

Infants with little or no pulmonary venous obstruction but with restrictive flow at the atrial level may do relatively well in the first few weeks of life. Within several months, however, tachypnea, respiratory distress, congestive heart failure, and pulmonary arterial hypertension commonly develop. Without intervention, most of these infants die by 1 year of age.[2]

When pulmonary venous obstruction and a restrictive interatrial connection are both absent, patients with PAPVC or TAPVC may have a mild clinical course similar to that of patients with a large ASD. Rarely, symptoms may not develop until well into the fourth or fifth decade of life.

Many centers advocate immediate surgical intervention for all infants with TAPVC. The operative mortality rate for patients treated in this manner is as high as 13%.[26,27] Few patients in these series had infracardiac venous return and, unfortunately, the operative mortality rate with infracardiac TAPVC remains high (14% to 67%).[26-28] Survival after surgical repair of isolated TAPVC has continued to improve, with operative mortality consistently <10%.[29] The mortality remains highest in young children and in patients with pulmonary venous obstruction or cardiac (type II) venous connection.[3] The prognosis for patients who have survived surgical correction is excellent. These postsurgical patients do have a high incidence of sinus node dysfunction and a low incidence of atrioventricular block, which merits ongoing monitoring for arrhythmia.[30]

In 2003 Valsangiacomo et al[31] published a retrospective review of 16 fetuses diagnosed prenatally with TAPVC or PAPVC. They reported an 88% mortality rate among live births, largely because of the presence of severe additional cardiac abnormalities.

Associated Anomalies

Approximately one third of patients with PAPVC or TAPVC have additional cardiac anomalies (Table 16–1).[15,32] Associated cardiac anomalies are

TABLE 16–1 Conditions Associated with Anomalous Pulmonary Venous Connection

Fetal		
Associated Cardiac Abnormalities	Chromosome Abnormalities	Syndromes
Atrioventricular septal defect	Partial trisomy 22 (cat-eye syndrome)	Asplenia
Coarctation	Turner syndrome (46,XO)	Bardet-Biedl syndrome
Dextrocardia		Fryns syndrome
Double-outlet right ventricle		Johanson-Blizzard syndrome
Hypoplastic left ventricle		Laurence-Moon syndrome
Interrupted aorta		Noonan syndrome
Persistent left SVC		Pentalogy of Cantrell
Pulmonary vein stenosis		Polysplenia
Right atrial isomerism		Scimitar syndrome
Single ventricle		
Tetralogy of Fallot		
Transposition of the great arteries		
Tricuspid atresia		

variable and include atrioventricular septal defect, single ventricle, transposition of the great arteries, a hypoplastic left heart, coarctation or interruption of the aorta, tetralogy of Fallot, tricuspid atresia, double-outlet right ventricle, and others. In addition, these patients may have abnormalities of visceral situs, specifically right atrial isomerism. Rarely, TAPVC has been associated with cat-eye syndrome.[33] Other associated syndromes and chromosomal anomalies are rare.[34] There is a strong correlation between supracardiac anomalous connection to the right SVC and other complex congenital cardiac anomalies.[4]

In a large autopsy series, anomalous pulmonary venous drainage was isolated in 62% of cases.[5]

References

1. Craig JM, Darling RC, Rothney WB: Total pulmonary venous drainage into the right side of the heart: Report of 17 autopsied cases not associated with other major cardiovascular anomalies. Lab Invest 1957; 6:44–64.
2. Borroughs JT, Edwards JE: Total anomalous pulmonary venous connection. Am Heart J 1960; 59:913–931.
3. Karamlou T, Gurofsky R, Al Sukhni E, et al: Factors associated with mortality and reoperation in 377 children with total anomalous pulmonary venous connection. Pediatr Cardiol 2007; 115:1591–1598.
4. Stanger P, Rudolph AM, Edwards JE: Cardiac malpositions: An overview based on the study of sixty-five necropsy specimens. Circulation 1977; 56:159–172.
5. Delisle G, Ando M, Calder AL, et al: TAPVC: Report of 93 autopsied cases with emphasis on diagnostic and surgical considerations. Am Heart J 1976; 91:99–122.
6. Gathman GE, Nadas AS: Total anomalous pulmonary venous connection. Clinical and physiologic observations of 75 pediatric patients. Circulation 1970; 42:143–154.
7. Jonas RA, Smolinsky A, Mayer JE, et al: Obstructed pulmonary venous drainage with TAPVC to the coronary sinus. Am J Cardiol 1987; 59:431–435.
8. Duff DF, Nihill MR, McNamara DG: Infradiaphragmatic total anomalous pulmonary venous return: Review of clinical and pathological findings and results of operation in 28 cases. Br Heart J 1977; 39:619–626.
9. Krabill KA, Lucas RV: Abnormal pulmonary venous connections. In: Moss AJ, Adams FH, Emmanouilides GC (eds): Heart Disease in Infants, Children and Adolescents. 5th ed. Baltimore, Williams & Wilkins, 1995, pp 841–849.
10. Yagel S, Kivilevitch Z, Achriron R: The fetal venous system: normal embryology, anatomy and physiology, and the development and appearance of anomalies. In: Yagel S, Silverman NH, Gembruch U (eds): Fetal Cardiology: Embryology, Genetics, Physiology, Echocardiographic Evaluation, Diagnosis and Perinatal Mangement of Cardiac Disease. London, Martin Dunitz, 2003, pp 321–332.
11. Grabitz RG, Joffres MR, Collins-Nakai RL: Congenital heart disease: Incidence in the first year of life. Alberta Heritage Pediatric Cardiology Program. Am J Epidemiol 1988; 128:381–388.
12. Flyer DC, Buckley LP, Hellenbrand WE, et al: Report of the New England Regional Infant Cardiac Program. Pediatrics 1980; 65(Suppl):375–461.
13. Lucas RV, Adams P, Anderson RC, et al: Total anomalous pulmonary venous connection to the portal venous system: A cause of pulmonary venous obstruction. AJR Am J Roentgenol Radium Ther Nucl Med 1961; 86:561–575.
14. Correa-Vallasenor A, Ferencz C, Boughman JA, et al: Total anomalous pulmonary venous return: Familial and environmental factors. Teratology 1991; 44:415–428.
15. Patel CR, Lane JR, Sallee D: In utero diagnosis of isolated obstructed supracardiac total anomalous pulmonary venous connection. J Ultrasound Med 2002; 21:573–576.
16. Allan LD, Chita SK, Sharland GK, et al: The accuracy of fetal echocardiography in the diagnosis of congenital heart disease. Int J Cardiol 1989; 25:279–288.
17. Bromley B, Estroff JA, Sanders SP, et al: Fetal echocardiography: Accuracy and limitations in a population at high and low risk for heart defects. Am J Obstet Gynecol 1992; 166:1473–1481.
18. Allan LD: Structural cardiac abnormalities of the venous atrial junction. In: Allan LD (ed): Manual of Fetal Echocardiography. Lancaster, UK, MTP Press, 1986, pp 75–79.
19. DiSessa TG, Emerson DS, Felker RE, et al: Anomalous systemic and pulmonary venous pathways diagnosed in utero by ultrasound. J Ultrasound Med 1990; 9:311–317.
20. Vople P, Campobasso G, DeRobertis V, et al: Two-and four-dimensional echocardiography with B-flow imaging and spatiotemporal image correlation in prenatal diagnosis of isolated total anomalous pulmonary venous connection. Ultrasound Obstet Gynecol 2007; 30:830–837.
21. Patel CR, Lane JR, Spector ML, et al: Totally anomalous pulmonary venous connection and

complex congenital heart disease: Prenatal echocardiographic diagnosis and prognosis. J Ultrasound Med 2005; 24:1191–1198.

22. Lincoln CR, Rigby ML, Mercanti C, et al: Surgical risk factors in total anomalous pulmonary venous connection. Am J Cardiol 1988; 61:608–611.

23. Yee ES, Turley K, Hsieh WR, et al: Infant total anomalous venous connection: Factors influencing timing of presentation and operative outcome. Circulation 1987; 76(3 pt 2):III83–III87.

24. Bullaboy CA, Johnson DH, Azar H, et al: Total anomalous pulmonary venous connection to portal system: A new therapeutic role for prostaglandin E. Pediatr Cardiol 1984; 5:115–116.

25. Talosi G, Katona M, Racz K, et al: Prostaglandin E1 treatment in patent ductus arteriosus dependent congenital heart defects. J Perinat Med 2004; 32:368–374.

26. Turley K, Tucker WY, Ullyot DJ, et al: Total anomalous pulmonary venous connection in infancy: Influence of age and type of lesion. Am J Cardiol 1980; 45:92–97.

27. Galloway AC, Campbell DN, Clark DR: The value of early repair for total anomalous pulmonary drainage. Pediatr Cardiol 1985; 6:77–81.

28. Mazzucco A, Rizzoli G, Fracasso A, et al: Experience with operation for total anomalous pulmonary venous connection in infancy. J Thorac Cardiovasc Surg 1983; 85:686–690.

29. Kanter KR. Surgical repair of total anomalous pulmonary venous connection: Semin Thorac Cardiovasc Surg Pediatr Card Surg Annu 2006; 40–44.

30. Tanel RE, Kirshbom PM, Paridon SM, et al: Long-term noninvasive arrhythmia assessment after total anomalous pulmonary venous connection repair. Am Heart J 2007; 153:267–274.

31. Valsangiacomo ER, Hornberger LK, Barrea C, et al: Partial and total anomalous pulmonary venous connection in the fetus: two-dimensional and Doppler echocardiographic findings. Ultrasound Obstet Gynecol 2003; 22:257–263.

32. Bonham-Carter RE, Capriles M, Noe Y: Total anomalous pulmonary venous drainage: A clinical and anatomical study of 75 children. Br Heart J 1969; 31:45–47.

33. Knoll JH, Asamoah A, Pletcher BA, et al: Interstitial duplication of proximal 22q: Phenotypic overlap with cat eye syndrome. Am J Med Genet 1995; 55:221–224.

34. Noonan JA: Syndromes associated with cardiac defects. In: Engle MA (ed): Pediatric Cardiovascular Disease. Philadelphia, FA Davis, 1981, pp 97–116.

CHAPTER 17

Double-Outlet Right Ventricle and Double-Outlet Left Ventricle

Julia A. Drose

OUTLINE

Definition

Double-Outlet Right Ventricle

Double-outlet right ventricle (DORV) refers to a spectrum of cardiac lesions unified by an abnormal ventriculoarterial connection.[1] DORV is most commonly defined as a condition in which more than 50% of both the aortic root and the pulmonary artery arise from the ventricle with right morphological features.[2-5] A ventricular septal defect (VSD) is usually, but not always, present.[5]

DORV was first described in 1703.[6] It was considered to be one type of transposition of the great arteries (TGA). In 1898, Vierordt referred to DORV as a partial transposition because only the aorta was actually transposed as the pulmonary artery originates appropriately from the right ventricle.[7]

In 1949, Taussig and Bing[8] described a patient with "complete transposition of the aorta and levoposition of the pulmonary artery." They described the first reported case in which both great arteries arose from the right ventricle, but the VSD was related to the pulmonary artery and not the aorta, as had been the case in all previous reports.[5] In 1952, Braun et al[9] described a case in which "the right ventricle serves as a double outlet ventricle." They classified it as a partial transposition of the Fallot type.

The term "double-outlet right ventricle" was first used by Witham[10] in 1957. He considered it to be a partial transposition complex in which both great arteries arose from the right ventricle. He divided his cases of DORV into two groups—the Fallot type and the Eisenmenger type—depending on whether pulmonary stenosis was present or absent.[7]

A classification system for DORV was first developed by Neufeld et al[11,12] in 1961. They separated cases into those with and those without pulmonary stenosis and included an additional category for those with "other intracardiac malformations."

They later subcategorized the group without pulmonary stenosis on the basis of the position of the VSD in relation to the crista supraventricularis and the great arteries.[13]

In 1972, Lev et al[14] classified DORV on the basis of the relationship of the VSD to the two great arteries, including subaortic, subpulmonary, doubly committed (involving both great vessels), or noncommitted (distant from either great artery). They advocated expanding the definition of DORV to include cases in which only two cusps and part of a third cusp of both semilunar valves originate from the right ventricle. Additionally, they considered the Taussig-Bing type of DORV as a spectrum ranging from cases in which both great arteries arise wholly from the right ventricle to those with pulmonary-mitral continuity, as in complete transposition.

In 1982, Van Praagh developed the most widely accepted classification of DORV, which included the following[2,5,15-21]:

- DORV with a subaortic VSD
- DORV with a subpulmonary VSD
- DORV with a doubly committed (both subaortic and subpulmonic) VSD
- DORV with a remote VSD (noncommitted) (Fig. 17–1)

Four types of great artery relationships at the level of the semilunar valves have been described in DORV[19]:

- Aorta right and posterior to the pulmonary artery (normal)
- Aorta right and lateral to the pulmonary artery (side by side)
- Aorta right and anterior to the pulmonary artery (dextromalposition)
- Aorta left and anterior to the pulmonary artery (levomalposition)

In 1978, Sridaromont et al[20] evaluated angiographically 72 patients with proven DORV to determine the location of a VSD when it was associated with various great artery relationships. They identified 16 possible combinations (Fig. 17–2).

Subaortic VSDs were the most common finding, occurring in 68% of cases. The most common combination was a subaortic VSD with side-by-side great vessels. This was seen in 46% of patients. A subaortic VSD with dextromalposition of the great vessels (right anterior aorta) was the next most common combination, occurring in 16% of patients. Subpulmonary VSDs were identified in

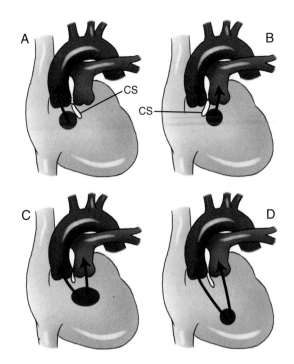

Figure 17–1 Diagram of the four types of VSD that occur in DORV. **A,** Subaortic VSD; note the anterior and leftward deviation of the conal septum *(CS)*, causing the aorta to override the VSD and the subpulmonary region to be narrowed. **B,** Subpulmonary VSD; note the posterior and rightward deviation of the conal septum, resulting in the pulmonary artery overriding the VSD and subaortic narrowing. **C,** Doubly committed VSD; the conal septum is absent and the VSD is large. **D,** Remote or noncommitted VSD in the muscular septum.

22% of cases, usually with dextromalposition of the great vessels (10%).

The combination of a subpulmonary VSD with side-by-side great vessels was found in 8% of patients. This type of DORV is commonly considered the classic Taussig-Bing heart (Fig. 17–3).[14] Pulmonary stenosis is not associated with this particular anomaly; therefore, the pulmonary artery is usually dilated. Anatomically, a subpulmonary VSD is usually located in a more anterior position than is a subaortic VSD.

Doubly committed VSDs were found in only 3% of patients. All patients had side-by-side great vessels. In this type of DORV, the VSD is usually in a superior position and closely related to both semilunar valves. It is often large.

Relationship of great arteries	Location of VSD (%)				
	Subaortic	Subpulmonary	Subaortic and subpulmonary	Remote	Total
Normal	3%	0	0	0	3%
Side-by-side	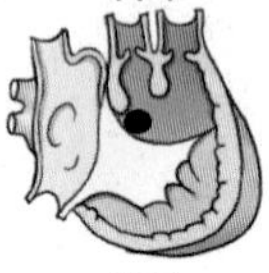 46%	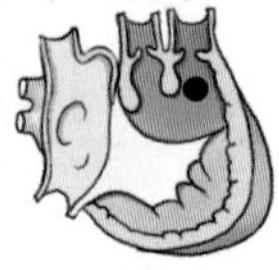 8%	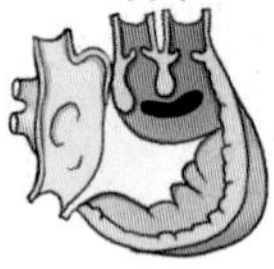 3%	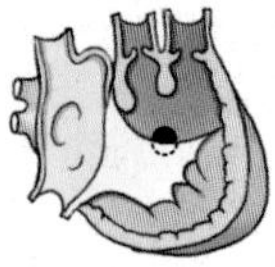 7%	64%
d-MGA	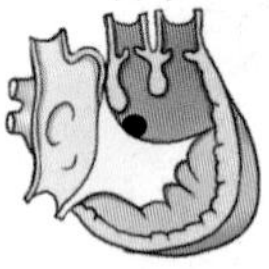 16%	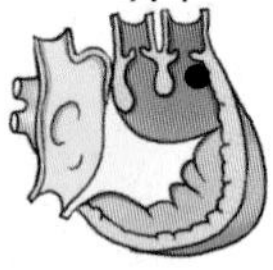 10%	0	0	26%
l-MGA	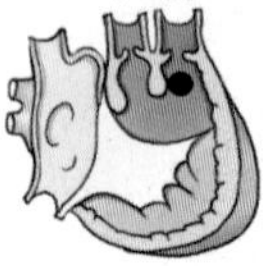 3%	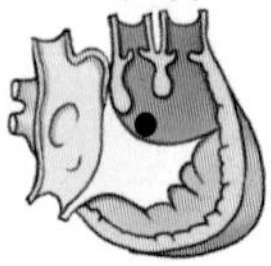 4%	0	0	7%
Total	68%	22%	3%	7%	

Figure 17–2   Relationship of the great arteries and location of the VSD in 70 patients with DORV. *A*, Aorta; *d-MGA*, dextromalposition of the great arteries; *l-MGA*, levomalposition of the great arteries; *P*, pulmonary artery. (Data from Hagler DJ: Double-outlet right ventricle. In: Emmanouilides GC, Riemenschneider TA, Allan HD, et al [eds]: Moss & Adams' Heart Disease in Infants, Children and Adolescents: Including the Fetus and Young Adult, 5th ed, vol 2. Baltimore, Williams & Wilkins, 1995, p 1248.)

Remote or noncommitted VSDs were identified in 7% of patients in this series. Similar to the doubly committed VSD, all were associated with side-by-side great vessels. The most common form recognized as a remote VSD is a complete atrioventricular canal defect with DORV.[7] This type can, however, be located in the anterior, middle, or posterior muscular septum.[22] DORV with a remote VSD is often associated with the heterotaxy syndromes. In a more recent study, Bradley et al[21] reviewed 393 cases of DORV. They also reported DORV with a subaortic VSD as being the most common form, occurring in 47% of cases. DORV with a noncommitted VSD was found in 26%, DORV with a subpulmonic VSD was found in 23%, and DORV with a doubly committed VSD was diagnosed in 4%.

DORV with an intact ventricular septum has also been reported.[20,23–26] It is, however, exceedingly rare. This type of DORV is usually associated with hypoplasia of the left ventricle and with anomalies of the mitral valve.

Although the Van Praagh system is still considered by many to be the traditional classification of DORV, many authors thought that it was not ideal because it is based solely on the anatomical relationship between the VSD and the great arteries and does not consider the surgical approach. In 2000, the Society of Thoracic Surgeons and the European Association of Cardiothoracic Surgery adopted four types of DORV on the basis of clinical presentation and treatment[27]:

- VSD-type: DORV with subaortic VSD
- Fallot-type: DORV with subaortic or double committed VSD and pulmonary outflow stenosis
- TGA-type (Taussig-Bing): DORV with a sub-pulmonary VSD
- Noncommitted VSD–type: DORV with a remote VSD

Double-Outlet Left Ventricle

Double-outlet left ventricle (DOLV) is far less common than DORV. It is defined as a malformation in which the aorta and the pulmonary artery both arise exclusively or predominantly from the ventricle with left morphological features.[28] Early reports of DOLV by Fragoyannis and Kardalinos[29] in 1962 and by Ruttenberg et al[30] in 1964 described the origin of both great arteries from the left ventricle, but these appeared to represent instances of a double-outlet ventricle with right ventricular morphological features with atrioventricular discordance. This sparked controversy as to the actual existence of DOLV. In 1970, however, Paul et al[31] reported the first autopsy proven case of DOLV with an intact ventricular septum. Van Praagh et al[32] published a review of 109 cases of DOLV in 1988, in which they described 26 different types.

Their classification was based on three primary criteria:

- The situs of the atria, the ventricles, and the great arteries: Normal situs (solitus), situs inversus, and situs ambiguous have all been reported.[33-37]
- The alignment or commitment of the atria, the ventricles, and the great vessels: Alignment can be concordant, discordant, double-inlet, or absent right or left atrioventricular connection.
- Location of the VSD or other associated cardiovascular anomalies

As in DORV, four basic anatomic locations of VSDs have been associated with DOLV[32]:

- Subaortic VSD
- Subpulmonic VSD
- Double-committed VSD
- Remote or noncommitted VSD

In the Van Praagh series, three main types of DOLV were observed. The most common type was DOLV with a subaortic VSD, which was observed

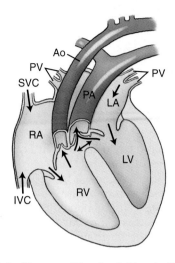

Figure 17–3 Diagram of the classic Taussig-Bing heart with a subpulmonary VSD and side-by-side great vessels. *Ao,* Aorta; *IVC,* inferior vena cava; *LA,* left atrium; *LV,* left ventricle; *PA,* pulmonary artery; *PV,* pulmonary veins; *RA,* right atrium; *RV,* right ventricle; *SVC,* superior vena cava.

in 48% of all cases and in 73% of cases with situs solitus and atrioventricular concordance (n = 71). This group of patients was further categorized on the basis of the great artery relationships (right anterior or left anterior aorta) and the presence or absence of aortic or pulmonary stenosis.[32]

The most common form of DOLV with a subaortic VSD had a right anterior or right lateral aorta (35 of 71 patients). Of these 35, 29 patients (83%) also had subvalvular and valvular pulmonary stenosis. This type of DOLV is also referred to as the tetralogy type of DOLV because it is often confused clinically and angiographically with tetralogy of Fallot as a result of the associated pulmonary stenosis.[28] The remaining six patients with a right anterior aorta and DOLV with subaortic VSD, but without pulmonary stenosis, were reported to have clinical and angiographic characteristics similar to complete transposition (dextro-transposition) of the great vessels.

The second most frequently occurring form of DOLV involved a subaortic VSD with a left anterior aorta and pulmonary stenosis. This type of DOLV was reported in 24% (17 of 71 patients) and was referred to as the transposition subtype of DOLV.

The great vessel orientation and clinical findings of the two entities are similar, with the degree of aortic override and commitment to the morphological left ventricle being the only clearly distinguishing feature.[28]

A subpulmonic VSD was the third most common form of DOLV in the Van Praagh series. It was observed in 11 (15%) of the 71 patients with normal situs. This type of VSD was described as high and anterior, involving the conus septum. The great vessel relationships in these cases were either normal or involved a right anterior aorta. Van Praagh postulated that this type of VSD results in significant malalignment of the aortic and pulmonary conus septum relative to the ventricular septum, often causing narrowing of the aortic outflow tract. This narrowing is accompanied by hypoplasia of the aortic annulus and aortic stenosis. In fact, 8 of the 11 patients with DOLV and a subpulmonary VSD also had aortic stenosis, whereas only 2 of the 11 individuals had pulmonary stenosis.

As with DORV, DOLV with a doubly committed VSD is rare, occurring in only 7 of the 109 cases (0.06%) reported in this series and in only 10% of the 71 patients identified with normal situs.

Doubly committed VSDs are described as very large in order to allow overriding of both the aorta and the pulmonary artery. The relationship of the great vessels at the semilunar valve level is usually side by side.

Unlike patients with DORV and a doubly committed VSD, these patients had marked underdevelopment of the subarterial conus septum; therefore, none of these patients had pulmonary stenosis.

Finally, a remote or noncommitted VSD is also a very unusual finding with DOLV. No patients were identified as having this type of VSD in the Van Praagh series; however, one patient described previously in the literature, with a noncommitted VSD and a left anterior aorta, was included in their data.

Embryology

Historically, DORV was thought to result from a failure of the normal spiraling of the aorta and pulmonary trunk, resulting in abnormal positioning. However, more recent research confirms that the primitive right ventricle is in fact a DORV, containing the conotruncus. If migration of the aortic side of the conotruncus toward the mitral valve is incomplete, the DORV anatomy persists.[38]

Another refinement of accepted embryology suggests that DOLV is actually caused by the misalignment and arrest of the ventricular septum.[39]

Regardless of the precise embryological events, it is correct to assume that DORV and DOLV represent a spectrum of complex defects that result from a failure of the normal sequence of events.

Occurrence Rate

DORV is considered a rare congenital malformation, occurring in approximately 0.033 to 0.09 per 1000 live births.[40-43] The frequency among abortuses and stillborn infants is reported to be 2.4%.[44] There does not appear to be an ethnic or a sex predilection in DORV.

The occurrence of DOLV is significantly less than that of DORV, although there are inadequate statistics available to allow a determination of its actual frequency.

Sonographic Criteria

As stated earlier, double-outlet ventricle refers to a heterogeneous group of lesions unified by an abnormal ventriculoarterial connection.[1] The clinical features of these defects may mimic several similar lesions. Therefore echocardiography is essential to correctly identify these malformations.

The surgical options available for correcting DORV and DOLV are as variable as the number of abnormal connections that make up this spectrum. Accurate diagnosis of these lesions in utero provides information necessary to determine the type of surgical repair most suitable.

The key to making the diagnosis of double-outlet ventricle in utero is visualization of both the aorta and pulmonary artery committed primarily to the right or left ventricle (Fig. 17–4).[5,43–46]

The echocardiographic views most amenable to making this diagnosis vary considerably in the fetus. Often, it is the long-axis views of the aorta or pulmonary artery, or both, that are most useful. A sweep through the ventricles and great vessels in a short-axis view may also be helpful.

The four-chamber view will usually appear normal in the setting of DORV or DOLV because chamber size may not be altered. Also, the VSD present is usually anterior. Therefore it is easier to appreciate in long-axis views.

Once it is determined that both great vessels arise predominantly from the same ventricle, the

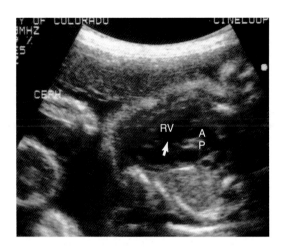

Figure 17–4   Subcostal four-chamber view in a fetus with DORV. Both the aorta *(A)* and pulmonary artery *(P)* are arising from the right ventricle *(RV)*. The pulmonary artery is small and atretic compared with the aorta. The VSD *(arrow)* is also appreciated from this view.

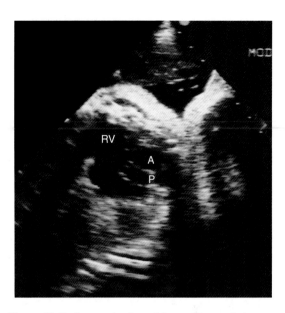

Figure 17–5   Long-axis view of the great vessels in a fetus with DORV. The aorta *(A)* and pulmonary artery *(P)* are both arising from the right ventricle *(RV)*. Note their parallel orientation.

orientation of these vessels should be investigated. In DORV, the most common relationship of the great vessels is side by side, with the aorta right and lateral to the pulmonary artery. When this occurs, the normal perpendicular course of the great vessels is lost. In the long-axis view, they appear to travel a parallel course (Fig. 17–5). In a short-axis view, the great vessels both appear as parallel or circular structures, as opposed to the normal orientation in which the pulmonary artery is draped over the aorta in a perpendicular fashion. (Fig. 17–6) These appearances are similar to complete transposition (dextrotransposition) of the great vessels. DORV is distinguished by appreciating both vessels originating from the right ventricle. With complete transposition alone, the aorta arises from the right ventricle and the pulmonary arises from the left ventricle. Tetralogy of Fallot may also appear similar to DORV, if considerable override of the aorta is present. However, with tetralogy of Fallot the aorta should still arise predominantly from the left ventricle.

Once orientation of the great vessels is determined, the location of the VSD should be evaluated. Most commonly, it will occur in a subaortic location in DORV. The spatial relationship between the great vessels and the VSD is an important surgical consideration. Unfortunately, the exact location may be very difficult to determine, particularly

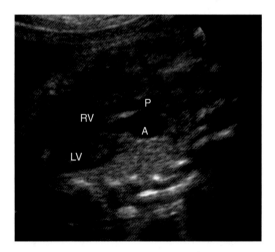

Figure 17–6   Short-axis view of the ventricles showing the bifurcating pulmonary artery *(P)* and the aorta *(A)* arising in a parallel orientation from the right ventricle *(RV)*. LV, Left ventricle.

in the fetus. Again, a combination of long- and short-axis views are necessary to carefully evaluate these relationships. Color and pulsed Doppler imaging can be used to confirm the presence of one or more VSDs. However, because of the nearly equal pressures in the fetal ventricles, smaller defects may show no appreciable flow.

Statistically, a subaortic VSD is also most likely to occur in DOLV. The aorta is usually located either right and anterior or right and lateral to the pulmonary artery.

In addition to confirming the diagnosis of double-outlet ventricle, the fetal echocardiogram can provide other important information necessary for treatment planning.

Many surgical decisions depend heavily on the presence or absence of associated abnormalities. A complete assessment should include the following:

- Apical and subcostal four-chamber views should be obtained to determine atrioventricular situs and to confirm the presence of two adequately sized ventricles.
- In addition to determining the location and position of the VSD relative to the great vessels, the size of the defect is also an important consideration. More than one VSD may be present. Color and pulsed Doppler imaging may be useful in confirming a defect seen on gray scale.
- Pulsed Doppler evaluation of the aorta and pulmonary artery, and measurements at the level of the aortic and pulmonic valves, should be undertaken to determine whether outflow tract obstruction (stenosis) or atresia are present.
- The three-vessel view is useful to compare the size of the aorta and pulmonary artery and to confirm antegrade flow in both.
- The presence of the mitral and tricuspid valves should be documented. If an atrioventricular septal defect is present, a single multileaflet valve may be seen.
- The aortic arch should be evaluated with both color and pulsed Doppler imaging to detect hypoplasia or the presence of a coarctation.

Because of the association of extracardiac abnormalities with DORV and DOLV, a thorough evaluation of the entire fetus should be undertaken.

Treatment

Severe cyanosis often occurs in the neonate with double-outlet ventricle with a subaortic or doubly committed VSD and pulmonary stenosis. This requires initial management with intravenous prostaglandin E_1 to maintain ductal patency until the time of surgical intervention. In double-outlet ventricle with a subaortic or doubly committed VSD without pulmonary stenosis, congestive heart failure may be immediately present, requiring diuretics and inotropic agents. Respiratory manipulation or mechanical ventilation may also be necessary.[5]

Double-outlet ventricle requires surgical intervention. The type of surgical procedure used is determined by the anatomy and physiology of the defect and the associated abnormalities.[5] In patients with a normal-sized mitral valve and left ventricle, a biventricular repair is feasible. If the left ventricle is small or if an abnormal atrioventricular valve is present, a single-ventricle repair is likely.[21]

The location of the VSD will also determine the type of surgical intervention attempted. Patients with noncommitted VSDs are more likely to undergo a single-ventricle repair, whereas a subaortic defect would lend itself to a biventricular repair.

The goals of complete biventricle repair include establishing unobstructed left ventricle–to–aorta continuity, establishing unobstructed right ventricle–to–pulmonary artery continuity, closing the VSD, and repairing associated lesions.[5] Closing the VSD associated with DOLV is usually a simpler procedure than it is in DORV.[47,48]

If early complete repair is not possible, lesion-specific palliative surgery (i.e., placement of a systemic-to-pulmonary shunt or pulmonary artery banding) may be necessary. Because of the complexity of intracardiac repair in some cases of double-outlet ventricle, some authors have advocated palliative procedures in infants who become symptomatic, reserving complete repair until 2 years of age.[7]

When biventricular repair is not possible, staging toward a Fontan procedure is warranted.[49-51] The Fontan procedure is usually a three-stage procedure that ultimately results in diverting the systemic venous flow directly into the pulmonary arteries. Reported complications after a Fontan procedure include thromboembolism, hepatic dysfunction, arrhythmia, and cyanosis.[52,53] Wilcox et al[54] reported 63 cases of DORV. Of these, 23 cases (36.5%) were determined to be inoperable. The hearts deemed inoperable had accompanying lesions such as multiple septal defects, a hypoplastic left ventricle, straddling valves, or other complex lesions that made the possibility of a successful surgical outcome unlikely. An autopsy series of 50 hearts with DORV found 26 (52%) to be inoperable because of the severity of the defects.[5]

In the Bradley series, biventricular repair, especially Rastelli-type reconstruction, was associated with higher late mortality rates and reintervention than was the Fontan repair.[21]

The mortality rate associated with surgical intervention in the neonate and infant is reported to be between 10% and 29%.[3,55-60] Complications reported after surgical repair include complete heart block, residual pulmonary stenosis, left ventricular failure, right ventricle failure, and residual shunts.[4,5,22] In some cases, reoperation may be necessary.

Prognosis

The prognosis for DORV varies with the presence of associated abnormalities.[61,62] Statistically, survival following surgical correction has increased over the past several years.[3] Kirklin et al[4] followed 127 patients undergoing surgical repair of DORV during an 18-year period (1967–1984). Because their early experience and repairs of all forms of DORV were included in this analysis, the actuarial survival rate at 12 years was only 38%. However, their more recent data showed an early (2-week) survival rate of 99% for DORV with subaortic VSD in 6-month-old infants and a 10-year survival rate of 97%. Results were similar for doubly committed VSDs but were lower in cases of subpulmonic VSDs. The 10-year survival rate for those with noncommitted or remote VSDs was dismal at only 22%.

Musumeci et al[63] reviewed 120 patients who had undergone surgical intervention for DORV between 1971 and 1986. These authors also reported a significant improvement in survival for those patients operated on most recently, particularly those with subpulmonic VSDs. This was attributed to refinement in surgical technique over the past several years.

Shen et al[64] reported a significant risk for late sudden death after repair of DORV. Of 89 patients operated on between 1965 and 1985, 16 (18%) succumbed to sudden death, half within 1 year of operation. Risk factors for sudden death included older age at the time of operation, perioperative ventricular tachycardia, and complete heart block. The year of repair did not correlate with the risk of sudden death.

In 2007, Gedikbasi et al[65] concluded that the overall prognosis for fetuses with DORV was poor, not only related to the primary lesion but also depending on associated abnormalities.

Associated Anomalies

DORV and DOLV are both associated with a variety of syndromes and chromosomal abnormalities. Additionally, the list of associated cardiac lesions is extensive (Tables 17–1 and 17–2). Pulmonary stenosis is the most commonly encountered associated cardiac anomaly, occurring in 65% to 70% of cases of DORV.[19,21,66,67] Other commonly associated cardiac lesions include a bicuspid pulmonary valve, atrial septal defect, atrioventricular septal defect, dextrocardia, anomalous pulmonary return, right aortic arch, and left superior vena cava.[68,69] TGA, coarctation of the aorta, mitral valve anomalies, and hypoplastic left heart syndrome are also frequently seen, suggesting abnormal hemodynamics in utero.[21,68,70]

A commonly observed association in DOLV is tricuspid atresia or stenosis in association with a hypoplastic right ventricle.[31,68,71]

A high association between DORV and infants of diabetic mothers has also been established.[72] The Baltimore-Washington Infant Study, which evaluated confirmed congenital heart disease in 2303 infants, found that overt diabetes was present in 138 (6%) mothers. The primary cardiac lesion in this subgroup of infants was DORV.[40,73]

Chromosome abnormalities are found in 28% of cases.[70] The most commonly reported chromosome abnormalities are 22q11 deletion (DiGeorge syndrome), trisomy 18, and trisomy 13.[65,70] Extracardiac anomalies occur in approximately 47% of cases, including central nervous system, genitourinary, and gastrointestinal abnormalities. Intrauterine growth restriction and single umbilical artery have also been reported.[43,65]

TABLE 17-1 Conditions Associated with Double-Outlet Right Ventricle				
Maternal		**Fetal**		
Condition	**Drug Use**	**Associated Cardiac Abnormalities**	**Chromosome Abnormalities**	**Syndromes**
Diabetes	Alcohol Isotretinoin (Accutane) Thalidomide Trimethadione	Absent pulmonary valve Absent inferior vena cava Aortic hypoplasia Aortic insufficiency Aortic stenosis Atrial septal defect Atrial stenosis Atrioventricular septal defect Bicuspid pulmonary valve Coarctation Common atrium Double-inlet left ventricle Double-chamber right ventricle Ebstein anomaly Hypoplasia of the right ventricle Hypoplastic left heart syndrome Left superior vena cava Mitral atresia Mitral stenosis Mitral insufficiency Partial anomalous pulmonary venous connection Pulmonary stenosis Quadricuspid aortic valve Right superior vena cava Right aortic arch Single ventricle Total anomalous pulmonary venous connection Tricuspid regurgitation Tricuspid stenosis Transposition Tetralogy of Fallot VSD	22q (DiGeorge syndrome) Trisomy 9 (mosaic) Trisomy 13 (Patau syndrome) Trisomy 18 (Edward syndrome)	Beemer lethal malformation syndrome CHARGE (coloboma, heart disease, atresia choanae, retarded growth and development or central nervous system anomalies, genital hypoplasia, and ear anomalies or deafness) syndrome Heterotaxy syndromes Polydactyly-chondrodystrophy Short rib polydactyly (non-Majewski type)

TABLE 17-2 Conditions Associated with Double-Outlet Left Ventricle				
Maternal		**Fetal**		
Condition	Drug Use	Associated Cardiac Abnormalities	Chromosome Abnormality	Syndrome
—	—	Atrial isomerism Aortic stenosis Atrioventricular septal defect Coarctation Common atrium Double-inlet left ventricle Ebstein anomaly Hypoplastic right ventricle Mitral atresia Pulmonary atresia Pulmonary stenosis Single ventricle Tricuspid atresia TGA Tetralogy of Fallot VSD	—	Short rib polydactyly (non-Majewski type)

References

1. Freedom RM, Smallhorn JF: Double-outlet right ventricle. In: Freedom RM, Benson LN, Smallhorn JF (eds): Neonatal Heart Disease. New York, Springer-Verlag, 1992, pp 453–470.
2. Anderson RH, Becker AE, Wilcox BR, et al: Surgical anatomy of double-outlet right ventricle—A reappraisal. Am J Cardiol 1983; 52:555–559.
3. Piccoli G, Pacifico AD, Kirklin JW: Changing results and concepts in the surgical treatment of double-outlet right ventricle: Analysis of 137 operations in 126 patients. Am J Cardiol 1983; 52:549–554.
4. Kirklin JW, Pacifico AD, Blackstone EH, et al: Current risks and protocols for operations for double-outlet right ventricle. J Thorac Cardiovasc Surg 1986; 92:913–930.
5. Thompson WE, Nichols DG, Ungerleider RM: Double-outlet right ventricle and double-outlet left ventricle. In: Nichols DG, Cameron DE, Greeley WJ, et al (eds): Critical Heart Disease in Infants and Children. St Louis, Mosby–Year Book, 1995, pp 623–646.
6. Van Praagh S, Davidoff A, Chin A, et al: Double outlet right ventricle: Anatomic types and developmental implications based on a study of 100 autopsied cases. Coeur 1982; 13:389–439.
7. Hagler DJ: Double-outlet right ventricle. In: Emmanouilides GC, Riemenschneider TA, Allan HD, et al (eds): Moss and Adams' Heart Disease in Infants, Children and Adolescents: Including the Fetus and Young Adult, 5th ed, vol 2.
Baltimore, Williams & Wilkins, 1995, pp 1246–1269.
8. Taussig HB, Bing RJ: Complete transposition of the aorta and a levoposition of the pulmonary artery: Clinical, physiological and pathological findings. Am Heart J 1949; 37:551–559.
9. Braun K, de Vries A, Feingold DS, et al: Complete dextroposition of the aorta, pulmonary stenosis, interventricular septal defect, and patent foramen ovale. Am Heart J 1952; 43:773–780.
10. Witham AC: Double-outlet right ventricle: A partial transposition complex. Am Heart J 1957; 53:928–939.
11. Neufield HN, DuShane JW, Edwards JE: Origin of both great vessels from the right ventricle. II: With pulmonary stenosis. Circulation 1961; 23:603–612.
12. Neufeld HN, DuShane JW, Wood EH, et al: Origin of both great vessels from the right ventricle. I: Without pulmonary stenosis. Circulation 1961; 23:399–412.
13. Neufeld HN, Lucas RV Jr, Lester RG, et al: Origin of both great vessels from the right ventricle without pulmonary stenosis. Br Heart J 1962; 24:393–408.
14. Lev M, Bharati S, Meng CC, et al: A concept of double-outlet right ventricle. J Thorac Cardiovasc Surg 1972; 64:271–281.
15. Hagler DJ, Ritter DG, Puga FJ: Double-outlet right ventricle. In: Adams FH, Emmanouilides GC, Riemenschneider TA (eds): Moss' Heart Disease in Infants, Children, and Adolescents, 4th ed, Baltimore, Williams & Wilkins, 1989, pp 442–460.

16. Lev M, Bharati S: Double-outlet right ventricle-association with other cardiovascular anomalies. Arch Pathol 1973; 81:24–35.

17. Macartney FJ, Rigby ML, Anderson RH, et al: Double-outlet right ventricle: Cross-sectional echocardiographic findings, their anatomical explanation, and surgical relevance. Br Heart J 1984; 52:164–177.

18. Sridaromont S, Feldt RH, Ritter DG, et al: Double-outlet right ventricle associated with persistent common atrioventricular canal. Circulation 1975; 52:933–942.

19. Sridaromont S, Feldt RH, Ritter DG: Double-outlet right ventricle: Hemodynamic and anatomic corrections. Am J Cardiol 1976; 38:85–94.

20. Sridaromont S, Ritter DG, Feldt RH, et al: Double-outlet right ventricle: Anatomic and angiocardiographic correlations. Mayo Clin Proc 1978; 53:555–577.

21. Bradley TJ, Karamlou T, Kulik A, et al: Determinants of repair type, reintervention and mortality in 393 children with double-outlet right ventricle. J Thorac Cardiovasc Surg 2007; 134:967–973.

22. Stellin G, Ho SY, Anderson RH, et al: The surgical anatomy of double-outlet right ventricle with concordant atrioventricular connection and noncommitted ventricular septal defect. J Thorac Cardiovasc Surg 1991; 102:849–855.

23. Zamora R, Moller JH, Edwards JE: Double-outlet right ventricle: Anatomic types and associated anomalies. Chest 1975; 68:672–677.

24. Ainger LF: Double-outlet right ventricle: Intact ventricular septum, mitral stenosis, and blind left ventricle. Am Heart J 1965; 70:521–525.

25. Davachi F, Moller JH, Edwards JF: Origin of both great vessels from right ventricle with intact ventricular septum. Am Heart J 1968; 75:790–794.

26. MacMahon HE, Lipa M: Double-outlet right ventricle with intact interventricular septum. Circulation 1964; 30:745–748.

27. Artrip JH, Sauer H, Campbell DN, et al: Biventricular repair in double outlet right ventricle: surgical results based on the STS-EACTS International Nomenclature classification. Eur J Cardiothorac Surg 2006; 545–550.

28. Hagler DJ, Edwards WD: Double-outlet left ventricle. In: Emmanouilides GC, Riemenschneider TA, Allan HD, et al (eds): Moss and Adams' Heart Disease in Infants, Children, and Adolescents: Including the Fetus and Young Adult, 5th ed, vol 2. Baltimore, Williams & Wilkins, 1995, pp 1270–1278.

29. Fragoyannis S, Kardalinos A: Transposition of the great vessels, both arising from the left ventricle (juxtaposition of the pulmonary artery): Tricuspid atresia, atrial septal defect and ventricular septal defect. Am J Cardiol 1962; 10:601–604.

30. Ruttenberg HD, Anderson RC, Elliot LP, et al: Origin of both great vessels from the arterial ventricle: A complex with ventricular inversion. Br Heart J 1964; 26:631–641.

31. Paul MH, Muster AJ, Sinha SN, et al: Double-outlet left ventricle with an intact ventricular septum: Clinical and autopsy diagnosis and developmental implications. Circulation 1970; 41:129–139.

32. Van Praagh R, Weinberg PM, Srebro JP: Double-outlet left ventricle. In: Adams FH, Emmanouilides GC, Riemenschneider TA (eds): Moss' Heart Disease in Infants, Children, and Adolescents, 4th ed. Baltimore, Williams & Wilkins, 1989, pp 461–485.

33. Akagawa H, Yoshioka F, Isomura T, et al: Surgical treatment of double-outlet left ventricle in situs inversus. Ann Thorac Surg 1984; 37:337–342.

34. Anderson R, Galbraith R, Gibson R, et al: Double-outlet left ventricle. Br Heart J 1974; 36:554–558.

35. Brandt PWT, Calder AL, Barratt-Boyes BG, et al: Double-outlet left ventricle: Morphology, cineangiocardiographic diagnosis and surgical treatment. Am J Cardiol 1976; 38:897–909.

36. Freedom RM, Culham JAG, Moes CAF: Angiocardiography of Congenital Heart Disease. New York, MacMillan, 1984, pp 588–592.

37. Urban AE, Anderson RH, Stark J: Double-outlet left ventricle associated with situs inversus and atrioventricular concordance. Am Heart J 1977; 84:91–95.

38. Lacour-Gayet F, Haun C, Ntalakoura K, et al: Biventricular repair of double outlet right ventricle with non-committed ventricular septal defect (VSD) by VSD rerouting to the pulmonary artery and arterial switch. Eur J Cardiothorac Surg 2002; 21:1042–1048.

39. Manner J, Seidl W, Steding G: Embryological observations on the formal pathogenesis of double-outlet left ventricle with a right-ventricular infundibulum. Thorac Cardiovasc Surg 1997; 45:172–177.

40. Mitchell SC, Korones SB, Berendes HW: Congenital heart disease in 56,109 births: Incidence and natural history. Circulation 1971; 43:323–332.

41. Ferencz C, Rubin JD, McCarter RJ: Congenital heart disease: Prevalence at livebirth. The Baltimore-Washington Infant Study. Am J Epidemiol 1985; 121:31–36.

42. Fyler DC: Report of the New England Regional Infant Cardiac Program. Pediatrics 1980; 65(Suppl):376–461.

43. Tongsong T, Chanprapaph P, Sittiwangkul R, et al: Antenatal diagnosis of double outlet of right ventricle without extracardiac anomaly: A report of 4 cases. J Clin Ultrasound 2007; 35:221–225.

44. Hoffman JIE: Incidence of congenital heart disease. II: Prenatal incidence. Pediatr Cardiol 1995; 16:155–165.

45. Sanders SP, Bierman FZ, Williams RG: Conotruncal malformations: Diagnosis in infancy

using subxiphoid 2-dimensional echocardiography. Am J Cardiol 1982; 50:1361–1367.

46. Snider AR, Serwer GA (eds): Abnormalities of ventriculoarterial connection. In: Echocardiography in Pediatric Heart Disease. St Louis, Mosby–Year Book, 1990, pp 190–194.

47. Lincoln C: Total correction of d-loop double-outlet right ventricle with bilateral conus, l-transposition, and pulmonic stenosis. J Thorac Cardiovasc Surg 1972; 64:435–440.

48. Patrick DL, McGoon DC: An operation for double-outlet right ventricle with transposition of the great arteries. J Cardiovasc Surg 1968; 9:537–542.

49. Fontan FM, Mounico FB, Baudet E, et al: "Correction" of tricuspid atresia: Two cases "corrected" using a new surgical technique. Ann Chir Thorac Cardiovasc 1971; 10:39–47.

50. Katogi T, Takenchi S, Katsumoto K, et al: Surgical correction of double outlet left ventricle associated with hypoplastic right ventricle: Direct anastomosis of right atrial appendage and pulmonary artery. Jpn Circ J 1979; 43:768–774.

51. Doty DB, Marvin WJ, Lauer RM: Modified Fontan procedure, methods to achieve direct anastomosis of right atrium to pulmonary artery. J Thorac Cardiovasc Surg 1981; 81:470–475.

52. Jacobs ML, Norwood WI. Fontan operation: Influence of modifications on morbidity and mortality. Ann Thorac Surg 1994; 58:945–952.

53. Ravn HB, Hjortdal VE, Stenbog EV, et al: Increased platelet reactivity and significant changes in coagulation markers after cavopulmonary connection. Heart 2001; 85:61–65.

54. Wilcox BR, Ho SY, Macartney FJ, et al: Surgical anatomy of double-outlet right ventricle with situs solitus and atrioventricular concordance. J Thorac Cardiovasc Surg 1981; 82:405–417.

55. Bical O, Hazan O, Lecompte Y, et al: Anatomic correction of transposition of the great arteries associated with ventricular septal defect: Midterm results in 50 patients. Circulation 1984; 70:891–897.

56. Judson JP, Danielson GK, Puga FJ, et al: Double-outlet right ventricle: Surgical results 1970–1980. J Thorac Cardiovasc Surg 1983; 85:32–40.

57. Mazzuco A, Faggion G, Stellin GEA: Surgical management of double-outlet right ventricle. J Thorac Cardiovasc Surg 1985; 90:29–34.

58. Quaegebeur JM: The optimal repair for the Taussig-Bing heart. J Thorac Cardiovasc Surg 1983; 85:276–277.

59. Yacoub MH, Radley-Smith R: Anatomic correction of the Taussig-Bing anomaly. J Thorac Cardiovasc Surg 1984; 88:380–388.

60. Gomes MMR, Weidman WH, McGoon DC, et al: Double-outlet right ventricle with pulmonic stenosis: Surgical considerations and results of operation. Circulation 1971; 43:889–894.

61. Nyberg DA, Emerson DS: Cardiac malformations. In: Nyberg DA, Mahony BS, Pretorius DH (eds): Diagnostic Ultrasound of Fetal Anomalies: Text and Atlas. Chicago, Year Book Medical, 1990, pp 300–341.

62. Franks R, Lincoln C: Surgical management of the double outlet right ventricle. In: Anderson RH, MacCartney FL, Shinebourne EA, et al (eds): Paediatric Cardiology, vol 5. London, Churchill Livingstone, 1983, pp 441–450.

63. Musumeci F, Shumway S, Lincoln C, et al: Surgical treatment for double-outlet right ventricle at the Brompton Hospital, 1973 to 1986. J Thorac Cardiovasc Surg 1988; 96:278–287.

64. Shen WK, Holmes DR, Porter CJ, et al: Sudden death after repair of double-outlet right ventricle. Circulation 1990; 81:128–136.

65. Gedikbasi AG, Oztarhan KO, Gul AG, et al: Double-outlet right ventricle: Prenatal diagnosis and fetal outcome. Ultrasound Obstet Gynecol 2007; 30:598–599.

66. Cameron AH, Acerete F, Quero M, et al: Double-outlet right ventricle: Study of 27 cases. Br Heart J 1976; 38:1124–1126.

67. Sondheimer HM, Freedom RM, Olley PM: Double-outlet right ventricle: Clinical spectrum and prognosis. Am J Cardiol 1977; 39:709–712.

68. Bharati S, Lev M: The Pathology of Congenital Heart Disease: A Personal Experience with More Than 6,300 Congenitally Malformed Hearts. Armonk, NY, Futura, 1996, pp 135–167.

69. Galindo A, Gutierrez-Larraya F, Escribano D, et al: Clinical significance of persistent left superior vena cava diagnosed in fetal life. Ultrasound Obstet Gynecol 2007; 30:152–161

70. Paladini D, Sglavo G, DeRobertis V, et al: Anatomy association and outcome of prenatally detected double-outlet right ventricle. Ultrasound Obstet Gynecol 2007; 30:408.

71. Freedom RM: Double-outlet left ventricle: Isolated atrioventricular discordance; anatomically corrected malposition of the great arteries; and syndrome of juxtaposition of the atrial appendages. In: Freedom RM, Benson LN, Smallhorn JF (eds): Neonatal Heart Disease. New York, Springer-Verlag, 1992, pp 561–562.

72. Stewart PA, Wladimiroff JW, Becker AE: Early prenatal detection of double outlet right ventricle by echocardiography. Br Heart J 1985; 54:340–342.

73. Ferencz C: A case-control study of cardiovascular malformations in liveborn infants: The morphogenetic relevance of epidemiologic findings. In: Clark EB, Takao A (eds): Developmental Cardiology: Morphogenesis and Function. Mount Kisco, NY, Futura, 1990, pp 523–539.

CHAPTER 18

Congenital Cardiac Masses

Tina M. Bachman

Heidi S. Barrett

Definition

Congenital cardiac tumors are rare. The occurrence rate in infants and children is approximately 0.027%.[1] Among the pediatric population, more than 90% of cardiac neoplasms are histologically benign. However, they have the potential for serious consequences if not detected in a timely manner, usually because of their conspicuous location.[1-4] The incidence of cardiac tumors in the fetus is approximately 0.14%.[4]

Rhabdomyoma is the most common tumor of both infancy and childhood, occurring in 60% of cases. Teratoma (25%), fibroma (12%), and hemangiomas (3%) occur less frequently.[5] Myxoma and neurofibroma have also been reported in childhood but are more commonly found in adults.[6-9]

Rhabdomyoma

Rhabdomyomas have been diagnosed in the fetus as early as 20 weeks' gestation.[4,10-20] They tend to be multiple (90%), occurring most frequently within the right or left ventricle or within the interventricular septum. They may occur within the myocardium, leading to a variety of arrhythmias (usually supraventricular tachycardia) or may grow within the cardiac chambers, which can lead to valvular obstruction.[11,21-26] Most congenital cardiac tumors are isolated anomalies; however, tuberous sclerosis has been reported in 60% to 80% of patients diagnosed with rhabdomyoma.[4,10,27] Tuberous sclerosis is a multisystem disease classically characterized by the triad of adenoma sebaceum, epilepsy, and mental retardation. It is a familial disease inherited as an autosomal dominant trait with variable penetrance and variable expressivity. Rarely, it may be a sporadic event.[28]

The clinical and hemodynamic findings of cardiac rhabdomyomas are related to the number, size, and position of the tumors.[29] In the fetus, if supraventricular tachycardia occurs, nonimmune hydrops fetalis and polyhydramnios may manifest. Decreased fetal growth has also been associated with rhabdomyoma.[11–18,30] Clinically, in addition to serious arrhythmias, severe cyanosis, mental retardation, seizures, cutaneous lesions, and visceral tumors may be observed in the neonate or infant.[9,24,26,31–33]

Spontaneous regression of cardiac rhabdomyomas in early childhood occurs in more than 80% of cases.[4,34] Although spontaneous regression has been observed, sudden death is not uncommon.[10,12,23–26,35,36]

Teratoma

Cardiac teratoma is the second most common tumor in the fetus; it accounts for up to 21% of benign cardiac tumors in infants and 14% of such tumors in children aged 1 to 15 years.[4,18,37] Intrapericardial teratomas are the second most common tumor reported prenatally. They are usually single, encapsulated tumors attached to the base of the heart.[38–42]

Intrapericardial teratomas are attached to the heart by a broad pedicle or stalk. Common sites of occurrence include the root of the aorta or pulmonary artery and the right ventricle and right atrium.[38–41,43–48] Less frequent locations include the left atrium, left ventricle, and superior vena cava.[38,41]

The size of intrapericardial teratomas is variable. Asymptomatic older children and adolescents are affected by very small lesions, whereas lesions reported in the neonate or infant have been three to four times the size of the heart.[40,41,49]

Intrapericardial teratomas in the fetus are almost always accompanied by a pericardial effusion.[41,44,46–47] Similar to rhabdomyomas, intrapericardial teratomas are space-occupying lesions that can cause hemodynamic compromise as a result of obstruction and compression of the heart. Sudden death has been reported in 66% of pediatric patients.[47] This is thought to result from acute rupture into the pericardial space, causing sudden cardiac tamponade, severe encroachment by the tumor on the heart and great vessels, infectious pericarditis, or a combination of these conditions.[38,47,50]

Fibroma

Prenatal diagnosis of cardiac fibroma on the basis of sonographic findings is unusual; however, a few cases have been described.[51] Cardiac fibromas are usually singular, nonencapsulated intramural lesions that most often involve the left ventricular free wall and interventricular septum.[52–60] They are usually located at the left ventricular apex. Other reported locations include the atria, the interatrial septum, and the right ventricular free wall, although this is an uncommon site.[52–54,57,61,62]

Fibromas may invade the conducting system because of their location, resulting in arrhythmias or sudden death.[37] As with all cardiac tumors, sequelae vary depending on the size and location of the tumor. Large fibromas may encroach on the intracavitary space, causing subaortic and subpulmonic obstruction.[63] Pedunculated fibromas that obstruct the outflow tracts have also been observed.

Clinical symptoms in the neonate include severe congestive heart failure and cyanosis.[52,54,56,63,64] Significant pericardial effusions have also been associated with fibromas.[29]

Hemangioma

Cardiac hemangiomas are rare, benign vascular tumors that account for 2% to 5% of all cardiac masses.[7,37,65–67] They can involve any chamber of the heart and have also been reported to invade the interventricular septum or atrioventricular node, resulting in rhythm disturbances.[65,67–69] Although hemangiomas are usually asymptomatic, growth occurring within the epicardium or pericardium may cause pericardial effusion and cardiac tamponade.[65–67,69] Prenatally, these polypoid masses may be diagnosed by demonstrating the main feeding vessel with color or power Doppler imaging.[70]

Myxoma

Cardiac myxomas are the most common primary cardiac tumor in adults.[3,68,71,72] Although they have been reported in the neonate, they are exceedingly rare.[73–77] They have not been reported in the fetus. Myxomas arise from the endocardium, occurring in the left atrium in 75% of patients and in the right atrium in 25%.[72,78,79] These tumors are usually singular lesions that are attached to the foramen ovale by a pedicle.[29,37] Attachment to the left atrial free wall has also been reported.[80]

The classic appearance of a cardiac myxoma is that of a large pedunculated tumor traversing back and forth through the atrioventricular valve.[71,81-87] Classified as benign, these tumors have a tendency for local recurrence and, rarely, malignant degeneration.[88-90]

Although more than 90% of myxomas occur sporadically, they have also been seen in children and adolescents with multiple lentigines syndrome.[91] These patients have pigmented skin lesions and endocrine neoplasms in addition to the cardiac tumor.[37]

Myxomas present with a classic triad of symptoms that includes hemodynamic obstruction, emboli, and systemic illness.[71,72,79,92,93] Rarely are patients asymptomatic. Most pediatric patients (80%) have symptoms of valvular obstruction.[87]

Large left-sided myxomas have been reported to obstruct pulmonary venous inflow, resulting in pulmonary edema, pulmonary arterial hypertension, and low cardiac output.[71,72,90] They may also cause left ventricular inflow obstruction and mimic mitral stenosis. Right atrial tumors impede systemic venous inflow and cause right ventricular failure and low cardiac output.[71-75] Myxomas may mimic neonatal cyanotic heart disease when an obstructive right-sided tumor causes right-to-left shunting at the atrial level.[73-76] Myxomas have also been associated with sudden death.[73,74]

Congenital Ventricular Diverticulum and Aneurysm

Other masses that occur in the fetal heart include congenital ventricular diverticulum (CVD) and congenital ventricular aneurysm (CVA). The terms CVD and CVA have been used in the literature interchangeably. However, they are two distinct entities with different histological and morphological characteristics.[94] Their true incidence is unknown because most cases are asymptomatic, but the prevalence of CVA has been suggested to be 0.5 in 100,000 births.[95]

The two entities have been variably classified according to four major criteria. These criteria include connection to the ventricular cavity, wall composition, wall motion, and association with intracardiac abnormalities or midline defects.[94-97] CVDs have a narrow connection to the ventricular cavity, whereas CVAs have a wide neck or broad connection to the ventricular cavity.[94-97] Histologically, CVDs are composed of the normal layers of the ventricular wall. Comparatively, CVAs tend to be fibrous with thinned myocardium or an outpouching through disrupted myocardium.[95,96] Because of the histological nature of these two entities, a CVD will contract during systole with the associated ventricle, whereas a CVA does not. This has been recognized as the most accurate parameter for diagnosis by ultrasonography.[94-96] The final classification is an association with intracardiac abnormalities or midline defects. Both CVDs and CVAs are usually isolated lesions; however, some associated cardiac anomalies have been reported with CVD.[98] Marijon et al[92] evaluated 16 cases of CVD. They identified two subgroups that were distinguished by location of the CVD in the ventricle. The apical CVD was a fingerlike contractile pouch with a narrow connection to the ventricle that was consistently associated with midline thoracoabdominal defects. Apical CVDs were always associated with cardiac rotation disorder or intracardiac abnormalities. In contrast, nonapical CVDs were described as a contractile pouch with a wider connection to the ventricle and were not associated with other abnormalities.[94]

Cardiac diverticula and aneurysms are thought to occur as a result of a focal weakening of the ventricular wall because of an interruption during embryogenesis, infection, or localized ischemia.[98]

Pseudomasses

A persistent or redundant eustachian valve can mimic an atrial mass.[99,100] The eustachian valve originates at the junction of the right atrium and the inferior vena cava.[99] It diverts blood flow from the inferior vena cava into two separate channels, allowing oxygenated blood from the ductus venosus to flow through the foramen ovale into the left atrium. Deoxygenated blood entering the inferior vena cava is directed through the tricuspid valve into the right ventricle.[99,100] In the first trimester, the eustachian valve is large, covering the mouth of the inferior and superior vena cavae.[99] As pregnancy progresses, the eustachian valve decreases in size and may disappear. It may also persist into adulthood. A wispy or circular structure should be recognized as a normal eustachian valve.

Echogenic intracardiac foci are small discrete structures found within the cardiac ventricles in the region of the papillary muscles or chordae tendinae. They are described as having echogenicity comparable to that of fetal bone and by autopsy correlated with areas of mineralization. They occur in the left ventricle 90% of the time but may also be identified in the right ventricle or bilaterally.[101-103] Echogenic foci are common in normal fetuses, occurring in 3% to 5% of the normal population.[102]

Echogenic foci should not be considered a cardiac mass. They are not associated with structural heart disease, nor do they cause any hemodynamic disturbance.[102,104] Previously, echogenic foci had been associated with chromosomal abnormalities such as Down syndrome.[102] More recent literature has cast doubt on this association.[101-105]

Sonographic Criteria

Most fetal cardiac masses are easily recognized on ultrasonography. The prenatal diagnosis of a cardiac tumor is usually an incidental finding on routine obstetrical ultrasonography.[106] The presence of an intracardiac mass in the fetus statistically suggests *rhabdomyoma*. Although it is impossible to make a histological diagnosis in utero, several sonographic criteria, including tumor number, size, location, and echogenicity, may help narrow the differential diagnosis (Table 18–1). The presence of multiple tumors is indicative of *rhabdomyoma*.* Sonographically, they appear as hyperechoic, heterogeneous masses of variable size. They are unencapsulated, well-circumscribed lesions.[10-18] Areas of fibrosis or calcification have been identified within them.[108]

Rhabdomyomas may occur anywhere in the heart but are most often located in the ventricular myocardium (Fig. 18–1).[4,109] Frequently the tumor appears to involve both sides of the interventricu-

---

*References 3, 8, 19, 20, 32, 37, 107.

lar septum.[59] Intracavitary extension is found in up to 50% of cases.[4] *Rhabdomyomas* may simulate a hypoplastic heart if the tumor becomes large enough to obliterate the ventricle (Fig. 18–2).

Rhabdomyomas obstructing the mitral or tricuspid valves have been reported to simulate atresia of the respective valve (Fig. 18–3).[1,23,26,110-120] They often obstruct valvular inflow or outflow, or both; therefore Doppler imaging of the valve or valves located near the mass is important.

Single pedunculated *rhabdomyomas* have been associated with subaortic stenosis and pulmonic valve stenosis.*

---

*References 31, 33, 110, 111, 121, 122.

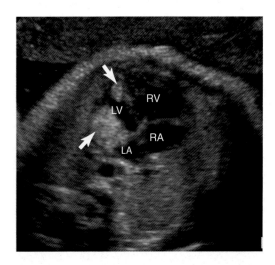

Figure 18–1 Apical four-chamber view showing two rhabdomyomas *(arrows)* within the left ventricle *(LV)*. *LA,* Left atrium; *RA,* right atrium; *RV,* right ventricle.

	Tumor Type				
TABLE 18–1	**Sonographic Criteria of Cardiac Tumors**				
Criteria	**Rhabdomyoma**	**Teratoma**	**Fibroma**	**Myxoma**	**Hemangioma**
Number	Multiple	Singular	Singular	Singular	Singular
Echotexture	Hyperechoic Homogeneous	Hyperechoic Cystic areas Calcifications	Hyperechoic or isoechoic	Hyperechoic Calcifications	Mixed
Most common location	Ventricles	Right side of the heart	Left ventricular free wall or septum	Left atrium	Any chamber
Size	Variable	Large	Variable	Variable	Variable

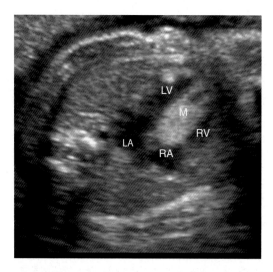

Figure 18–2 Four-chamber view showing a rhabdomyoma *(M)* invading the right ventricle *(RV)*. *LA*, Left atrium; *LV*, left ventricle; *RA*, right atrium.

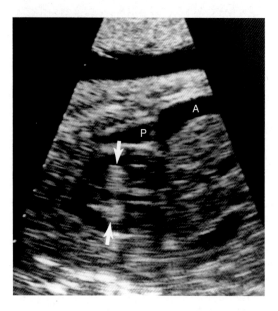

Figure 18–3 Coronal image of a fetus with bilateral cardiac rhabdomyomas *(arrows)*. The tumors are located at the level of the tricuspid and mitral valves. A pleural effusion *(P)* and ascites *(A)* are also seen.

Fetuses with cardiac *rhabdomyomas*, or any cardiac mass, can present with almost any type of arrhythmia; therefore M-mode or pulsed Doppler imaging should be used to document a normal rhythm or to differentiate an arrhythmia.

Because of the strong association of *rhabdomyoma* with tuberous sclerosis, the fetus should be evaluated for other stigmata of this syndrome, including tumors of the brain, liver, or kidneys and renal cysts.[10,123–127]

A family history of tuberous sclerosis or evidence of other organ system involvement is fairly indicative of *rhabdomyoma*. However, a negative family history should not preclude the diagnosis because spontaneous mutations do occur.[29]

The majority of *rhabdomyomas* may significantly decrease in size or disappear toward the end of the third trimester, whereas other tumor types should not.[4,29] However, despite this decrease in size, fetal loss may occur as a result of arrhythmia or congestive heart failure.[4]

Teratomas are usually singular lesions that appear heterogeneous, lobulated, and encapsulated on ultrasonography.[38,39,43–46,48,128] They may contain cystic areas or echogenic foci.[43,45–48] They are usually detected in the pericardial cavity attached to the aorta or pulmonary artery.[4] Doppler interrogation is necessary to evaluate the hemodynamic consequences of the tumor. Tumor extension into the superior vena cava has also been reported.[38] A stalk or pedicle may be seen attaching the tumor to the heart.[39–41,43–47]

The most distinguishing feature of an intrapericardial *teratoma* may be its size. These tumors may attain huge proportions, causing severe rotation or compression of the heart. A pericardial effusion is often present.[4]

Fibromas are also singular, nonencapsulated lesions. They usually occur within the interventricular septum or left ventricular free wall.[6,56–58,64] Their echotexture is usually homogeneous but sometimes can show central necrosis with calcification and cystic degeneration.[129] They can also be isoechoic with the surrounding myocardium and may mimic a massively hypertrophied ventricle.[59] Although *fibromas* are intramural tumors, they can reach significant proportions that obliterate the intracavitary space.[52–54,61–63]

Hemangiomas are solitary, well-defined masses that can occur in any chamber of the heart.[65] They are usually of mixed echogenicity and are variable in size.[66,67,130]

The sonographic appearance of a cardiac *myxoma* is that of a singular, hyperechoic tumor that is most often located within the atrium, usually the left. Calcifications are not uncommon. When a cardiac tumor is seen prolapsing from the atrium to the ventricle, this is virtually pathognomonic of a myxoma. Mitral or tricuspid valve stenosis and semilunar valve obstruction have been reported in cases of cardiac *myxomas*.*

Sonographically a *CVD* has a narrow connection to the ventricle and contracts during systole. *CVD* usually extend into the pericardial space (Fig. 18–4). A *CVA* has a wide connection to the ventricle and is noncontractile during systole.[94-97] They may extend into the pericardial space or into the cardiac chamber (Figs. 18–5 and 18–6). *CVD* and *CVA* can be associated with fetal arrhythmia, pericardial effusion, and fetal hydrops.[95-97] Apical *CVD* has an association with midline thoracoabdominal defects and intracardiac abnormalities.[94] Most *CVDs* are associated with the right ventricle.[98]

In summary, there may be some sonographic findings that help in differentiating cardiac masses in the fetus. However, regardless of tumor type, a global echocardiographic evaluation should be conducted.

---

*References 3, 71, 72, 76, 84, 85, 131.

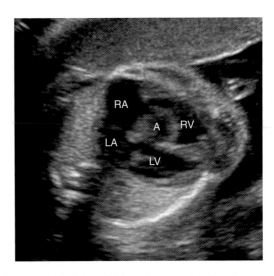

Figure 18–5 Subcostal four-chamber view in a fetus with a congenital ventricular aneurysm *(A)* that can be seen within the right ventricle *(RV)* at the level of the tricuspid valve. Note the severe levorotation of the fetal heart. *LA,* Left atrium; *LV,* left ventricle; *RA,* right atrium.

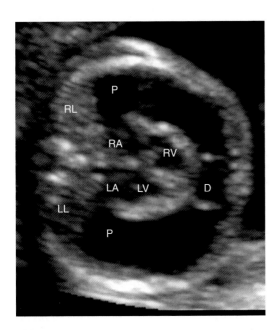

Figure 18–4 Subcostal four-chamber view in a fetus with a congenital ventricular diverticulum *(D)* arising from the right ventricle *(RV)*. A large pericardial effusion *(P)* can be seen surrounding the heart and compressing the right *(RL)* and left *(LL)* lungs. *LA,* Left atrium; *LV,* left ventricle; *RA,* right atrium.

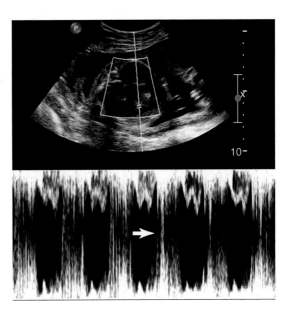

Figure 18–6 Pulsed Doppler imaging of the congenital ventricular aneurysm seen in Figure 18–5 showing massive tricuspid regurgitation *(arrow)* occurring as a result of the location of the aneurysm.

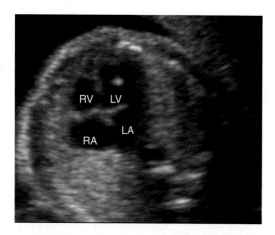

Figure 18–7 Apical four-chamber view showing an echogenic focus within the left ventricle *(LV)* at the level of the papillary muscle. The echogenicity is similar to that of the fetal spine. *LA,* Left atrium; *RA,* right atrium; *RV,* right ventricle.

All cardiac masses have the potential to cause an arrhythmia. Therefore M-mode or pulsed Doppler imaging should always be obtained to identify the presence and type of arrhythmia. Additionally, all tumors may cause obstruction, stenosis, or insufficiency of any cardiac valve they are located near, warranting color or pulsed Doppler evaluation of all valves. Finally, all cardiac masses can result in congestive heart failure. A fetus identified with a cardiac mass should always be evaluated for signs of nonimmune hydrops fetalis, such as ascites, pleural effusion, or pericardial effusion.

Echogenic foci in the ventricles should not be mistaken for a cardiac tumor. As stated previously, they are areas of mineralization of the papillary muscle or chordae tendinae that appear as echogenic as fetal bone. They are often more readily seen in an apical four-chamber view because of the angle of insonation. They occur predominately in the left ventricle, but it is not uncommon to observe them in the right ventricle or in both ventricles (Fig. 18–7).

Treatment

Appropriate management of a cardiac mass is based on size, location, and hemodynamic effect of the tumor. Therefore echocardiographic information obtained both in utero and immediately after birth is crucial.

Conservative management may be undertaken in the asymptomatic patient.[6,12,30,132–134] This is particularly applicable in *rhabdomyoma,* in which tumor regression has been well documented.[8,22,30,31,133–137]

Masses causing significant hemodynamic compromise resulting from obstruction or those invading the myocardium and causing a life-threatening arrhythmia require prompt surgical intervention.* In critically ill neonates with severe right or left ventricular obstruction, prostaglandin E is often used to maintain patency of the ductus arteriosus until surgery is performed.[29]

When severe obstruction or obliteration has occurred as a result of tumor involvement, valve replacement is often necessary.[138] Giamberti et al[138] reported successful replacement of the aortic root with a pulmonary allograft in a case of severe subvalvular and valvular aortic stenosis resulting from a *rhabdomyoma.*

Partial excision may provide significant relief of inflow or outflow tract obstruction if attempts at complete extirpation would severely damage the remaining myocardium.[6,31,32] Several authors have reported successful outcomes of subtotal excision of an individual tumor with removal of only the problematic portion.[27,31,32,140] In cases of severe extensive myocardial invasion, heart transplantation has been performed.[4,77,132,141,142]

Surgical removal of *myxomas* usually involves excision of the mass and wide resection of the point of attachment on the interatrial septum.[29,143] Careful examination of the heart is performed to remove concurrent sites of myxomatous tissue. Later development of peripheral arterial aneurysms has been reported in patients undergoing surgical excision of a *myxoma.*[71,79,144–148]

Surgical removal of *intrapericardial teratomas* and decompression of concomitant pericardial effusion has resulted in high survival rates in symptomatic infants and neonates. In utero diagnosis has allowed prompt postnatal surgical intervention before significant cardiac distress develops.[44]

In older children, even when they are asymptomatic, once an intrapericardial *teratoma* is diagnosed, it is removed. This is due to the propensity of these tumors to cause sudden death or, rarely, to undergo malignant degeneration.† Surgical treatment of a *teratoma* usually involves tumor

---

*References 13, 22, 23, 26, 109, 116, 134.
†References 38, 39, 41, 45, 59, 149.

excision and removal of the tumor pedicle from the aorta or pulmonary artery.[38–40,48,150]

As stated previously, malignant cardiac tumors are exceedingly rare in infants. If malignancy is present, treatment includes surgery in addition to combined irradiation and cytotoxic therapy.[21,59,150,151] In utero treatment of cardiac masses is confined to maternal administration of antiarrhythmic agents in cases of fetal arrhythmia. Drug therapy has proven successful even when hydrops fetalis is present.[10]

Treatment with respect to *CVD* and *CVA* remains unclear. When symptomatic or when associated with other cardiac abnormalities, surgical removal is recommended.[12] Prenatal pericardiocentesis has been performed in certain cases.[97,98] Other treatments include antibiotic prophylaxis, thromboembolism prevention, and treatment of any associated symptoms such as arrhythmia or congestive heart failure.[152] Small diverticula, when asymptomatic, may not require surgical repair.[98]

Prognosis

The prognosis for fetuses with cardiac tumors is generally dependent on size and location rather than on histological characteristics. A high rate of intrauterine death is associated with *rhabdomyoma*, particularly in the setting of multiple tumors.[9] Infants with *rhabdomyomas* generally have a good prognosis following tumor regression or surgical intervention.[108,109,134,153,154] For infants also affected with tuberous sclerosis, however, the prognosis is poor.[9,155–157] The high mortality rate may be a direct result of the *rhabdomyoma* or a result of other associated sequelae.[10,59] Left untreated, 60% of infants with *rhabdomyomas* will die within the first year of life.[9]

The prognosis for apical *CVD* is dependent on the associated intracardiac malformations but is generally good after repair. In contrast, *CVAs* tend to have a poor prognosis, with frequent fatal cardiovascular complications in the neonatal period.[94]

Left untreated, cardiac tumors that cause flow obstruction carry a mortality rate of approximately 90%.[21,135,158] Cardiac malformations may coexist with a cardiac mass, also diminishing the chances of a good prognosis.[59,159] Sudden death associated with all types of cardiac masses has been reported.*

---

*References 6, 11, 12, 23–26, 35, 36, 160, 161.

Associated Anomalies

Most cardiac masses are isolated entities, the exception being the association of *rhabdomyoma* with tuberous sclerosis[7,34] and an association of apical CVD with pentalogy of Cantrell.[94]

Cardiac *myxomas* have been reported in children and adolescents with LAMB (lentigines, atrial myxoma, mucocutaneous myxoma, and blue naevi) and NAME (naevi, atrial myxoma, myxoid neurofibromata, and ephelides) syndromes.[4,91,109] Familial cases usually present with multiple tumors, whereas sporadic cases are usually solitary.[4]

Some cardiac tumors are associated with additional congenital cardiac disease.

Russell et al[158] reported one case of Ebstein anomaly and one case of a hypoplastic tricuspid valve in conjunction with cardiac *rhabdomyomas*. A cardiac *myxoma* was seen in a child with a double-outlet right ventricle, and pulmonary atresia was seen in association with a case of a cardiac fibroma.

Marijon et al[92] reported an association of apical *CVD* with three cases of tetralogy of Fallot, two cases of ventricular septal defects, and one case of tricuspid atresia.

References

1. Nadas AS, Ellison RC: Cardiac tumors in infancy. Am J Cardiol 1968; 21:363–366.
2. Chan HS, Sonley MJ, Moes CAF, et al: Primary and secondary tumors of childhood involving the heart, pericardium and great vessels: A report of 75 cases and review of the literature. Cancer 1985; 56:825–836.
3. McAllister HA Jr: Primary tumors of the heart and pericardium. Pathol Annu 1979; 14:325–355.
4. Uzun O, Wilson DG, Vuganic GM, et al: Cardiac tumours in children. Orphan J Rare Dis 2007; 2:1–4.
5. Lacey SR, Donofrio MT: Fetal cardiac tumors: Prenatal diagnosis and outcome. Pediatr Cardiol 2007; 28:61–67.
6. Bini RM, Westaby S, Bargeron LM Jr, et al: Investigation and management of primary cardiac tumors in infants and children. J Am Coll Cardiol 1983; 2:351–357.
7. McAllister HA Jr, Fenoglio JJ Jr: Tumors of the cardiovascular system. In: Hartman WH, Cowan WE (eds): Atlas of Tumor Pathology. Washington, DC, Armed Forces Institute of Pathology, 1978, pp 1–141.

8. Marx GR, Bierman FZ, Matthews E, et al: Two-dimensional echocardiography diagnosis of intracardiac masses in infancy. J Am Coll Cardiol 1984; 3:827–832.

9. D'Addario V, Pinto V, DiNaro E, et al: Prenatal diagnosis and postnatal outcome of cardiac rhabdomyomas. J Perinat Med 2002; 30:170–175.

10. Dennis MA, Appareti K, Manco-Johnson ML: The echocardiographic diagnosis of multiple fetal cardiac tumors. J Ultrasound Med 1985; 4:327–329.

11. Birnbaum SE, McGahan JP, Hanos GG, et al: Fetal tachycardia and intramyocardial tumors. J Am Coll Cardiol 1985; 6:1358–1361.

12. Deeg KH, Voigt HJ, Hofbeck M, et al: Prenatal ultrasound diagnosis of multiple cardiac rhabdomyomas. Pediatr Radiol 1990; 20:291–292.

13. Journel H, Roussey M, Plais MH, et al: Prenatal diagnosis of familial tuberous sclerosis following detection of cardiac rhabdomyoma by ultrasound. Prenat Diagn 1986; 6:283–289.

14. Guereta LG, Burgueros M, Elorza MD, et al: Cardiac rhabdomyoma presenting as fetal hydrops. Pediatr Cardiol 1986; 7:171–174.

15. Watanabe T, Hojo Y, Kozaki T, et al: Hypoplastic left heart syndrome with rhabdomyoma of the left ventricle. Pediatr Cardiol 1991; 12:121–122.

16. Harding CO, Pagon RA: Incidence of tuberous sclerosis in patients with cardiac rhabdomyoma. Am J Med Genet 1990; 37:443–446.

17. Platt LD, Devore GR, Horenstein J, et al: Prenatal diagnosis of tuberous sclerosis: The use of fetal echocardiography. Prenat Diagn 1987; 7:407–411.

18. Gresser CD, Shime J, Rakowski H, et al: Fetal cardiac tumor: A prenatal echocardiographic marker for tuberous sclerosis. Am J Obstet Gynecol 1987; 156:689–690.

19. Brand JM, Friederg DZ: Spontaneous regression of a primary cardiac tumor presenting as fetal tachyarrythmias. J Perinatol 1992; 12:48–50.

20. Schaffer RM, Cabbad M, Minkoff H, et al: Sonographic diagnosis of fetal cardiac rhabdomyoma. J Ultrasound Med 1986; 5:531–533.

21. Murphy MC, Sweeney MS, Putnam JB Jr, et al: Surgical treatment of cardiac tumors: A 25 year experience. Ann Thorac Surg 1990; 49:612–615.

22. Farooki ZQ, Ross RD, Paridon SM, et al: Spontaneous regression of cardiac rhabdomyoma. Am J Cardiol 1991; 67:897–899.

23. Van der Hauwaert LF: Cardiac tumors in infancy and childhood. Br Heart J 1971; 33:125–132.

24. Allen JD, Blieden L, Stone FM, et al: Echocardiographic demonstration of a right

ventricular tumor in a neonate. J Pediatr 1974; 84:854–855.

25. Yamashita H, Nagaoka H, Matsushia R, et al: Cardiac rhabdomyoma: A clinicopathologic and electron microscopic study. Am J Cardiol 1976; 38:241–250.

26. Shaher RM, Mintzer J, Farina M, et al: Clinical presentation of rhabdomyoma of the heart in infancy and childhood. Am J Cardiol 1972; 30:95–103.

27. Corno A, de Simone G, Catena G, et al: Cardiac rhabdomyoma: Surgical treatment in the neonate. J Thorac Cardiovasc Surg 1984; 87:725–731.

28. Romero R, Pilu G, Jeanty P, et al: The heart. In: Romero R, Pilu G, Jeanty P, et al (eds): Prenatal Diagnosis of Congenital Anomalies. Norwalk, CT, Appleton & Lange, 1988, pp 125–194.

29. Marx GR: Cardiac tumors. In: Emmanouilides GC, Riemenschneider TA, Allen HD, et al (eds): Moss and Adams' Heart Disease in Infants, Children, and Adolescents: Including the Fetus and Young Adult, 5th ed, vol 2. Baltimore, Williams & Wilkins, 1995, pp 1773–1786.

30. Smythe JF, Dyck JD, Smallhorn JF, et al: Natural history of cardiac rhabdomyoma in infancy and childhood. Am J Cardiol 1990; 66:1247–1249.

31. Foster ED, Spooner EW, Farina MA, et al: Cardiac rhabdomyoma in the neonate: Surgical management. Ann Thorac Surg 1984; 37:249–253.

32. Arciniegas E, Hakimi M, Farooki ZQ, et al: Primary cardiac tumors in children. Surgery 1980; 79:582–591.

33. Fischer DR, Beerman LB, Park SC, et al: Diagnosis of intracardiac rhabdomyoma by two dimensional echocardiography. Am J Cardiol 1984; 53:978–997.

34. Smythe J, Dyck J, Freedom RM, et al: Rhabdomyoma in childhood. Am J Cardiol 1990; 66:1247–1249.

35. Simopoulos AP, Breslow A: Tuberous sclerosis in the newborn. Arch Pediatr Adolesc Med 1983; 3:313–316.

36. Yamashita H, Nagaoka H, Matsushia R, et al: Cardiac rhabdomyoma associated with tuberous sclerosis: An autopsy case of newborn infant died of cardiac failure. Acta Pathol Jpn 1987; 37:645–653.

37. Hall RA, Kron IL: Cardiac tumors. In: Mavroudis C, Backer CL (eds): Pediatric Cardiac Surgery. St Louis, Mosby–Year Book, 1994, pp 539–549.

38. Lintermans JP, Schoevaertds JC, Fiasse L, et al: Intrapericardial teratoma: A curable cause of cardiac tamponade in infancy. Clin Pediatr 1973; 12:316–318.

39. Arciniegas E, Hakimi M, Farooki ZQ: Intrapericardial teratoma in infancy. J Thorac Cardiovasc Surg 1980; 79:306–311.

40. Legnami FA, Corwin RD: Intrapericardial teratoma: A report of a case. Am Heart J 1963; 65:674–677.

41. Reynolds JL, Donahue JK, Pearce CW: Intrapericardial teratoma: A cause of acute pericardial effusion in infancy. Pediatrics 1969; 43:71–78.

42. MacDonald S, Fay JE, Lynn RB: Intrapericardial teratoma: A continuing challenge. Can J Surg 1983; 26:81–82.

43. Farooki ZQ, Arciniegas E, Hakimi M, et al: Real-time echocardiographic features of intrapericardial teratoma. J Clin Ultrasound 1982; 10:125–128.

44. De Getter B, Kretz JF, Nisand I, et al: Intrapericardial teratoma in a newborn infant: Use of fetal echocardiography. Ann Thorac Surg 1983; 35:664–666.

45. Agozzino L, Vosa C, Arciprete P, et al: Intrapericardial teratoma in the newborn: Review of literature and report of successful surgery in infant with intrapericardial teratoma. Int J Cardiol 1984; 5:21–28.

46. Cyr DR, Guntheroth WG, Nyberg DA, et al: Prenatal diagnosis of an intrapericardial teratoma: A cause for nonimmune hydrops. J Ultrasound Med 1988; 7:87–90.

47. White JJ, Kaback MM, Haller JA Jr: Diagnosis and excision of an intrapericardial teratoma in an infant. J Thorac Cardiovasc Surg 1968; 55:704–710.

48. Weber HS, Kleinman CS, Hellenbrand WE, et al: Development of a benign intrapericardial tumor between 20 and 40 weeks of gestation. Pediatr Cardiol 1988; 9:153–156.

49. Banfield F, Dick M II, Behrendt DM, et al: Intrapericardial teratoma: A new and treatable cause of hydrops fetalis. Arch Pediatr Adolesc Med 1980; 134:1174–1175.

50. Marsten JL, Cooper AG, Ankeney JL: Acute cardiac tamponade due to perforation of a benign mediastinal teratoma into the pericardial sac: Review of cardiovascular manifestations of mediastinal teratomas. J Thorac Cardiovasc Surg 1966; 51:700–707.

51. Kim TH, Kim YM, Han MY, et al: Perinatal sonographic diagnosis of cardiac fibroma with MR imaging correlation. AJR Am J Roentgenol 2002; 178:727–729.

52. Gonzalez-Crussi F, Eberts TJ, Mirkin DL: Congenital fibrous hamartoma of the heart. Arch Pathol Lab Med 1978; 102:491–493.

53. Tahernia AC, Bricker JY, Ott DA, et al: Intracardiac fibroma in an asymptomatic infant. Clin Cardiol 1990; 13:506–512.

54. Marin-Garcia J, Fitch CW, Shenefelt RE: Primary right ventricular tumor (fibroma) simulating cyanotic heart disease in a newborn. J Am Coll Cardiol 1984; 3:868–871.

55. Feldman PS, Meyer MW: Fibroelastic hamartoma (fibroma) of the heart. Cancer 1976; 38:314–323.

56. Kutayli F, Malouf J, Slim M, et al: Cardiac fibroma with tumor involvement of the mitral valve: Diagnosis by cross-sectional echocardiography. Eur Heart J 1988; 9:563–566.

57. Brown IW, McGoldrick JP, Robles A, et al: Left ventricular fibroma: Echocardiographic diagnosis and successful surgical excision in three cases. J Cardiovasc Surg 1990; 31:536–540.

58. Filiatrault M, Beland MJ, Neilson KA, et al: Cardiac fibroma presenting with clinically significant arrhythmias in infancy. Pediatr Cardiol 1991; 12:118–120.

59. Freedom RM, Benson LN: Cardiac Neoplasms. In: Freedom RM, Benson LN, Smallhorn JF (eds): Neonatal Heart Disease. London, Springer-Verlag, 1992, pp 723–729.

60. Schwartz J, Saldivar V, Fermin T, et al: Interventricular fibroma and cystic renal dysplasia in a newborn. Pediatr Pathol 1984; 2:187–195.

61. Fernando SSE: Cardiac fibroma (fibrous hamartoma) of infancy: Two case reports. Pathology 1979; 11:111–117.

62. Abend M, Tirosh E, Grishkan A, et al: Congenital cardiac fibroma: An unusual presentation. Eur J Pediatr 1982; 139:207–209.

63. Folger GM Jr, Peters HJ: Nodular fibroelastosis (fibroelastic hamartoma): A tumorous malformation of the heart. Am J Cardiol 1968; 21:420–427.

64. Takahashi K, Imamura Y, Ochi T, et al: Echocardiographic demonstration of an asymptomatic patient with left ventricular fibroma. Am J Cardiol 1984; 53:981–982.

65. Breglia RA: Primary tumors of the heart. Congress Cardiol 2001; 49:1–20.

66. Laga S, Gewilling MH, Van Schoubroeck D: Imminent fetal cardiac tamponade by right atrial hemangioma. Pediatr Cardiol 2006; 27:633–635.

67. Schratz LM, Martin GR: Fetal cardiac tumors. In: Yagel S, Silverman NH, Gembruch U (eds): Fetal Cardiology. London, Taylor-Francis, 2003, pp 313–320.

68. Prichard RW: Tumors of the heart: Review of the subject and report of 150 cases. Arch Pathol 1951; 51:98–128.

69. Kober G, Magedanz A, Mohrs O, et al: Non-invasive diagnosis of a pedunculated left

ventricular hemangioma. Clin Res Cardiol 2007; 96:227–231.

70. Tongsong T, Sirichotiyakul S, Sittiwangkul R, et al: Prenatal sonographic diagnosis of a cardiac hemangioma with postnatal spontaneous regression. Ultrasound Obstet Gynecol 2004; 24:207–209.

71. Talley JD, Wenger NK: Atrial myxoma: Overview, recognition, and management. Compr Ther 1987; 13:12–18.

72. Zitnik RS, Giuliani ER: Clinical recognition of atrial myxoma. Am Heart J 1970; 80:689–700.

73. Dianzumba SS, Char G: Large calcified right atrial myxoma in a newborn: Rare cause of neonatal death. Br Heart J 1982; 48:177–179.

74. Hals J, Ek J, Sandnes K: Cardiac myxoma as the cause of death in an infant. Acta Paediatr Scand 1990; 79:999–1000.

75. Sanyal SK, de Leuchtenberg N, Rojas RH, et al: Right atrial myxoma in infancy and childhood. Am J Cardiol 1967; 20:263–269.

76. Baslsara RK, Pelias AJ: Myxoma of right ventricle presenting as pulmonic stenosis in a neonate. Chest 1983; 83:145–146.

77. Butto F, Shachar GB, Najmabadi H, et al: Massive cardiac tumor presenting as severe cyanosis in a newborn [letter]. Pediatr Cardiol 1994; 15:103–105.

78. Osano M, Yashiro K, Oikawa T, et al: Intramural fibroma of the heart: A case report. Pediatrics 1969; 43:605–608.

79. Crawford FA Jr, Selby JH Jr, Watson D, et al: Unusual aspects of atrial myxoma. Ann Surg 1978; 188:240–244.

80. Johnson ML, Sieker HO, Behar VS, et al: Echocardiographic diagnosis of a left atrial myxoma found attached to the free left atrial wall. J Clin Ultrasound 1973; 1:75–81.

81. Bhat PS, Subramanyan R, Venkitachalam CG, et al: Biatrial myxomas—A case report. Indian Heart J 1984; 36:75–77.

82. Oetgen WJ, Umfrid RP III, Hamilton KM, et al: Two-dimensional echocardiography in the diagnosis of left atrial myxoma in a child. South Med J 1982; 75:1125–1127.

83. Abramowitz R, Majdan JF, Plzak LF, et al: Two-dimensional echocardiographic diagnosis of separate myxomas of both the left atrium and left ventricle. Am J Cardiol 1984; 53:379–380.

84. Roudaut R, Pouget P, Videau P, et al: Right atrial myxoma in an asymptomatic child: Echocardiographic diagnosis. Eur Heart J 1980; 1:453–459.

85. Liu HY, Panidis I, Soffer J, et al: Echocardiographic diagnosis of intracardiac myxomas: Present status. Chest 1983; 84:62–67.

86. Salcedo EE, Adams KV, Lever HM, et al: Echocardiographic findings in 25 patients with left atrial myxoma. J Am Coll Cardiol 1983; 1:1162–1166.

87. Gray IR, Williams WG: Recurring cardiac myxoma. Br Heart J 1985; 53:645–649.

88. Read RC, White HJ, Murphy ML, et al: The malignant potentiality of left atrial myxoma. J Thorac Cardiovasc Surg 1974; 68:857–868.

89. Robertson R: Primary cardiac tumours: Surgical treatment. Am J Surg 1957; 94:183–193.

90. Steinke WE, Perry LW, Gold HR, et al: Left atrial myxoma in a child. Pediatrics 1972; 49:580–589.

91. Goodwin JF, Lond MD: Diagnosis of left atrial myxoma. Lancet 1963; 1:464–468.

92. Marijon E, Ou P, Fermont L, et al: Diagnosis and outcome in congenital ventricular diverticulum and aneurysm. J Thorac Cardiovasc Surg 2006; 131:433–437.

93. Sharma JR, Oforl-Amanfo G, Marboe D, et al: Congenital left ventricular aneurysm with pericardial effusion: Surgical management and follow-up. Pediatr Cardiol 2002; 23:458–461.

94. Prefumo F, Bhide A, Thilaganathan B, et al: Fetal congenital cardiac diverticulum with pericardial effusion: Two cases with different presentations in the first trimester of pregnancy. Obstet Gynecol 2005; 25:405–408.

95. Del Rio M, Martinez JM, Bennasar M, et al: Prenatal diagnosis of a right ventricular diverticulum complicated by pericardial effusion in the first trimester. Ultrasound Obstet Gynecol 2005; 25:409–411.

96. McAuliffe FM, Hornberger LK, Johnson J, et al: Cardiac diverticulum with pericardial effusion: Report of two new cases treated by in-utero pericardiocentesis and a review of the literature. Ultrasound Obstet Gynecol 2005; 25:401–404.

97. Ramirez JA, Fernandez-Castro C, Otero Chouza M, et al: Persistent and redundant eustachian valve simulating atrial tumor: Prenatal diagnosis. Ultrasound Obstet Gynecol 2007; 29:704–707.

98. Ghi T, Perolo A, Prandstraller D, et al: Antenatal sonography of eustachian valve aneurysm. Ultrasound Obstet Gynecol 2002; 20:206–208.

99. Arda S, Saym NC, Varol FG, et al: Isolated fetal intracardiac hyperechogenic focus associated with neonatal outcome and triple test results. Arch Gynecol Obstet. Printed on-line March 13, 2007.

100. Bethune M: Management options for echogenic intracardiac focus and choroids plexus cysts. Austral Radiol 2007; 51:324–329.

101. Wax JR, Cartin A, Pinette MG, et al: Sonographic grading of fetal intracardiac echogenic foci in a

population at low risk of aneuploidy. J Clin Ultrasound 2002; 31:31–38.

102. Wax JR, Royer D, Mather J, et al: A preliminary study of sonographic grading of fetal intracardiac echogenic foci: Feasibility, reliability and association with aneuploidy. Ultrasound Obstet Gynecol 2000; 16:123–127.

103. Gazit AZ, Singh GK, Shumway J, et al: Fetal cardiac rhabdomyoma: A sheep or a wolf? J Matern Fetal Neonat Med 2007; 20:343–348.

104. Smith-Bindman R, Hosmer W, Feldstein VA, et al: Second trimester ultrasound to detect fetuses with Down Syndrome. JAMA 2001; 285:1044–1055.

105. Sharratt GP, Lacson AG, Cornel G, et al: Echocardiography of intracardiac filling defects in infants and children. Pediatr Cardiol 1986; 7:189–194.

106. Taber RE, Lam CR: Diagnosis and surgical treatment of intracardiac myxoma and rhabdomyoma. J Thorac Cardiovasc Surg 1960; 40:337–354.

107. Kirklin JW, Baratt-Boyes BG: Cardiac Surgery. New York, Churchill Livingstone, 1993, pp 1627–1653.

108. Rees AH, Elbl FE, Minhas KV, et al: Echocardiographic evidence of left ventricular tumor in a neonate. Chest 1978; 73:433–435.

109. Howanitz EP, Teske DW, Qualman SJ, et al: Pedunculated left ventricular rhabdomyoma. Ann Thorac Surg 1986; 41:443–444.

110. Bass JL, Breningstall GN, Swaiman KF: Echocardiographic incidence of cardiac rhabdomyoma in tuberous sclerosis. Am J Cardiol 1985; 55:1379–1382.

111. Chao AS, Chao A, Wang TH, et al: Outcome of antenatally diagnosed cardiac rhabdomyoma: Case series and a meta-analysis. Ultrasound Obstet Gynecol 2008; 3:289–295.

112. Duncan WJ: Left ventricular rhabdomyoma. Pediatr Cardiol 1983; 4:170–171.

113. Farooki ZQ, Henry JG, Arciniegas E, et al: Ultrasonic pattern of ventricular rhabdomyoma in two infants. Am J Cardiol 1974; 34:842–844.

114. Fenoglio JJ, McAllister HA, Ferrans VJ: Cardiac rhabdomyoma: A clinicopathologic and electron microscopic study. Am J Cardiol 1976; 38:241–251.

115. Golding R, Reed G: Rhabdomyoma of the heart. N Engl J Med 1967; 276:957–960.

116. Kuehl KS, Perry LW, Chandra R, et al: Left ventricular rhabdomyoma: a rare cause of subaortic stenosis in the newborn infant. Pediatrics 1970; 46:464–468.

117. Lababidi Z, Wu JR, Walls J, et al: Neonatal cyanosis caused by cardiac rhabdomyomas. Am Heart J 1984; 108:624–627.

118. Mair DD, Titus JL, Davis GD, et al: Cardiac rhabdomyoma simulating mitral atresia. Chest 1977; 71:102–105.

119. Shrivastava S, Jack JJ, White RS, et al: Diffuse rhabdomyomatosis of the heart. Arch Pathol Lab Med 1977; 101:78–80.

120. Mahoney L, Schieken RM, Doty D: Cardiac rhabdomyoma simulating pulmonic stenosis. Cathet Cardiovasc Diagn 1979; 5:385–388.

121. Spooner EW, Farina MA, Shaher RM, et al: Left ventricular rhabdomyoma causing subaortic stenosis—The two-dimensional echocardiographic appearance. Pediatr Cardiol 1982; 2:67–71.

122. Gomez MR: Varieties of expression of tuberous sclerosis. Neurofibromatosis 1988; 1:330–338.

123. Wilding G, Green HL, Longo DL, et al: Tumors of the heart and pericardium. Cancer Treat Rev 1988; 15:165–181.

124. Arens R, Feingold M: Denouement and discussion. Arch Pediatr Adolesc Med 1988;142:1083–1084.

125. Fryer AE, Connor JM, Povey S, et al: Evidence that the gene for tuberous sclerosis is on chromosome 9. Lancet 1987; 1:659–662.

126. Williams R, Taylor D: Tuberous sclerosis. Surv Ophthalmol 1985; 30:143–154.

127. Seguin JR, Coulon PI, Perz M, et al: Echocardiographic diagnosis of an intrapericardial teratoma in infancy. Am Heart J 1987; 113:1239–1240.

128. Kagan KO, Schmidt M, Kuhn U, et al: Ventricular outflow obstruction, valve aplasia, bradyarrhythmia, pulmonary hypoplasia and non-immune fetal hydrops because of a large rhabdomyoma in a case of unknown tuberous sclerosis: A prenatal diagnosed cardiac rhabdomyoma with multiple symptoms. Br J Obstet Gynaecol 2004; 111:1478–1480.

129. Hou CF, Chao A, Wang CJ, et al: Atrial hemangioma: a rare cause of hydrops fetalis and intrauterine fetal death. Eur J Obstet Gynecol Reprod Biol 2007; 130:271–272.

130. Chandraratna PAN, San Pedro S, Elkins RC, et al: Echocardiographic, angiocardiographic, and surgical correlations in right ventricular myxoma simulating valvular pulmonic stenosis. Circulation 1977; 55:619–622.

131. Scully RE, Mark EF, McNeely BU: Case records of the Massachusetts General Hospital: Weekly clinicopathological exercises. N Engl J Med 1983; 308:206–214.

132. Alkalay AL, Ferry DA, Lin B, et al: Spontaneous regression of cardiac rhabdomyoma in tuberous sclerosis. Clin Pediatr 1987; 26:532–535.

133. Matsuoka Y, Nakati T, Kawaguchi K, et al: Disappearance of a cardiac rhabdomyoma

complicating congenital mitral regurgitation as observed by serial two-dimensional echocardiography. Pediatr Cardiol 1990; 11:98–101.

134. Smith HC, Watson GH, Patel RG, et al: Cardiac rhabdomyomata in tuberous sclerosis: Their course and diagnostic value. Arch Dis Child 1989; 64:196–200.

135. Khattar H, Goerin R, Fouron JD, et al: Heart tumors in children: Report of three cases with favorable spontaneous courses. Arch Mal Coeur 1975; 68:419–429.

136. Stijns M, Lintermans J, Tremouroux M, et al: Spontaneous disappearance of aortic subvalvular obstruction in young infants with tuberous sclerosis. Pediatr Cardiol 1982; 3:88–89.

137. Jacobs JP, Konstantakos AK, Holland FW: Surgical treatment for cardiac rhabdomyomas in children. Ann Thorac Surg 1994; 58:1552–1555.

138. Giamberti A, Giannico S, Squiteri C, et al: Neonatal pulmonary autograft implantation for cardiac tumor involving aortic valve. Ann Thorac Surg 1995; 59:1219–1221.

139. Gutierrez de Loma J, Villagra F, Perez de Leon J, et al: Rhabdomyoma of the heart: Surgical treatment. J Cardiovasc Surg 1982; 23:149–154.

140. Demkow M, Sorenson K, Whitehead BF: Heart transplantation in an infant with rhabdomyoma. Pediatr Cardiol 1995; 16:204–206.

141. Altunbasak S, Demirtas M, Tunali N, et al: Primary rhabdomyosarcoma of the heart presenting with increased intracranial pressure. Pediatr Cardiol 1996; 17:260–264.

142. Smith CR: Septal superior exposure of the mitral valve: The transplant approach. J Thorac Cardiovasc Surg 1992; 103:623–628.

143. Markel ML, Armstrong WF, Waller BF, et al: Left atrial myxoma with multicentric recurrence and evidence of metastases. Am Heart J 1986; 111:409–413.

144. Leonhardt ETG, Kullenberg KPG: Bilateral atrial myxomas with multiple arterial aneurysms— syndrome mimicking polyarteritis nodosa. Am J Med 1977; 62:792–794.

145. Attum AA, Johnson GS, Masri Z, et al: Malignant clinical behavior of cardiac myxomas and "myxoid imitators." Ann Thorac Surg 1987; 44:217–222.

146. New PFJ, Price DL, Carter B: Cerebral angiography in cardiac myxoma: Correlation of angiographic and histopathologic findings. Radiology 1970; 96:335–345.

147. St. John Sutton MG, Mercier LA, Giuliani ER, et al: Atrial myxomas: A review of clinical experience in 40 patients. Mayo Clin Proc 1980; 55:371–376.

148. Farooki ZQ, Hakimi M, Arciniegas E, et al: Echocardiographic features in a case of intrapericardial teratoma. J Clin Ultrasound 1978; 6:108–110.

149. Deenadayalu RP, Tuuri D, Dewall RA, et al: Intrapericardial teratoma and bronchogenic cyst. J Thorac Cardiovasc Surg 1974; 67:945–952.

150. Vergnon JM, Vincent M, Perinetti M, et al: Chemotherapy of metastatic primary cardiac sarcomas. Am Heart J 1985; 110:682–684.

151. Brachlow A, Sable C, Smith S, et al: Fetal diagnosis and postnatal follow-up of an asymptomatic congenital left ventricular diverticulum. Pediatr Cardiol 2002; 23:658–660.

152. Goldman S, Lortscher R, Pappas G: Surgical treatment for rhabdomyoma of the right atrium causing arrhythmias. J Thorac Cardiovascular Surg 1985; 89:802–804.

153. Bertolini P, Meisner H, Pack SU, et al: Special considerations on primary cardiac tumors in infancy and childhood. Thorac Cardiovasc Surg 1990; 38(2 Suppl):164–167.

154. Kedder L: Congenital glycogenic tumors of the heart. Arch Pathol 1950; 49:55–62.

155. Shepherd CW, Gomez MR, Lie JT, et al: Causes of death in patients with tuberous sclerosis. Mayo Clin Proc 1991; 66:792–796.

156. Fyler DC: Cardiac tumors. In: Fyler DC (ed) Nadas' Pediatric Cardiology. Philadelphia, Hanley and Belfus, 1992, pp 727–730.

157. Fischer DR, Beerman LB, Park SC, et al: Diagnosis of intracardiac rhabdomyoma by two-dimensional echocardiography. Am J Cardiol 1984; 53:978–979.

158. Russell GA, Dhasmana JP, Berry PJ, et al: Coexistent cardiac tumours and malformations of the heart. Int J Cardiol 1989; 22:89–98.

159. Geva T, Santini F, Pear W, et al: Cardiac rhabdomyoma: Rare cause of fetal death. Chest 1991; 99:139–142.

160. Soltan MH, Keohane C: Hydrops fetalis due to congenital cardiac rhabdomyoma. Br J Obstet Gynaecol 1981; 88:771–773.

161. Kieny R, de Geeter B, Kretz JG, et al: Cardiac tumors in infancy: Recent aspects. Thorac Cardiovasc Surg 1983; 31:169–171.

CHAPTER 19

Cardiosplenic Syndromes

Teresa M. Bieker

Definition

Cardiosplenic syndromes are disorders of lateralization characterized by the symmetrical development of normally asymmetrical organs or organ systems. A constellation of cardiac, vascular, and visceral abnormalities make up these syndromes. Situs ambiguous, heterotaxy syndrome, right and left isomerism, and situs ambiguous are synonyms for these defects.

Asplenia and *polysplenia* are the two most common forms of cardiosplenic syndromes. These two subtypes are usually considered separate entities; however, there is considerable overlap in the associated abdominal and complex cardiac malformations.

Visceral heterotaxy represents approximately 30% of cardiac malpositions in infants and 45% of the deaths associated with these conditions.[1]

Asplenia is characterized by bilateral right sidedness or right atrial isomerism. Typical features of this syndrome include bilateral right atrial appendages, bilateral morphological right lungs (trilobed), an absent spleen, a midline liver, and multiple cardiac anomalies.[2-6] The stomach, liver, and gallbladder are likely to be in a situs ambiguous or inversus position.[7] A malpositioned inferior vena cava, which may be anterior or juxtaposed to the aorta, and abnormal pulmonary venous return are frequently seen.[2,8,9]

The incidence of cardiac abnormalities associated with asplenia is high. Atrioventricular septal defects are reported in approximately 85% to 95% of cases.[10-12] Common atrium (90%), transposition of the great arteries (80%), pulmonary atresia or stenosis (80%), double-outlet right ventricle (80%), and total anomalous pulmonary venous return (70%) are also commonly associated with asplenia (Table 19–1).[7,10,12]

Asplenia was first described by Ivemark in 1955.[6,8] From a review of 69 cases, he postulated that because the atrioventricular canal and the conotruncus undergo division simultaneous with the development of the splenic primordia, a single embryological insult could adversely affect both cardiac and splenic development. Asplenia also bears the name Ivemark syndrome.[7]

Polysplenia is defined as bilateral left sidedness or left atrial isomerism. Bilateral morphological left (bilobed) lungs, abnormal visceral and venous anatomy, and cardiac abnormalities are all

TABLE 19–1 Incidence of Cardiovascular Abnormalities in Asplenia and Polysplenia Syndromes

	Asplenia	Polysplenia
Atrial septal defect	90%	80%
Atrioventricular septal defect	85%	40%
Azygous continuation of the inferior vena cava	Rare	70%
Bilateral superior vena cava	50%	40%
Dextrocardia	40%	40%
Double-outlet right ventricle	80%	40%
Left pulmonary isomerism	Rare	60%
Partial anomalous pulmonary venous connection	Rare	40%
Pulmonary stenosis, pulmonary atresia	80%	30%
Right pulmonary isomerism	70%	10%
Single ventricle	50%	10%
Subaortic stenosis	Rare	40%
Total anomalous pulmonary venous connection	70%	Rare
Transposition of the great arteries	80%	30%

Data from Gutgesell HP: Cardiac malposition and heterotaxy. In: Garson A, Bricker JT, McNamara DG (eds): The Science and Practice of Pediatric Cardiology, vol 2. Philadelphia, Lea & Febiger, 1990, p 1292.

associated with polysplenia. The visceral abnormalities, as the name polysplenia would imply, include multiple spleens.

In the majority of cases, the stomach, liver, and gallbladder are situs ambiguous; however, situs inversus and solitus are also possible.[7] The gallbladder is frequently absent, and dextrocardia or mesocardia is found in 55% of patients.[13] Additionally, absence of the intrahepatic inferior vena cava with collateral drainage through the azygous or hemiazygous vein has been reported in 65% to 94% of patients with polysplenia.[14–16]

Cardiac defects occur in 90% to 95% of cases of polysplenia. Although they are typically less severe than those found in asplenia (see Table 19–1), they are still the leading cause of death associated with this syndrome.[17–19]

A common atrium occurs in approximately 80% of cases. Left-sided cardiac obstruction appears to occur more frequently in polysplenia than in asplenia. However, other cardiac anomalies that are prevalent in asplenia (such as total anomalous pulmonary venous connection) are rarely associated with polysplenia. Complete heart block has been reported in 50% of fetuses with the polysplenia syndrome.[13] Other anomalies include atrioventricular septal defects (60%–70%) and transposition of the great arteries (20%).[12]

Polysplenia and asplenia are two separate, distinct entities. The majority of cases of left isomerism are discovered during fetal life, whereas right isomerism is typically diagnosed postnatally.[7]

Embryology

Cardiosplenic syndromes are not a specific disease but a spectrum of abnormalities that involve the abdominal viscera and the cardiovascular system. From an embryological standpoint, polysplenia and asplenia syndromes are thought to be the result of a midline developmental field defect.[2,20] Opitz and Gilbert[21] defined developmental fields as units of the embryo in which the development of complex structures are determined and controlled in a spatially coordinated, temporally synchronous, and epimorphically hierarchical manner. This means that an insult to this delicate space-time balance may give rise to complex malformations, including errors in symmetry or laterality. An embryogenic insult occurring between the twenty-eighth and thirty-fifth days of gestation has been postulated to result in the spectrum of developmental abnormalities that is considered asplenia or polysplenia.[22–24]

The specific embryology of many of the associated cardiac abnormalities is discussed in the chapters dealing with each malformation. Generally, it appears that the sequence of cardiac development is arrested in patients with cardiosplenic syndromes during the fifth week of gestation.[23–25]

In normal development, growth of the endocardial cushions and septation of the conotruncus occur at this time. Additionally, during this embryological period lobation of the lungs and rotation of the gut begin. The connection between the atria and the pulmonary venous plexus is established by 30 to 32 days of gestation.[10,22]

The spleen arises from the left side of the dorsal mesogastrium at about day 32 of gestation. As stated previously, the result of this early insult is disruption of the normal asymmetrical development of many of these organs.

It should be borne in mind that, although the syndrome of right atrial isomerism is usually associated with asplenia, this is not invariable, and a normal spleen has been reported in some cases.[26] Conversely, patients with polysplenia syndrome and left atrial isomerism have been found to have a solitary spleen.

There is clearly considerable overlap in the cardiac abnormalities associated with these two syndromes, but the most specific marker of the polysplenia syndrome appears to be azygos continuation of the inferior vena cava.[2,17,19,27–38] This finding has rarely been reported in cases of asplenia.

Abnormalities of systemic and pulmonary venous connections occur in both syndromes. Additionally, hearts with right atrial isomerism exhibit a higher incidence of abnormal ventriculoarterial connections, with double-outlet right ventricle and transposition of the great arteries occurring in more than 75% of cases.[26] Conversely, hearts with left atrial isomerism demonstrate a normal ventriculoarterial connection in approximately 70% of reported cases.[17]

Most cases of polysplenia and asplenia syndromes are sporadic. However, familial occurrence of these syndromes has been described.[39–42] The coexistence of asplenia and polysplenia in sibships has also been reported.[40,42,43] The occurrence of these sibships, together with the findings of consanguinity in some sporadic cases, suggests autosomal recessive inheritance with reduced penetrance.[44–46]

Occurrence Rate

The occurrence rate for heterotaxy syndromes is 1 in 10,000 live births or in 0.8% of all patients with congenital heart disease.[47,48]

A predominance of left isomerism over right isomerism in utero has been well documented.[7,16,49]

In contrast, postnatally right atrial isomerism appears more common than left atrial isomerism.[2,11,50–52]

It has been postulated that, although the severity and complexity of congenital heart disease is greater in right atrial isomerism, the increased incidence of complete heart block in conjunction with atrioventricular valve insufficiency associated with left atrial isomerism often leads to congestive heart failure, hydrops fetalis, and death in utero.[49]

The occurrence rate in siblings of patients with asplenia is reported to be approximately 5%.[40,44,52–56] A tendency for asplenia syndrome to occur more frequently in males and for polysplenia syndrome to occur more often in females has been suggested.[2,26] Also, right atrial isomerism tends to be more common then left isomerism in the Asian population.[7,48]

Sonographic Criteria

The in utero sonographic findings associated with asplenia and polysplenia are multiple. Right or left atrial isomerism is a difficult diagnosis to make in the fetus.

The most consistent indicators of polysplenia appear to be an interrupted inferior vena cava with a large azygous vein continuation into the superior vena cava and heart block in the presence of structural heart disease. Yildirim et al[16] observed these findings in 94% of their cases.

Sheley et al[13] reviewed the prenatal sonographic findings in eight fetuses with polysplenia. Interruption of the inferior vena cava with azygous continuation was seen in all eight patients. The authors diagnosed this finding by identifying what they termed the double-vessel sign: two vessels of similar size in a paraspinous location posterior to the heart. Compared with the normal relationship, which shows only the aorta posterior to the heart (Fig. 19–1), interruption of the inferior vena cava results in collateral flow through the azygous vein, which becomes enlarged and readily visible (Fig. 19–2). Therefore two vessels are seen at the level of the heart in a paraspinous location (Fig. 19–3). The azygous veins in their study ranged in diameter from 6 to 12 mm. They did report one false-positive diagnosis of inferior vena cava interruption with azygous continuation in a fetus with asplenia. At autopsy, a large left-sided superior vena cava in this fetus as the likely explanation for the sonographic finding.

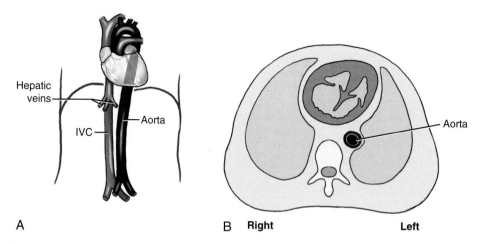

Figure 19–1   Diagram of a normal inferior vena cava. **A,** Frontal view showing normal drainage of the inferior vena cava *(IVC)* into the right atrium. **B,** Transverse view shows only a single vessel posterior to the heart, representing the aorta.

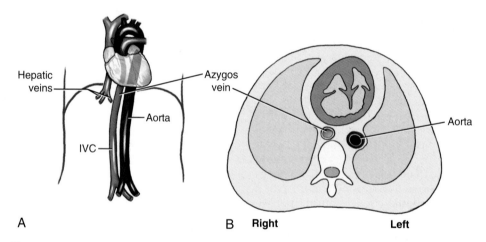

Figure 19–2   Diagram of an interrupted inferior vena cava *(IVC)* with azygous continuation. **A,** Frontal view shows interruption of the inferior vena cava. Collateral flow through the azygous vein drains into the superior vena cava. **B,** Transverse view shows both the aorta and the dilated azygous vein posterior to the heart.

Azygous continuation of an interrupted inferior vena cava may also be visualized in a sagittal view of the fetus. In this projection it will appear as a long vessel running parallel with the aorta, extending to the superior vena cava (Fig. 19–4).

Because the cardiosplenic syndromes are basically abnormalities of situs, the first step when beginning a fetal echocardiographic evaluation is to confirm the location of the heart within the chest. Both dextrocardia and mesocardia have been reported (Figs. 19–5 and 19–6).[57]

Evaluation for right or left atrial isomerism should also be attempted. This is a difficult diagnosis to make in utero. The presence of normal or abnormal venous inflow into the atria may provide insight.

Color Doppler imaging may be useful in trying to identify the pulmonary veins entering the left atrium, thus excluding total anomalous pulmonary venous connection (Fig. 19–7). The pulmonary veins are always totally anomalously connected whenever atrial isomerism is present (Fig. 19–8).[58]

Colloridi et al[59] described right atrial morphological characteristics as "pyramidal" and left atrial morphological characteristics as "fingerlike" (Fig. 19–9). They reported three cases of right atrial isomerism diagnosed in utero at 23, 28, and 34 weeks' gestation, respectively, by identifying two atria in a four-chamber view, both having this

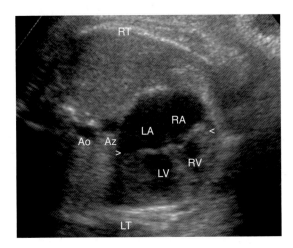

Figure 19–3 Apical four-chamber view in a fetus with an interrupted inferior vena cava with azygous continuation and an atrioventricular septal defect *(arrowheads)*. Both the aorta *(Ao)* and the dilated azygous vein *(Az)* can be seen posterior to the heart. *LA,* Left atrium; *LT,* left chest; *LV,* left ventricle; *RA,* right atrium; *RT,* right chest; *RV,* right ventricle.

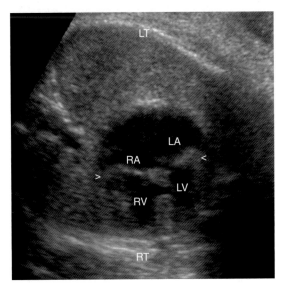

Figure 19–5 Dextrocardia, with the fetal cardiac apex pointing to the right side of the fetal chest in a fetus with polysplenia. An complete atrioventricular septal defect with a single atrioventricular valve *(arrowheads)* is also appreciated. *LA,* Left atrium; *LT,* left chest; *LV,* left ventricle; *RA,* right atrium; *RT,* right chest; *RV,* right ventricle.

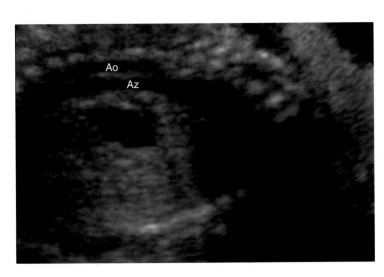

Figure 19–4 Sagittal image of the fetal abdomen and chest showing the dilated azygous vein *(Az)* running parallel to the aorta *(Ao)* and extending above the heart to join the superior vena cava.

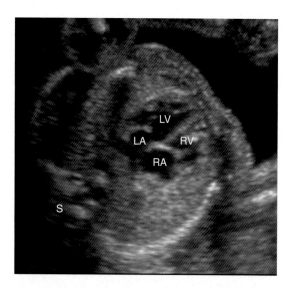

Figure 19–6   Four-chamber view in a fetus with mesocardia, showing the cardiac apex pointing directly midline. *LA,* Left atrium; *LV,* left ventricle; *RA,* right atrium; *RV,* right ventricle; *S,* spine.

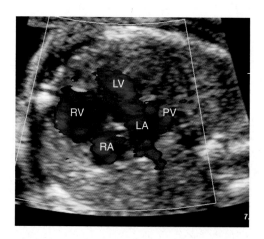

Figure 19–7   Four-chamber view in a normal fetus using color Doppler imaging to show normal blood flow of the two superior pulmonary veins *(PV)* entering the left atrium *(LA). LV,* Left ventricle; *RA,* right atrium; *RV,* right ventricle.

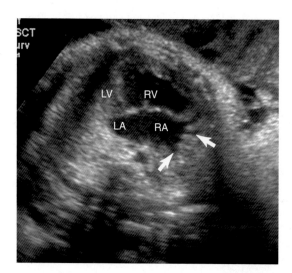

Figure 19–8   Apical four-chamber view in a fetus with total anomalous pulmonary venous return, showing the pulmonary veins *(arrows)* abnormally entering the right atrium *(RA). LA,* Left atrium; *LV,* left ventricle; *RV,* right ventricle.

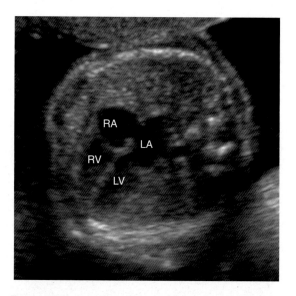

Figure 19–9   Normal apical four-chamber view showing the morphological "fingerlike" characteristic of the left atrium *(LA)* and the more "pyramidal" shape of the right atrium *(RA). LV,* Left ventricle; *RV,* right ventricle.

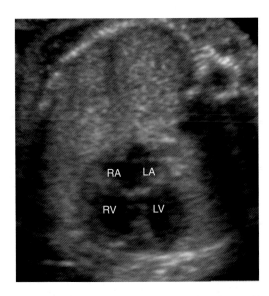

Figure 19–10 Apical four-chamber view in a fetus with an atrioventricular septal defect characterized by a single multileaflet atrioventricular valve, an atrial septal defect, and a ventricular septal defect. *LA,* Left atrium; *LV,* left ventricle; *RA,* right atrium; *RV,* right ventricle.

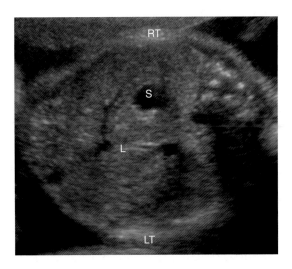

Figure 19–11 Transverse image of the fetal abdomen in the same fetus as Figure 19–10. Polysplenia is identified with the fetal stomach *(S)* on the morphological right side and the fetal liver *(L)* located midline. *LT,* Left chest; *RT,* right chest.

pyramidal shape. However, configuration of the atria can be variable. This makes diagnosis based on morphology alone difficult.

The right and left ventricles should be evaluated to confirm that they are morphologically correct and properly connected to their corresponding atria. Finally, the aorta and pulmonary artery should be identified to make sure that they are of normal caliber and properly related.

From a cardiac standpoint, the most likely in utero finding is an atrioventricular septal defect (Fig. 19–10). This is best appreciated from either an apical or subcostal four-chamber view. Most atrioventricular septal defects associated with these entities are complete, resulting in one multileaflet atrioventricular valve.[50]

If an atrioventricular defect is detected, a thorough search for other indicators of these syndromes should be instigated. Specifically, the fetal abdomen should be evaluated for visceral situs abnormalities such as a fetal stomach on the right side (Fig. 19–11).

The combination of atrioventricular septal defect with heart block is considered virtually pathognomonic for polysplenia syndrome.[13,18,60,61] In the absence of the cardiosplenic syndromes, prenatal diagnosis of an atrioventricular septal

defect should suggest the likelihood of Down syndrome or other chromosome abnormality. A common atria and single ventricle have also been reported with cardiosplenic syndromes. Color Doppler imaging in an apical or subcostal four-chamber view may help confirm these entities.

Several defects of the great vessels also occur with both asplenia and polysplenia. Double-outlet right ventricle and transposition of the great arteries are reported most often.[13] Pulmonary stenosis and pulmonary atresia are almost always present with asplenia. Subaortic stenosis occurs in polysplenia but is rare in asplenia. The potential for any of these entities necessitates assessment of the great vessels for size discrepancies and color or pulsed Doppler interrogation, or both, to document stenosis or occlusion.

Finally, evaluation of the inferior vena cava to detect interruption as described earlier, and evaluation of the superior vena cava to identify bilaterality, which is often associated, is warranted.[58]

Noncardiac abnormalities associated with the cardiosplenic syndromes, aside from situs abnormalities, may include duodenal atresia, esophageal abnormalities, malrotation of the bowel and mesentery, absence of the gallbladder, and biliary atresia.[8,13,58,62]

Sheley et al[13] reported absence of the gallbladder in 50% of their cases with polysplenia.[13]

Genitourinary, skeletal, and central nervous system abnormalities have also been reported.[17]

The absence of the spleen in the fetus with asplenia or the presence of multiple spleens in the fetus with polysplenia may help confirm the diagnosis of cardiosplenic syndrome. Although identification of the fetal spleen in normal fetuses has been described, an abnormal location may make identification more difficult.[62,63]

Finally, because the presence of heart block in the setting of congenital heart disease may cause congestive heart failure in the fetus, the presence or absence of hydrops fetalis or polyhydramnios should be documented.

Treatment

The presence and complexity of cardiac defects usually determines the treatment and outcome for infants born with polysplenia or asplenia. Confirmation of asplenia in the neonate often includes testing for the presence of inclusions in the erythrocytes—the Howell-Jolly bodies. Their presence may be suggestive of splenic hypofunction. Other methods of documenting asplenia include abdominal ultrasonography or computed tomography or magnetic resonance imaging of the abdomen.

Most patients with polysplenia have normal splenic function, although patients with tiny rudimentary nodules of splenic tissue may also have splenic hypofunction.

Most infants born with asplenia have pulmonary outflow tract obstruction and are therefore dependent on ductal flow to provide pulmonary perfusion.[11] This requires the emergent infusion of prostaglandin E_1 to maintain ductal patency. Infants with asplenia are also given prophylactic antibiotics because of an increased possibility of sepsis.[44,64]

Waldman et al[65] reported that asplenic children who survived the first month of life were at greater risk of dying from sepsis than from their heart disease.

From a surgical standpoint, the complexity of cardiac malformations associated with asplenia usually precludes a biventricular repair.[26] In the absence of a grossly incompetent common atrioventricular valve, the initial surgical management is to construct a systemic-to-pulmonary connection. If obstructive pulmonary venous drainage is present, it must also be repaired. All surgeries are considered palliative to relieve symptoms. Total correction is typically not attempted.[16]

Because of the propensity for obstructed pulmonary venous connections to occur in conjunction with an insufficient atrioventricular valve and small-caliber pulmonary arteries, initial medical and surgical mortality rates in the neonate are high, and even fewer infants become acceptable candidates for a Fontan procedure.[26]

Sadiq et al[66] reported 11 infants with right atrial isomerism between 1 and 14 days of life. Pulmonary outflow tract obstruction was present in all patients. Nine patients had anomalous pulmonary venous drainage, which was obstructive in seven patients (64%); four had supracardiac and three had infracardiac drainage. Ten (91%) patients had transposition of the great arteries, four (36%) with a double-outlet right ventricle. All 11 patients had a complete atrioventricular septal defect, and 7 (64%) had a common atrium.

Of the seven patients with obstructed pulmonary venous drainage, five died postoperatively. One patient survived the initial surgery and follow-up surgery 2 weeks later but died at the age of 2 years following a modified Fontan operation. The remaining patient survived the initial surgery as well as subsequent surgeries at 6 months and 1 year of age. Of the remaining four patients in their series, only two survived and are now 1.8 and 6.8 years past initial palliation.[66]

Neonates with polysplenia pose different risks. Many also have complex forms of atrioventricular septal defects but may also have a small left ventricle, subaortic stenosis, and pulmonary artery hypertension.

Surgical repair of the atrioventricular septal defect is usually attempted initially. The complex cardiac defects that often preclude successful surgical intervention in cases of asplenia, such as total anomalous pulmonary venous connection and pulmonary artery obstruction, are not as common in polysplenia. However, the association of polysplenia with other organ system anomalies, such as extrahepatic biliary atresia, may present special problems.

Peoples et al[17] reported 41 cases of polysplenia resulting in death. Ten of the deaths occurred during or immediately after cardiac operation.

The presence of complete heart block in infants with polysplenia or asplenia also poses a significant threat to survival. Implantation of a permanent pacemaker following structural repair may be necessary in these cases.[36]

Prognosis

Patients with asplenia have a poor prognosis, with 79% to 94% dying before 1 year of age.[2,10,52,67] Phoon and Neill[68] reported a median survival of 2.6 months. Deaths occurred earlier in females than in males and in blacks than in whites, although the differences were not statistically significant. When both total anomalous pulmonary venous connection and pulmonary atresia were present, survival decreased to 1 month.

An additional study by Sadiq et al[66] reported on the outcome of 20 consecutive children with asplenia who underwent cardiac surgery between 1987 and 1993. The overall survival rate was 45%, 18% in patients requiring surgery in the first month of life, and 78% in patients requiring surgery after the first month of life.

The 1-year survival rate (39%) for infants with polysplenia is slightly higher than for those with asplenia.[52] Peoples et al[17] reviewed 117 cases of death related to polysplenia. Approximately one third of the patients died before 1 month of age, and half died by 4 months of age. Only one fourth of patients remained alive by 5 years, and by mid adolescence only 10% of patients were alive. In addition, patients with complete atrio-ventricular canal and complete heart block carry an increased risk for fetal death.[7]

Differences in survival between patients with asplenia and polysplenia syndromes may be related to the types of cardiac lesions as well as the risk of infection associated with asplenia. Specifically, the greater mortality rate with total anomalous pulmonary venous connection and pulmonary atresia (associated with asplenia) may account for a substantial number of early deaths because these lesions are found less frequently in polysplenia.[2,68]

Unfortunately, despite recent surgical advancements, the prognosis for infants diagnosed with cardiosplenic syndrome remains poor, particularly when the cardiac abnormalities cause symptoms in early infancy.

Associated Anomalies

The cardiac and extracardiac malformations that make up the cardiosplenic syndromes are numerous (Table 19–2).

Of 172 necropsied patients with asplenia reviewed by Phoon et al,[50] 39% had at least one extracardiac defect, excluding lung lobation and heterotaxic defects. A total of 29% had one

TABLE 19–2 Conditions Associated with Asplenia and Polysplenia

Asplenia		Polysplenia	
Cardiac	Noncardiac	Cardiac	Noncardiac
Aortic atresia	Absent spleen	Aortic atresia	Absent gallbladder
Aortic stenosis	Agenesis of the corpus callosum	Aortic stenosis	Agenesis of the corpus callosum
Atrial septal defect	Bilateral trilobed lungs	Atrial septal defect	Atrioventricular septal defect
Atrioventricular septal defect	Cleft palate	Coarctation	Azygous drainage of inferior vena cava
Coarctation	Duodenal atresia	Common atrium	Bilateral bilobed lungs
Dextrocardia	Esophageal atresia	Complete heart block	Biliary atresia
Double-outlet right ventricle	Gut malrotation	Cor triatriatum	Central nervous system anomalies
Hypoplastic left heart syndrome	Malpositioned inferior vena cava	Double-outlet right ventricle	Cleft palate
Mitral stenosis	Midline liver	Hypoplastic left heart syndrome	Dextrocardia
Partial anomalous pulmonary connection	Spina bifida	Right aortic arch	Genitourinary anomalies
Pulmonary atresia		Transposition of the great arteries	Gut malrotation
Pulmonary stenosis		Truncus arteriosus	Malpositioned stomach
Right atrial hypoplasia		Univentricular heart	Mesocardia
Right atrial isomerism			Polysplenia
Tetralogy of Fallot			Skeletal anomalies
Total anomalous pulmonary venous connection			Spina bifida
Transposition			
Univentricular heart			
Ventricular septal defect			

additional extracardiac defect; 4% had two such defects; 3.5% had three defects; and one patient each (0.6%) had four, five, and seven additional extracardiac defects.[50]

Chromosomal anomalies, including monosomies, trisomy 13 and 18, microdeletion of chromosome 22q11, and translocations, have been associated with heterotaxy syndromes.[12,47]

References

1. Van Praagh S, Kreutzer J, Alday L, et al: Systemic and pulmonary venous connections in visceral heterotaxy, with emphasis on the diagnosis of the atrial situs: A study of 109 postmortem cases. In: Clark EB, Takao A (eds): Developmental Cardiology: Morphogenesis and Function. Mount Kisko, NY, Futura,1990, pp 671–727.
2. Van Mierop LHS, Gessner IH, Schiebler GL: Asplenia and polysplenia syndrome. Birth Defects 1972; 8:74–82.
3. Plowman DEM: Congenital absence of spleen associated with cardiac abnormalities. BMJ 1957; 1:147–148.
4. Freedom RM: The asplenia syndrome: A review of significant extracardiac structural abnormalities in 29 necropsied patients. J Pediatr 1972; 81:1130–1133.
5. Putschar WGJ, Manion WC: Congenital absence of the spleen and associated anomalies. Am J Clin Pathol 1956; 26:429–470.
6. Ivemark BI: Implications of agenesis of the spleen on the pathogenesis of cono-truncus anomalies in childhood. Acta Paediatr 1955; 44:7–110.
7. Berg C, Geipel A, Smrcek J, et al: Prenatal diagnosis of cardiosplenic syndromes: a 10-year experience. Ultrasound Obstet Gynecol 2003; 22:451–459.
8. Salomon LJ, Baumann C, Delezoide AL, et al: Abnormal abdominal situs: what and how should we look for? Prenat Diagn 2006; 26:282–285.
9. Patel CR, Lane JR, Muise KL: In utero diagnosis of obstructed supracardiac total anomalous pulmonary venous connection in a patient with right atrial isomerism and asplenia. Ultrasound Obstet Gynecol 2001; 17:268–271.
10. Gutgesell HP: Cardiac malposition and heterotaxy. In: Garson A, Bricker JT, McNamara DG (eds): The Science and Practice of Pediatric Cardiology, vol II. Philadelphia, Lea & Febiger, 1990, pp 1280–1303.
11. Neill CA, Zuckerberg AL: Syndromes and congenital heart defects. In: Nichols DG, Cameron DE, Greeley WJ, et al: Critical Heart Disease in Infants and Children. St Louis, Mosby–Year Book, 1995, pp 987–1012.
12. Marino B, Digilio MC: Congenital heart disease and genetic syndromes: Specific correlation between cardiac phenotype and genotype. Cardiovasc Pathol 2000; 9:303–315.
13. Sheley RC, Nyberg DA, Kapur R: Azygous continuation of the interrupted inferior vena cava: A clue to prenatal diagnosis of the cardiosplenic syndromes. J Ultrasound Med 1995; 14:381–387.
14. Chuang BP, Mena CE, Hoskins PA: Congenital anomalies of the inferior vena cava: Review of embryogenesis and presentation of a simplified classification. Br J Radiol 1974; 47:206–213.
15. Mayo J, Gray R, St. Louis E, et al: Review: Anomalies of the inferior vena cava. AJR Am J Roentgenol 1983; 140:339–345.
16. Yildirim SV, Tokel K, Varan B, et al: Clinical investigations over 13 years to establish the nature of the cardiac defects in patients having abnormalities of lateralization. Cardiol Young 2007; 17:275–282.
17. Peoples WM, Moller JH, Edwards JE: Polysplenia: A review of 146 cases. Pediatr Cardiol 1983; 4:129–137.
18. Stanger P, Rudolph AM, Edwards JE: Cardiac malpositions: An overview based on study of sixty-five necropsy specimens. Circulation 1977; 56:159–172.
19. Moller JH, Nakib A, Anderson RC, et al: Congenital cardiac disease associated with polysplenia: A developmental complex of bilateral "left-sidedness." Circulation 1967; 36:789–799.
20. de la Monte SM, Hutchins GM: Brief clinical report: Sisters with polysplenia. Am J Med Genet 1985; 21:171–173.
21. Opitz JM, Gilbert EF: CNS anomalies and the midline as a "developmental field." Am J Med Genet 1982; 12:443–455.
22. Neill CA: Development of the pulmonary veins. With reference to the embryology of anomalies of pulmonary venous return. Pediatrics 1988; 82:698–706.
23. Sadler TW: Cardiovascular system. In: Sadler TW (ed): Langman's Medical Embryology, 6th ed. Baltimore, Williams & Wilkins, 1990, pp 179–227.
24. Streeter GL: Developmental horizons in human embryos: Description of age groups XV, XVI, XVII, and XVIII, being the third issue of a survey of the Carnegie Collection. Contrib Embryol 1948; 32:133.
25. Corliss CE: Patten's Human Embryology: Elements of Clinical Development. New York, McGraw-Hill, 1976, 389–451.
26. Freedom RM, Smallhorn JF: Syndromes of right or left atrial isomerism. In: Freedom RM, Benson LN, Smallhorn JF (eds): Neonatal Heart Disease. London, Springer-Verlag, 1992, pp 545–560.

27. Campbell M, Deuchar DC: Absent inferior vena cava, symmetrical liver, splenic agenesis, and situs inversus, and their embryology. Br Heart J 1967; 29:268–275.

28. Caruso G, Becker AE: How to determine atrial situs? Considerations initiated by 3 cases of absent spleen with a discordant anatomy between bronchi and atria. Br Heart J 1979; 41:559–567.

29. Hastreiter AR, Rodriguez-Coronel A: Anomalous inferior vena cava with azygos continuation, high (sinus venosus) atrial septal defect and alterations of sinoatrial rhythm. Am J Cardiol 1968; 21:575–581.

30. Hastreiter AR, Rodriguez-Coronel A: Discordant situs of thoracic and abdominal viscera. Am J Cardiol 1968; 22:111–118.

31. Huhta JC, Smallhorn JF, Macartney FJ: Cross-sectional echocardiographic diagnosis of azygos continuation of the inferior vena cava. Cathet Cardiovasc Diagn 1984; 10:221–232.

32. Macartney FJ, Zuberbuhler JR, Anderson RH: Morphological considerations pertaining to recognition of atrial isomerism: Consequences for sequential chamber localization. Br Heart J 1980; 44:657–667.

33. Maksem JA: Polysplenia syndrome and splenic hypoplasia associated with extrahepatic biliary atresia. Arch Pathol Lab Med 1980; 104:212–214.

34. Merrill WH, Pieroni DR, Freedom RM, et al: Diagnosis of infrahepatic interruption of the inferior vena cava. Johns Hopkins Med J 1973; 133:329–338.

35. Tonkin ILD, Tonkin AK: Visceroatrial situs abnormalities: Sonographic and computed tomographic appearance. Am J Radiol 1982; 138:509–515.

36. Garcia OL, Mehta AV, Pickoff AS, et al: Left isomerism and complete atrioventricular block: A report of six cases. Am J Cardiol 1981; 48:1103–1107.

37. Partridge J: The radiological evaluation of atrial situs. Clin Radiol 1979; 30:95–103.

38. Vaughan TJ, Hawkins IF Jr, Elliott LP: Diagnosis of polysplenia syndrome. Radiology 1971; 101:511–518.

39. Chitayat D, Lao A, Wilson D, et al: Prenatal diagnosis of asplenia/polysplenia syndrome. Am J Obstet Gynecol 1988; 158:1085–1087.

40. Zlotogora J, Elian E: Asplenia and polysplenia syndromes with abnormalities of lateralization in a sibship. J Med Genet 1981; 18:301–302.

41. McChane RH, Hersh JH, Russell LJ, et al: Ivemark's "asplenia" syndrome: A single gene disorder. South Med J 1989; 82:1312–1313.

42. Devriendt K, Casaer A, Van Cauter A, et al: Asplenia syndrome and isolated total anomalous

43. Niikawa N, Kohsaka S, Mizumoto M, et al: Familial clustering of situs inversus totalis, and asplenia and polysplenia syndromes. Am J Med Genet 1983; 16:43–47.

44. Katcher AL: Familial asplenia, other malformations, and sudden death. Pediatrics 1980; 65:633–635.

45. Layton WM, Manasek FJ: Cardiac looping in early iv/iv mouse embryos. In: Van Praagh R, Takao A (eds): Etiology and Morphogenesis of Congenital Heart Disease. Mt Kisko, NY, Futura, 1980, pp 109–126.

46. Casey B, Devoto M, Jones KL, et al: Mapping a gene for familial situs abnormalities to human chromosome Xq24-q27.1. Nat Genet 1993; 5:403–407.

47. Piacentini G, Digilio MC, Sarkozy A, et al: Genetics of congenital heart diseases in syndromic and non-syndromic patients: new advances and clinical implications. J Cardiovasc Med (Hagestertown) 2007; 8:7–11.

48. Lin JH, Chang CI, Wang JK, et al: Intrauterine diagnosis of heterotaxy syndrome. Am Heart J 2002; 143:1002–1008.

49. Phoon CK, Villegas MD, Ursell PC, et al: Left atrial isomerism detected in fetal life. Am J Cardiol 1996; 77:1083–1088.

50. Phoon CK, Neill CA: Asplenia syndrome: Insight into embryology through an analysis of cardiac and extracardiac anomalies. Am J Cardiol 1994; 73:581–587.

51. Phoon CK, Neill CA: Polysplenia syndrome: Embryological considerations and comparison with asplenia syndrome [abstract]. Pediatr Res 1995; 37:31A.

52. Rose V, Izukawa T, Moes CAF: Syndromes of asplenia and polysplenia: A review of cardiac and non-cardiac malformations in 60 cases with special reference to diagnosis and prognosis. Br Heart J 1975; 37:840–852.

53. Simpson J, Zellweger H: Familial occurrence of Ivemark syndrome with splenic hypoplasia and asplenia in sibs. J Med Genet 1973; 10:303–304.

54. Torgersen J: Genetic factors in visceral asymmetry and in the development and pathologic changes of lungs, heart and abdominal organs. Arch Pathol 1949; 47:566–593.

55. Anderson RH, Macartney FJ, Shinebourne EA, et al: Paediatric Cardiology. Edinburgh, Churchill Livingstone, 1987, pp 473–496.

56. Chen SC, Monteleone PL: Familial splenic anomaly syndrome. J Pediatr 1977; 99:160–161.

57. DeVore GR, Sarti DA, Siassi B, et al: Prenatal diagnosis of cardiovascular malformations in the fetus with situs inversus viscerum during the

second trimester of pregnancy. J Clin Ultrasound 1986; 14:454–457.

58. Lin AE, Ticho BS, Houde K, et al: Heterotaxy: associated conditions and hospital-based prevalence in newborns. Genet Med 2000; 2:157–172.

59. Colloridi V, Pizzuto F, Ventriglia F, et al: Prenatal echocardiographic diagnosis of right atrial isomerism. Prenat Diagn 1994; 14:299–302.

60. Crawford D, Chapman M, Allan L: The assessment of persistent bradycardia in prenatal life. Br J Obstet Gynaecol 1985; 92:941–944.

61. Machado MV, Crawford DC, Anderson RH, et al: Atrioventricular septal defect in prenatal life. Br Heart J 1988; 59:352–355.

62. Brown DL, Emerson DS, Shulman LP, et al: Predicting aneuploidy in fetuses with cardiac anomalies: Significance of visceral situs and noncardiac anomalies. J Ultrasound Med 1993; 3:153–161.

63. Schmidt W, Yarkoni S, Jeanty P, et al: Sonographic measurements of the fetal spleen: Clinical implications. J Ultrasound Med 1985; 4:667–672.

64. Horgan JG, Lock JH, Cioffi-Ragan D: Horseshoe adrenal in Ivemark (asplenia) syndrome. J Ultrasound Med 1995; 14:785–786.

65. Waldman JD, Rosenthal A, Smith AL, et al: Sepsis and congenital asplenia. J Pediatr 1977; 90:555–559.

66. Sadiq M, Stumper O, De Giovanni JV, et al: Management and outcome of infants and children with right atrial isomerism. Heart 1996; 75:314–319.

67. Stewart RA, Becker AE, Wladimiroff JW, et al: Left atrial isomerism associated with asplenia: Prenatal echocardiographic detection of complex congenital cardiac malformations. J Am Coll Cardiol 1984; 4:1015–1020.

68. Phoon CK, Neill CA: Asplenia syndromerisk factors for early unfavorable outcome. Am J Cardiol 1994; 73:1235–1237.

CHAPTER 20

Fetal Cardiomyopathies

Marisa R. Lydia
Julia A. Drose

OUTLINE

Definition

A cardiomyopathy is a disorder of heart muscle that may be a primary disorder or may be associated with structural anomalies or pericardial disease. Cardiomyopathies account for approximately 2% of congenital heart disease in live-born infants.[1,2] The in utero occurrence is reported to be between 8% and 11%.[3] There are three different presentations in the fetus. The congestive, or dilated, form is most common and presents with dilated, poorly contracting chambers, atrioventricular regurgitation, and, often, associated hydrops fetalis (pleural and pericardial effusions, ascites, and skin thickening). The second most common type of cardiomyopathy is the hypertrophic form. Hypertrophic cardiomyopathies are recognized by markedly thickened ventricular walls and septum. The third form, a restrictive cardiomyopathy, is unusual in the fetus, manifesting primarily as endocardial fibroelastosis.[4,5]

Physiology

Fetal cardiomyopathies are caused by a broad spectrum of underlying disorders (Table 20–1). There is not always correlation between presentation (i.e., dilated versus hypertrophic) and cause; however, it is helpful to use basic physiological principles to understand, identify, and perhaps treat the underlying disorder.

Dilated Cardiomyopathies

In general, dilated cardiomyopathies can be divided into two categories. The first contains cardiomyopathies resulting from high-output failure caused by severe fetal anemias, or volume overload from massive arteriovenous shunting.

Severe fetal anemias result in high-output failure when the fetal heart increases cardiac output by increasing heart rate or stroke volume, or both, to meet peripheral oxygen requirements. As a result, cardiac work and oxygen demand increase and eventually exceed myocardial oxygen supply. Myocardial ischemia leads to poor cardiac function and contractility with chamber dilation (Fig. 20–1).

TABLE 20–1 Causes of Primary Cardiomyopathies		
Dilated	**Hypertrophic**	**Restrictive**
High-output failure	Infants of diabetic mothers	Endocardial fibroelastosis
Anemia	Noonan syndrome	Maternal lupus erythematosus
Rh isoimmunization	Glycogen storage disease	
Alpha-thalassemia	Twin-twin transfusion	
Glucose-6-phosphate-dehydrogenase		
deficiency		
Hemophilia A		
Volume overload		
Arteriovenous malformation		
Hemangioendotheliomas		
Sacrococcygeal teratomas		
Vein of Galen malformation		
Twin-twin transfusion		
Acardiac twin		
Direct myocardial damage		
Infection		
Coxsackie virus		
TORCH		
Parvovirus		
Fetal tachycardia		
Fetal hypoxia		
Supraventricular tachycardia		
Maternal lupus erythematosus		
Fetal bradycardia		

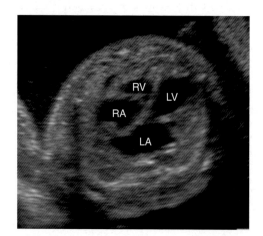

Figure 20–1 Apical four-chamber view in a fetus with a dilated cardiomyopathy resulting from anemia. The left atrium *(LA)*, left ventricle *(LV)*, right atrium *(RA)*, and right ventricle *(RV)* are all enlarged.

Anemia-associated cardiomyopathies include immune hydrops fetalis, homozygous alpha-thalassemia, glucose-6-phosphate-dehydrogenase deficiency, and hemophilia A.[6] Immune hydrops fetalis occurs when maternal serum immunoglob-ulin (Ig) G antibodies are formed against antigens on fetal red blood cells. Maternal serum antibodies are formed from the mixing of maternal and fetal blood during parturition of a prior pregnancy, placental abruption, amniocentesis, spontaneous or therapeutic abortion, blood transfusion, or placental intervillous hemorrhage. Maternal IgG crosses the placenta, enters the fetal circulation, and binds to fetal red blood cell antigens. Fetal hemolysis and hemolytic anemia may then occur.

A nonimmune mediated anemia, homozygous alpha-thalassemia, accounts for approximately 10% of cases of nonimmune hydrops fetalis in North America.[6] In this condition, fetal red blood cells contain Bart hemoglobin. This hemoglobin irreversibly binds to oxygen, resulting in the inability of red blood cells to deliver oxygen to fetal tissues. Homozygous alpha-thalassemia is uniformly fatal to the fetus. If the pregnancy is allowed to progress, there is a significant risk of preeclampsia and maternal microcytic anemia.

High-output failure may also ensue when cardiac output is increased because of massive arteriovenous shunting. Increased venous return to the heart results in increased stroke volume, which, as in the case of severe anemia, eventually leads to increased cardiac work and myocardial oxygen demand.

Hemangioendotheliomas of the liver, sacrococcygeal teratomas, intracranial teratomas, vein of Galen arteriovenous malformations, and other congenital shunts may present with dilated cardiomyopathy caused by high-output failure from volume overload (Figs. 20–2 and 20–3).[6-11]

Direct myocardial damage, another cause of dilated cardiomyopathy, includes fetal infection, tachycardia-induced cardiomyopathies, and fetal anoxia.[12]

Direct myocardial damage with resultant heart failure may occur with fetal infection (Fig. 20–4).[13,14] Coxsackie virus; toxoplasmosis, rubella, cytomegalovirus, and herpes simplex (TORCH) agents; and parvovirus are most often responsible. Maternal penicillin therapy for syphilis may reverse syphilitic fetal myocarditis, congestive heart failure, and hydrops fetalis.[14] Although identification of viral agents may be particularly difficult, cultures and serological tests, as well as associated sonographic findings (i.e., intracranial or hepatic calcifications, hepatosplenomegaly, echogenic bowel), may confirm suspected cases.

Myopathy induced by arrhythmia (tachyarrhythmia or bradyarrhythmia) is the most common cause of nonimmune hydrops fetalis in North America.[15] Fetal supraventricular tachycardia is the most common sustained fetal arrhythmia. It

may present with congestive cardiomyopathy when the rapid heart rate results in such shortened diastole that myocardial perfusion (the majority of which occurs in diastole) is markedly diminished (Fig. 20–5). Myocardial ischemia and

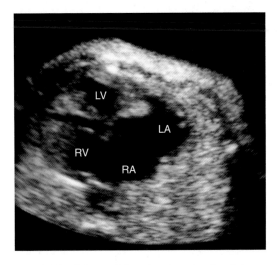

Figure 20–2 Subcostal four-chamber view in a fetus with Klippel-Trenaunay-Weber syndrome exhibiting a dilated cardiomyopathy resulting from multiple congenital arteriovenous fistulas of the right leg and multiple microscopic cutaneous hemangiomas. *LA*, Left atrium; *LV*, left ventricle; *RA*, right atrium; *RV*, right ventricle.

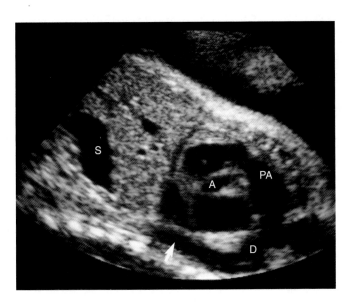

Figure 20–3 Short-axis view of the great vessels in the fetus with Klippel-Trenaunay-Weber syndrome seen in Figure 20–2. The pulmonary artery *(PA)*, ductus arteriosus *(D)*, and descending aorta *(arrow)* are all dilated. *A*, Aortic root; *S*, stomach.

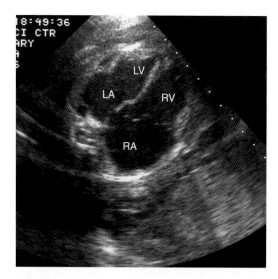

Figure 20–4 Four-chamber view in a fetus with cytomegalovirus showing a severely dilated cardiomyopathy that occupies the majority of the fetal chest. *LA,* Left atrium; *LV,* left ventricle; *RA,* right atrium; *RV,* right ventricle.

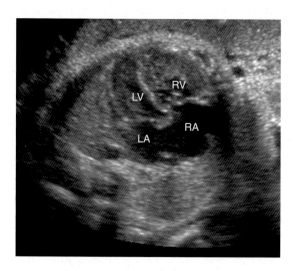

Figure 20–6 Apical four-chamber view in the fetus with a hypertrophic cardiomyopathy. The interventricular septum and right and left ventricular walls are thickened. *LA,* Left atrium; *LV,* left ventricle; *RA,* right atrium; *RV,* right ventricle.

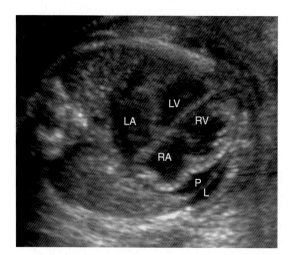

Figure 20–5 Subcostal four-chamber view in a fetus with a congestive cardiomyopathy caused by supraventricular tachycardia. A pericardial effusion *(P)* and a pleural effusion *(L)* are also seen. *LA,* Left atrium; *LV,* left ventricle; *RA,* right atrium; *RV,* right ventricle.

direct myocardial cell damage may ensue.[9] Fetal supraventricular tachycardia is one of the few potentially treatable causes of congestive heart failure and therefore is important to recognize to initiate appropriate therapy.[16,17]

Fetal asphyxia can result in direct myocardial damage and cardiac decompensation.[18,19] The fetus responds to hypoxia by vasoconstriction, bradycardia, and hypertension. Hypotension, myocardial ischemia, and myocardial cell injury occur with worsening asphyxia, resulting in subsequent cardiac decompensation.

Hypertrophic Cardiomyopathies

Hypertrophic cardiomyopathies present with thickened ventricular walls from increased myocardial cell size, resulting in decreased ventricular compliance (Fig. 20–6). This may lead to poor diastolic filling of the heart (diastolic dysfunction), which, in turn, results in diminished cardiac output.

Biventricular hypertrophy occurs in most recipient twins in twin-twin transfusion syndrome (TTTS) (Fig. 20–7).[20,21] In this syndrome, monochorionic twins share (usually at the level of the cotyledons) a placental arteriovenous circulation. Blood is transferred through the interconnected placental circulation from a donor twin on the arterial side to a recipient twin on the venous side. This results in an oligohydramniotic, anemic donor twin and a plethoric, polyhydramniotic and often hydropic recipient twin. Although the

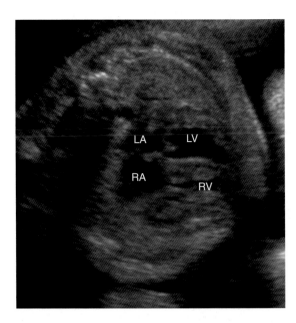

Figure 20–7 Subcostal four-chamber view in the recipient twin in twin-twin transfusion syndrome. The ventricular walls and the interventricular septum show marked hypertrophy. *LA,* Left atrium; *LV,* left ventricle; *RA,* right atrium; *RV,* right ventricle.

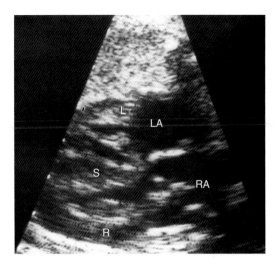

Figure 20–8 Subcostal four-chamber view in the fetus of a diabetic mother. The interventricular septum *(S)* is disproportionately thickened in relation to the right *(R)* and left *(L)* ventricular walls. *LA,* Left atrium; *RA,* right atrium.

cardiomegaly found in the recipient twin has long been thought to result from volume overload, no significant difference in cardiac output, when adjusted to fetal weight, is found between donor and recipient.[20] The fact that the cardiomegaly present in the recipient twin exhibits myocardial hypertrophy rather than ventricular dilation implies that the pathogenesis is more complex. Therapies used to treat TTTS in utero, such as amnio reduction or anastomosis ablation, do not seem to improve cardiac function. In fact, the hypertrophic cardiomyopathy associated with TTTS often persists and worsens as gestation progresses.[22] Donor twins are affected with cardiovascular disease much less frequently.[20]

Fetal hypertrophic cardiomyopathy can also occur as a result of maternal insulin-dependent diabetes. The incidence of hypertrophic cardiomyopathy in infants of diabetic mothers has been reported to be from 33% to 84%.[23–27] In this condition, the ventricular septum can be disproportionately thickened in relation to the ventricular free walls (Fig. 20–8), similar to the asymmetrical septal hypertrophy (ASH) (unrelated to diabetes) seen in children and adults. Concentric hypertrophy may

also occur. Infants of diabetic mothers may also have fetal hyperinsulinemia, macrosomia, and organomegaly. There is conflicting opinion in the literature regarding the pathophysiologic mechanisms of these changes.[24,27–28] One theory is that maternal hyperglycemia induces production of fetal insulin. The anabolic effect of endogenous fetal insulin subsequently causes macrosomia and organomegaly, including ASH.

Generally, ASH is progressive throughout gestation. Fetuses may therefore appear normal in second-trimester examinations and subsequently exhibit sonographic findings of diabetic hypertrophic cardiomyopathy on follow-up examination. ASH is usually asymptomatic in the fetus and neonate, with spontaneous postnatal resolution.[29,30] Rarely, hypertrophic cardiomyopathy is a primary disorder of hypertrophic myocardium, as is seen in Noonan syndrome and glycogen storage disease.[3,6,31]

Restrictive Cardiomyopathies

Restrictive cardiomyopathies decrease cardiac output because of impaired diastolic filling.[32] In the fetus, this is primarily due to abnormal fibroelastic proliferation within the endocardium (endocardial fibroelastosis). This abnormal tissue decreases endocardial compliance, with resultant diastolic dysfunction and decreased cardiac output. Endocardial fibroelastosis results from pathological deposition of collagen and elastin within the endocardium.[33] It accounts for approximately 1% to 4% of cases of congenital heart disease and occurs in 1 of every 5000 to 6000 births.[34] It is divided into primary and secondary forms.

Primary endocardial fibroelastosis occurs when no associated structural cardiac anomaly is found. It may be a result of fetal infection such as Coxsackie virus or of an autoimmune process such as lupus erythematosus. In this setting, transplacental passage of maternal anti-Ro and anti-La antibodies induce inflammation and fibrosis of the myocardium.[33,35,36]

Secondary endocardial fibroelastosis is usually associated with obstructive lesions, predominantly left sided, such as aortic stenosis or atresia.[36] In this setting, obstruction to blood flow causes the fibrin build up, which is then deposited in the endocardium.[33,34] The sonographic appearance is classically ventricular enlargement and a strongly echogenic endocardium (Fig. 20–9). Contracted forms have been reported without ventricular enlargement, and there is at least one report of a dilated endocardial fibroelastosis progressing to a contracted form. Therapy includes digoxin and diuretics, but the prognosis is poor. Most fetuses die in utero or in the early neonatal period.[37-41]

Sonographic Criteria

With the caveat that many but not all fetal cardiomyopathies present with an enlarged heart, the sonographic diagnosis of cardiomyopathy is best approached by initially answering two questions: Is the heart large, and if so, why? It is important to distinguish a large heart in a normal-sized thorax from a normal-sized heart in a small thorax. This can be accomplished by tracing the cardiac and chest circumferences on a transverse image of the fetal chest (Fig. 20–10). The chest circumference can then be compared with the age-related gestational norms (Table 20–2). If the chest circumference is appropriate for gestational age, and the heart appears subjectively large, cardiomyopathy should be suspected.

Cardiac circumference (CC) to thoracic circumference (TC) or cardiac area (CA) to thoracic area (TA) ratios can be calculated to confirm the diagnosis. The normal CC-to-TC ratio is approximately 0.5; the normal CA-to-TA ratio is approximately 0.33.[42]

Once a cardiomyopathy is considered, chamber size and wall thickness should be assessed.

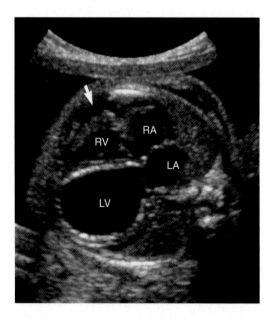

Figure 20–9 Subcostal four-chamber view in a fetus with endocardial fibroelastosis of the left ventricle *(LV)*. The echogenic endocardium can be seen surrounding the ventricle. A pericardial effusion *(arrow)* is also noted. *RV,* Right ventricle; *RA,* right atrium; *LA,* left atrium.

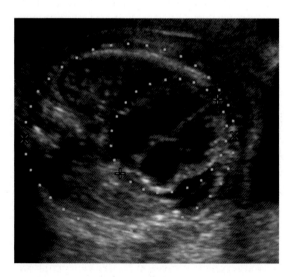

Figure 20–10 Measuring the fetal heart and fetal chest circumferences to assess cardiac size on a transverse view of the fetal chest.

TABLE 20–2 Fetal Thoracic Circumference Measurements*

Gestational Age (wk)	No.	Predictive Percentiles								
		2.5	5	10	25	50	75	90	95	97.5
16	6	5.9	6.4	7.0	8.0	9.1	10.3	11.3	11.9	12.4
17	22	6.8	7.3	7.9	8.9	10.0	11.2	12.2	12.8	13.3
18	31	7.7	8.2	8.8	9.8	11.0	12.1	13.1	13.7	14.2
19	21	8.6	9.1	9.7	10.7	11.9	13.0	14.0	14.6	15.1
20	20	9.5	10.0	10.6	11.7	12.8	13.9	15.0	15.5	16.0
21	30	10.4	11.0	11.6	12.6	13.7	14.8	15.8	16.4	16.9
22	18	11.3	11.9	12.5	13.5	14.6	15.7	16.7	17.3	17.8
23	21	12.2	12.8	13.4	14.4	15.5	16.6	17.6	18.2	18.8
24	27	13.2	13.7	14.3	15.3	16.4	17.5	18.5	19.1	19.7
25	20	14.1	14.6	15.2	16.2	17.3	18.4	19.4	20.0	20.6
26	25	15.0	15.5	16.1	17.1	18.2	19.3	20.3	21.0	21.5
27	24	15.9	16.4	17.0	18.0	19.1	20.2	21.3	21.9	22.4
28	24	16.8	17.3	17.9	18.9	20.0	21.2	22.2	22.8	23.3
29	24	17.7	18.2	18.8	19.8	21.0	22.1	23.1	23.7	24.2
30	27	18.6	19.1	19.7	20.7	21.9	23.0	24.0	24.6	25.1
31	24	19.5	20.0	20.6	21.6	22.8	23.9	24.9	25.5	26.0
32	28	20.4	20.9	21.5	22.6	23.7	24.8	25.8	26.4	26.9
33	27	21.3	21.8	22.5	23.5	24.6	25.7	26.7	27.3	27.8
34	25	22.2	22.8	23.4	24.4	25.5	26.6	27.6	28.2	28.7
35	20	23.1	23.7	24.3	25.3	26.4	27.5	28.5	29.1	29.6
36	23	24.0	24.6	25.2	26.2	27.3	28.4	29.4	30.0	30.6
37	22	24.9	25.5	26.1	27.1	28.2	29.3	30.3	30.9	31.5
38	21	25.9	26.4	27.0	28.0	29.1	30.2	31.2	31.9	32.4
39	7	26.8	27.3	27.9	28.9	30.0	31.1	32.2	32.8	33.3
40	6	27.7	28.2	28.8	29.8	30.9	32.1	33.1	33.7	34.2

From Chitkara U, Rosenberg J, Chervenak FA, et al: Prenatal sonographic assessment of fetal thorax: Normal values. Am J Obstet Gynecol 1987; 156:1071.
*Measurements in centimeters.

Two-dimensional assessment of ventricular chamber dimensions and wall thickness are performed using the subcostal four-chamber view. All measurements should be taken just distal or inferior to the atrioventricular valves.[43] Chamber dimensions are measured from endocardial-to-endocardial surface at end-diastole when the chambers are at their maximum dimension (Fig. 20–11). Ventricular wall thickness is measured from epicardial-to-endocardial surface, also at end-diastole when wall thickness is at its minimum (Fig. 20–12). The atria should be measured at end-systole when their dimensions are at their maximum (Fig. 20–13). A short-axis view of the ventricles is also useful for assessing chamber size and wall thickness. Nomograms comparing chamber size and wall thickness with gestational age are available (see Chapter 2). Severely dilated cardiomyopathies are often apparent without the need of measurement. A rule of thumb for normal ventricular wall and interventricular septal thickness is <5 mm throughout gestation.

M-mode imaging is also useful to measure chamber size and wall thickness.[44,45] End-diastolic measurements for ventricular wall and septal wall thickness are made between the endocardial surfaces just distal to the atrioventricular valves in either a subcostal four-chamber view or a short-axis view of the ventricles (Fig. 20–14). End-diastolic measurements of chamber size are measured at the same level (Fig. 20–15). Measurements derived by two-dimensional imaging versus M-mode imaging are reported to be statistically similar (see Chapter 2).[46]

M-mode imaging is also useful in assessing ventricular compliance, which is often impaired

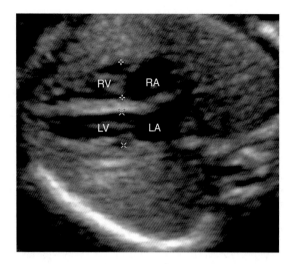

Figure 20–11 Measuring ventricular size on a subcostal four-chamber view. The right *(RV)* and left *(LV)* ventricle measurements *(calipers)* are taken from endocardial to endocardial surface, just inferior to the tricuspid and mitral valves. *LA,* Left atrium; *RA,* right atrium.

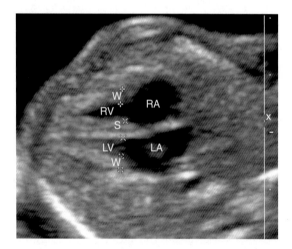

Figure 20–12 Measuring the ventricular walls *(W)* and interventricular septum *(S)* on a subcostal four-chamber view. Measurements are taken just inferior to the mitral and tricuspid valves. *LA,* Left atrium; *LV,* left ventricle; *RA,* right atrium; *RV,* right ventricle.

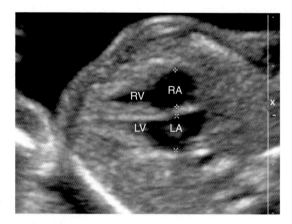

Figure 20–13 Measuring the right *(RA)* and left *(LA)* atria on a subcostal four-chamber view. Measurements are taken at the largest dimensions *(calipers)* of the atria. *LV,* Left ventricle; *RV,* right ventricle.

in the setting of all types of cardiomyopathy (Fig. 20–16).

One of the earliest sonographic findings of cardiomyopathy is impaired systolic function, which may be present in the absence of apparent chamber dilation or hypertrophy.[47] Systolic function is best assessed by evaluating ventricular systolic shortening as determined by the ventricular shortening fraction:

$$SF = \frac{(EDD - ESD)}{EDD}$$

where SF is shortening fraction, EDD is end-diastolic dimension, and ESD is end-systolic dimension.

Approximate normal right and left ventricular shortening fractions are 0.25 and 0.30, respectively.[43] Serial shortening fractions can be particularly useful in following individual patients for progression or resolution of disease.

Atrioventricular regurgitation is often seen with severe cardiomyopathy.[15,19,44] In the dilated form, ventricular dilation with associated dilation of the valve annulus causes incomplete valve closure during systole, leading to regurgitation. With the hypertrophic or restrictive forms, the inability of blood to exit the ventricle can result in a reversal of flow back into the atria. Atrioventricular regurgitation can be identified with either color or spectral Doppler analysis (Fig. 20–17, *A* and *B*).

Because cardiomyopathies can often occur as a result of congenital cardiac disease, a complete fetal echocardiogram should always be performed. All four valves should be evaluated with pulsed and color Doppler imaging to identify stenosis or atresia. If either of these are present with dilated

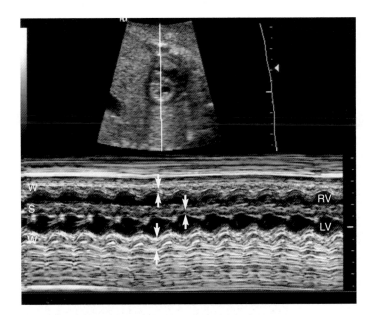

Figure 20–14 Use of M-mode imaging through a short-axis view of the ventricles to measure the ventricular walls *(W)* and interventricular septal thickness *(S)*. *LV,* Left ventricle; *RV,* right ventricle.

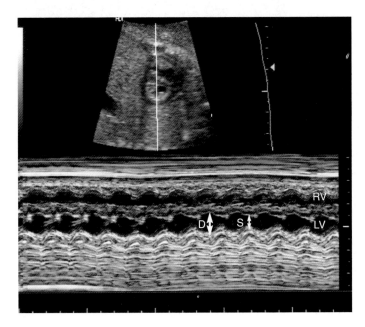

Figure 20–15 Use of M-mode imaging through a short-axis view of the ventricles to measure ventricular chamber size at end-diastole *(D)* and systole *(S)*. *LV,* Left ventricle; *RV,* right ventricle.

ventricular chambers, endocardial fibroelastosis may be appreciated. If the ventricular walls are hypertrophic, with an associated stenosis, it should be borne in mind that the hypertrophy may be the result of a pressure overload from the stenosis (secondary form) or the hypertrophy may be causing the stenosis (primary form) by obstructing the outflow tracts (Figs. 20–18 and 20–19). This functional obstruction caused by hypertrophic cardiomyopathy is seen in TTTS.

All fetuses with a diagnosis of cardiomyopathy should also be assessed for evidence of arrhythmia, the presence of nonimmune hydrops, and associated findings of fetal infection.

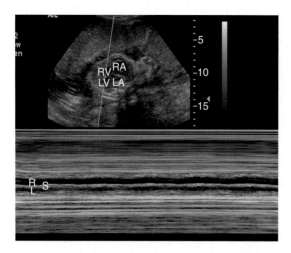

Figure 20–16 M-mode imaging through the ventricles showing decreased contractility of the right *(R)* and left *(L)* ventricles in a fetus with a dilated cardiomyopathy. *LA,* Left atrium; *RA,* right atrium.

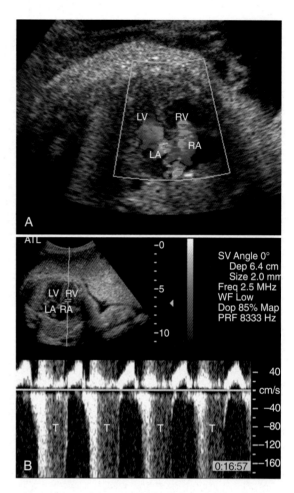

Figure 20–17 Tricuspid regurgitation in a fetus with a dilated cardiomyopathy seen with color Doppler **(A)** and pulsed Doppler **(B)** imaging. *LA,* Left atrium; *LV,* left ventricle; *RA,* right atrium; *RV,* right ventricle; *T,* regurgitant flow.

Treatment

In utero treatment of cardiomyopathies is restricted to controlling the underlying cause, for example, maternal diabetes or fetal anemia, or attempting to correct a resulting arrhythmia. Supraventricular tachycardia has been successfully controlled in utero by using digoxin and other antiarrhythmic agents.[16,17] There have also been reports of the successful use of maternal corticosteroids or plasmapheresis in treating fetuses that have complete heart block of mothers with systemic lupus erythematosus.[48,49] In utero balloon angioplasty has been attempted in some cases of aortic stenosis.[50] As stated previously, in utero treatments of TTTS do not seem to improve cardiac outcome.[51] Cardiac transplant has been attempted in rare cases.[12]

Prognosis

The prognosis for fetal cardiomyopathies is variable given the broad spectrum of underlying causes. In general, the presence of nonimmune hydrops fetalis is a poor prognostic sign. Fetal cardiomyopathies caused by structural cardiac disease may fare better than primary occurrences.[12] Overall mortality rates for fetuses affected with a dilated cardiomyopathy range from 25% to 82%.[3,23] Hypertrophic cardiomyopathies, including TTTS, have a reported mortality rate of 52%, with the majority of deaths occurring in utero.[3] Primary restrictive cardiomyopathies exhibiting endocardial fibroelastosis are usually accompanied by nonimmune hydrops fetalis and carry a mortality rate of 83%.[35]

Associated Anomalies

Outflow tract obstructions, usually aortic or pulmonary stenosis, can result in or be caused by hypertrophic cardiomyopathies.[34,37–39] Sustained fetal arrhythmias may be the underlying cause of dilated cardiomyopathies. Maternal conditions such as diabetes mellitus (hypertrophic), lupus erythematosus (restrictive), and infection (dilated)

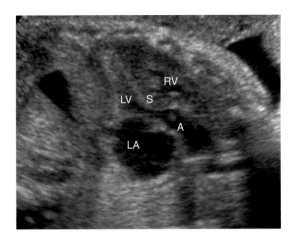

Figure 20–18 Long-axis view of the aorta in the recipient twin in TTTS. The right ventricle *(RV)* is hypertrophied, causing the interventricular septum *(S)* to obstruct outflow through the aorta *(A)*. *LA,* Left atrium; *LV,* left ventricle.

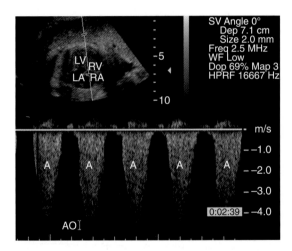

Figure 20–19 Pulsed Doppler imaging of the aorta of the same fetus in Figure 20–18. Blood flow velocity is markedly increased *(A)* through the aorta, consistent with aortic stenosis. *LA,* Left atrium; *LV,* left ventricle; *RA,* right atrium; *RV,* right ventricle.

also carry an association. Fetal cardiomyopathies are not usually associated with chromosomal abnormalities; however, rare occurrences have been reported.[52] An association with Noonan syndrome has been established.[3]

References

1. Ferencz C, Rubin JD, McCarter RJ, et al: Congenital heart disease: Prevalence at live birth. The Baltimore-Washington Infant Study. Am J Epidemiol 1985; 121:31–36.
2. Bianchi DW, Crombleholme TW, D'Alton ME: Cardiomyopathy. Fetology 2000; 45:357–363.
3. Pedra S, Smallhorn JF, Ryan G, et al: Fetal Cardiomyopathies: Pathogenic mechanisms, hemodynamic findings, and clinical outcome. Circulation 2002; 106:585–591.
4. Simpson JM: Cardiomyopathy in the fetus. Fetal Cardiol 2003; 24:291–298.
5. Zielinksy P: Diseases of the myocardium, endocardium, and pericardium during fetal life. Fetal Cardiol 2003; 23:281–290.
6. Silverman NH, Schmidt KG: Ultrasound evaluation of the fetal heart. In: Calen P (ed): Ultrasonography in Obstetrics and Gynecology, 3rd ed. Philadelphia, WB Saunders, 1994, pp 315–316.
7. Walton JM, Rubin SZ, Soucy P, et al: Fetal tumors associated with hydrops: The role of the pediatric surgeon. J Pediatr Surg 1993; 28:1151–1153.
8. Sherer DM, Abramowicz JS, Eggers PC, et al: Prenatal ultrasonographic diagnosis of intracranial teratoma and massive craniomegaly associated with high-output cardiac failure. Am J Obstet Gynecol 1993; 168:97–99.
9. Bond SJ, Harrison MR, Schmidt KG, et al: Death due to high output cardiac failure in fetal sacrococcygeal teratoma. J Pediatr Surg 1990; 25:1287–1291.
10. Gonen R, Fong K, Chaisson DA: Prenatal sonographic diagnosis of hepatic hemangioendothelioma with secondary nonimmune hydrops fetalis. Obstet Gynecol 1989; 73:485–487.
11. Holgrove W, Flake AW, Langer JC: The fetus with sacrococcygeal teratoma. In: Harrison MR, Gobus MS, Filly RA (eds): The Unborn Patient: Prenatal Diagnosis and Treatment. Philadelphia, WB Saunders, 1990, pp 460–469.
12. Yinon Y, Yagel S, Hegesh J, et al: Fetal cardiomyopathy—In utero evaluation and clinical significance. Prenat Diagn 2007; 27:23–28.
13. Drose JA, Dennis MA, Thickman D: Infection in utero: US findings in 19 cases. Radiology 1991; 178:369–374.
14. Barton JR, Thorpe EM Jr, Shaver DC, et al: Nonimmune hydrops fetalis associated with maternal infection with syphilis. Am J Obstet Gynecol 1992; 167:56–58.
15. Gembruch U, Rede DA, Bald R, et al: Longitudinal study in 18 cases of fetal supraventricular tachycardia: Doppler echocardiographic findings

and pathophysiologic implications. Am Heart J 1993; 125:1290–1301.

16. Wiggins JW, Bowes W, Clewell W, et al: Echocardiographic diagnosis and intravenous digoxin management of fetal tachyarrhythmias and congestive heart failure. Arch Pediatr Adolesc Med 1986; 140:202–204.

17. Arnoux P, Seyral P, Llurens M, et al: Amiodarone and digoxin for refractory fetal tachycardia. Am J Cardiol 1987; 59:166–170.

18. Shime J, Gresser CD, Rakowski H: Quantitative two-dimensional echocardiographic assessment of fetal cardiac growth. Am J Obstet Gynecol 1986; 154:292–300.

19. Weil SR, Huhta JC: Sonographic differential diagnosis of fetal cardiac abnormalities. Semin Ultrasound CT MRI 1993; 14:298–318.

20. Barrea C, Alkazaleh R, Ryan G, et al: Prenatal cardiovascular manifestations in the twin-to-twin transfusion syndrome recipients and the impact of therapeutic amnio reduction. Am J Obstet Gynecol 2005; 192:892–902.

21. Achiron R, Rabinovitz R, Aboulafia Y, et al: Intrauterine assessment of high-output cardiac failure with spontaneous remission of hydrops fetalis in twin-twin transfusion syndrome: Use of two-dimensional echocardiography, Doppler ultrasound and color flow mapping. J Clin Ultrasound 1992; 20:271–277.

22. Fisk NM, Galea P. Twin-twin transfusion—As good as it gets? N Engl J Med 2004; 35:182–184.

23. Boldt T, Andersson S, Eronen M. Etiology and outcome of fetuses with functional heart disease. Acta Obstet Gynecol Scand 2004; 83:531–535.

24. Sheehan PQ, Rowland TW, Shah BL, et al: Maternal diabetic control and hypertrophic cardiomyopathy in infants of diabetic mothers. Clin Pediatr 1986; 25:266–271.

25. Walther FJ, Siassi B, King J, et al: Cardiac output in infants of insulin-dependent diabetic mothers. J Pediatr 1985; 107:109–114.

26. Rizzo G, Arduini D, Romanini C: Accelerated cardiac growth and abnormal cardiac flow in fetuses of type I diabetic mothers. Obstet Gynecol 1992; 80:369–376.

27. Cooper MJ, Enderlein MA, Tarnoff H, et al: Asymmetric septal hypertrophy in infants of diabetic mothers: Fetal echocardiography and the impact of maternal diabetic control. Arch Pediatr Adolesc Med 1992; 146:226–229.

28. Weber HS, Botti JJ, Baylen BG: Sequential longitudinal evaluation of cardiac growth and ventricular diastolic filling of fetuses of well controlled diabetic mothers. Pediatr Cardiol 1994; 15:184–189.

29. Zielinsky P, Hagemann L, Daudt L, et al: The fetus with hypertrophic cardiomyopathy related to maternal diabetes: A pre- and postnatal analysis of the associated factors. J Am Coll Cardiol 1992; 19:342A.

30. McMahon JN, Berry PJ, Joffe HS: Fetal hypertrophic cardiomyopathy in an infant of a diabetic mother. Pediatr Cardiol 1990; 11:211–212.

31. Mendex HMM, Opitz JM: Noonan syndrome: A review. Am J Med Genet 1985; 21:493–506.

32. Simchen MJ, Toi A, Silver M, et al: Fetal cardiac calcifications: report of four prenatally diagnosed cases and review of the literature. Ultrasound Obstet Gynecol 2006; 27:325–330.

33. Raboisson MJ, Fouron JC, Sonesson SE, et al: Fetal Doppler echocardiographic diagnosis and successful steroid therapy of Luciani-Wenckebach phenomenon and endocardial fibroelastosis related to maternal anti-Ro and anti-La antibodies. J Am Soc Echocardiogr 2005; 18:375–380.

34. Rustico MA, Benetton A, Bossani R, et al: Early fetal endocardial fibroelastosis and critical aortic stenosis: A case report. Ultrasound Obstet Gynecol 1995; 5:202–205.

35. Nield LE, Silverman ED, Taylor GP: Maternal anti-Ro and anti-La antibody-associated endocardial fibroelastosis. Circulation 2002; 105:843–848.

36. Trastour C, Bafghi A, Delotte J, et al: Early prenatal diagnosis of endocardial fibroelastosis. Ultrasound Obstet Gynecol 2005; 26:303–306.

37. Ben-Ami M, Shalev E, Romano S, et al: Midtrimester diagnosis of endocardial fibroelastosis and atrial septal defect: A case report. Am J Obstet Gynecol 1986; 155:662–663.

38. Sharland GK, Chaita SK, Fagg NL, et al: Left ventricular dysfunction in the fetus: Relation to aortic valve anomalies and endocardial fibroelastosis. Br Heart J 1991; 66:419–424.

39. Carceller AM, Maroto E, Fouron JC: Dilated and contracted forms of primary endocardial fibroelastosis: A single fetal disease with two stages of development. Br Heart J 1990; 63:311–313.

40. Revel A, Ariel L, Rein AJ, et al: Fetal endocardial fibroelastosis. J Clin Ultrasound 1994; 22:355–356.

41. Veille JC, Sivakoff M: Fetal echocardiographic signs of congenital endocardial fibroelastosis. Obstet Gynecol 1988; 72:219–222.

42. Veille JC, Sivakoff M, Nemeth M: Evaluation of human fetal cardiac size and function. Am J Perinatol 1990; 7:54–59.

43. Tan J, Silverman NH, Hoffman JI, et al: Cardiac dimensions determined by cross-sectional echocardiography in the normal human fetus from 18 weeks to term. Am J Cardiol 1992; 70:1459–1467.

44. Devore GR, Siassi B, Platt LD: M-mode assessment of ventricular size and contractility during the second and third trimesters of pregnancy in the normal fetus. Am J Obstet Gynecol 1984; 150:981–988.

45. Allan LD, Joseph MC, Boyd EG: M-mode echocardiography in the developing human fetus. Br Heart J 1982; 47:573–583.

46. Cartier MS, Davidoff A, Warneke LA, et al: The normal diameter of the fetal aortic and pulmonary artery: Echocardiographic evaluation in utero. AJR Am J Roentgenol 1987; 149: 1003–1007.

47. Schmidt KG, Birk E, Silverman NH, et al: Echocardiographic evaluation of dilated cardiomyopathy in the human fetus. Am J Cardiol 1989; 63:599–605.

48. Friedman DM: Fetal echocardiography in the assessment of lupus pregnancies. Am J Reprod Immunol 1992; 28:164–167.

49. Buyon JP, Swersky SH, Fox HE, et al: Intrauterine therapy for presumptive fetal myocarditis with acquired heart block due to systemic lupus erythematosus. Arthritis Rheum 1987; 30:44–49.

50. Tworetzky W, Wilkins-Haug L, Jennings RW: Balloon dilation of severe aortic stenosis in the fetus: Potential for prevention of hypoplastic left heart syndrome: Candidate selection, technique and results of successful intervention. Circulation 2004; 110: 2125–2131.

51. Ville Y, Hyett J, Hecher K, et al: Preliminary experience with endoscopic laser surgery for severe twin-twin transfusion syndrome. N Engl J Med 1995; 332:224–227.

52. Larkins LD, MacPherson SS, Kilby R: Prenatal diagnosis and prenatal imaging features of fetal monosomy 1p36. Prenat Diagn 2007;27:874–878.

CHAPTER 21

Fetal Arrhythmias

Karrie L. Villavicencio

OUTLINE

Definition

Fetal cardiac arrhythmias occur in up to 1% to 3% of all pregnancies and account for 10% to 20% of referrals to fetal cardiologists.[1-4] The majority of fetal arrhythmias are benign; however, they can be an important cause of fetal morbidity and death.[5] The normal fetal heart rate is regular and between 100 and 180 beats per minute.[6] Fetal arrhythmias are therefore defined as those that are irregular or outside the normal range. Clinically, fetal arrhythmias can be classified as those with an irregular but overall normal rate, tachycardia, and bradycardia.[7] The approach to diagnosing prenatal arrhythmias is significantly different from

that used in the postnatal period because of the difficulty in distinguishing fetal electrocardiographic (ECG) signals from maternal cardiac signals.

Fetal magnetocardiography allows precise measurement of fetal intracardiac intervals in the diagnosis of fetal arrhythmias; however, the clinical utility of this technique is limited by lack of availability in most centers. Currently, fetal echocardiography remains the primary modality for diagnosing and evaluating fetal arrhythmias.

Embryology

Spontaneously depolarizing cells, which give the heart its unique characteristic of automaticity, are present early in gestation in all parts of the developing heart. Rhythmic contraction of the fetal heart begins 21 to 22 days after conception and is present before the conduction system is established.[8] The conduction system of the fetal heart is functionally mature by 16 weeks of gestation.[9] The heart rate changes throughout gestation. Initially, the rate is slow (82 beats per minute), increasing to 177 beats per minute at 63 days and then decreasing to 147 beats per minute at 15 weeks of gestation.[10,11] After 34 weeks of gestation, fetal heart rate patterns are related to fetal rest and activity.[12] Fetal heart rate control is through the parasympathetic and sympathetic nervous systems.[13] The conduction system of the heart consists of the sinus node, atrioventricular node, bundle of His, and Purkinje fibers. The pacemaker of the heart is the sinus node. The electrical signal travels down specialized conduction tissue through the atria to the atrioventricular node, where conduction of the signal is slowed. The signal is then sent through the bundle of His to the Purkinje fibers, which initiate ventricular contraction.

Occurrence Rate

The number of fetuses referred for evaluation of arrhythmias varies among institutions. Fouron[14] reported that approximately 14% of the 1450 fetuses seen annually at St Justine Hospital were referred for arrhythmia. Over a 5-year study period at that institution, 584 of the 940 fetuses referred for apparent arrhythmia were in sinus rhythm at the time of their echocardiographic examinations. Among the 356 fetuses with sustained fetal arrhythmias, premature atrial or ventricular contractions were noted in 86%, tachycardia in 8%, and bradycardia in 5%.[14] Copel et al[15] reported that 10% to 12% of the referrals for fetal echocardiography at Yale are due to fetal arrhythmias; of the 595 fetuses referred to Yale for irregular heart rhythm over a 10-year period, 55% had normal rhythms, 43% had extrasystoles, and 2.4% had hemodynamically significant arrhythmias.

Irregular Fetal Rhythms

Irregular heart rhythms are generally detected during routine obstetrical auscultation of the fetal heart, most commonly between 28 and 32 weeks' gestation, but can be noted as early as 17 weeks. Premature atrial contractions (PACs) account for the majority of irregular fetal rhythms.[1,2] PACs in the fetus are generally idiopathic; however redundancy of the foramen ovale flap (Fig. 21–1) has been reported to possibly contribute to initiation of an ectopic atrial focus.[16]

Maternal consumption of nicotine, caffeine, or alcohol has also been implicated.[17] Isolated ectopic beats are associated with congenital heart defects in up to 1% to 2% of cases.[2]

PACs generally present as irregular pauses detected by routine obstetrical auscultation and are usually transient and benign.[18–20] They may increase as pregnancy progresses. Premature beats become significant when they occur with appropriate timing to initiate sustained tachycardia.[21] Progression to sustained tachycardia can occur in up to 2% to 3% of cases of frequent atrial ectopy, either in utero or in the first 3 to 4 weeks of life.[22,23] Those cases in which there are multiple blocked atrial ectopic beats causing a low ventricular rate appear to be at higher risk of progressing to tachycardia than do those with a normal ventricular

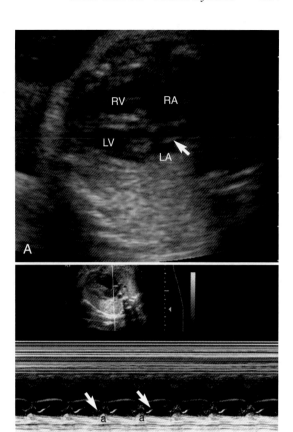

Figure 21–1 **A,** Redundant foraminal flap *(arrow)* moving toward the left atrial wall *(LA)* shown from the subcostal four-chamber view. *LV,* Left ventricle; *RA,* right atrium; *RV,* right ventricle. **B,** M-mode cursor traversing the foraminal flap *(arrows),* showing it striking the left atrial wall *(a).*

rate.[2] The risk increases to approximately 10% with complex ectopy, including couplets or triplets.[24] Progression of PACs to sustained tachycardia is generally mediated by anatomic bypass tracts and leads to supraventricular tachycardia (SVT), but atrial flutter may also occur.[23] Less commonly, premature ventricular contractions (PVCs) may cause an irregular fetal heart rhythm; the ratio of occurrence of PACs to PVCs in utero is approximately 10:1.[5] PVCs may be difficult to distinguish from PACs in utero. A premature ventricular beat that is not preceded by a premature atrial beat should be interpreted as a PVC. The presence of atrioventricular valve regurgitation concurrent with the ectopic beat, less prominent flow reversal in the inferior vena cava by Doppler imaging, and a longer compensatory pause can be helpful to differentiate PVCs from PACs.[2-4] The presence of PVCs may be benign but warrants exclusion of myocardial disease, intracardiac tumors, and any evidence of cardiac decompensation.

Tachyarrhythmia

Fetal tachycardia is defined as a sustained heart rate that exceeds 180 beats per minute. The fetal myocardium is intrinsically more susceptible to sustained tachycardia as a result of impaired diastolic relaxation and compliance. The inherent diastolic dysfunction of the fetal myocardium is thought to be at least in part due to immature structure and function of the sarcoplasmic reticulae.[25,26] The most common forms of fetal tachycardia are SVT (66%–90%) and atrial flutter (10%–30%).[27]

Fetal SVT is characterized by a regular fast rate with a 1:1 ratio of atrioventricular conduction. The heart rate in SVT is monotonous with no variation in the atrial or ventricular rate, in contrast to sinus tachycardia in which there is heart rate variability. Sinus tachycardia is generally a result of maternal or fetal distress, and identifying the underlying cause is of primary importance.[28]

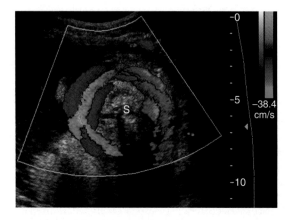

Figure 21-2 *Transverse image of the fetal cervical spine (S) using color Doppler imaging to show the umbilical cord wrapped around the fetal neck.*

Atrial flutter and fibrillation are rare fetal arrhythmias characterized by very fast atrial rates, often 300 to 500 beats per minute, with an irregular slower ventricular rate resulting from variable conduction delay, generally 2:1 or 3:1 block.[29] Atrial flutter is associated with structural heart defects, chromosomal anomalies, or other pathological states in 30% of cases.[5]

Ventricular tachycardia is extremely rare in fetal life. It can, however, be present in association with long QT syndrome, which is a genetic syndrome involving ion channel abnormalities and increased risk of sudden death. Magnetocardiography has been the only definitive way to measure the QT interval in the fetus[30,31]; given the limited availability of this technique, the diagnosis is generally made in the postnatal period. Fetuses with long QT syndrome often present with sinus bradycardia between periods of tachycardia, which may facilitate determination of the diagnosis.[32,33]

Bradyarrhythmia

Fetal bradycardia is defined as a sustained heart rate less than 100 beats per minute. The most common causes of fetal bradycardia are blocked premature atrial beats, atrioventricular block, and sinus bradycardia.[5] Transient bradycardia is common and is often associated with fetal vagotonia due to pressure on the maternal abdomen from the ultrasound probe, which resolves with removal of the transducer. Cord compression, which may occur when the umbilical cord is located around the fetal neck, may also result in a transient bradycardia (Fig. 21–2).

Bradycardia may be due to nonconducted premature atrial beats (blocked PACs). Most commonly this occurs with atrial bigeminy in which every other beat is premature and is blocked in the atrioventricular node, causing the ventricular rate to appear slow. Blocked PACs are usually benign and self-limited. The most important cause of sustained fetal bradycardia is complete atrioventricular block. Fetal heart block can be detected as early as the first trimester, endovaginally, with two-dimensional and color Doppler flow imaging.[34] Complete heart block occurs in 1:20,000 newborns,[34] but the overall incidence of fetal heart block is unknown. In complete heart block there is complete dissociation between the atrial and ventricular beats. It is important to distinguish pathological bradycardia resulting from complete heart block from benign blocked PACs. In complete heart block, the atrial rate is regular, whereas in blocked PACs the atrial rate is irregular, with every other beat occurring prematurely.

Complete heart block may be associated with structural heart defects involving the atrioventricular junction (atrioventricular discordance as in congenitally corrected transposition of the great arteries) or visceral heterotaxy syndrome with left atrial isomerism.[35-37] Alternatively, complete heart block may be immune mediated in the setting of maternal connective tissue disorders such as systemic lupus erythematosus or Sjögren syndrome with elevated anti-SS-A or anti-SS-B antibodies. These antibodies may cross the placenta as early as 16 weeks' gestation and cause inflammatory injury of the fetal atrioventricular node.[21] Cardiac structure is generally but not always normal in the setting of immune-mediated complete atrioventricular block. These fetuses may also have autoimmune myocarditis from damage to cardiac contractile elements.

Fetal sinus bradycardia is marked by a regular slow rate with 1:1 atrioventricular conduction and may be due to cardiac structural defects (primarily left atrial isomerism) or prolonged QT syndrome or may be an isolated finding. Sinus bradycardia is usually the result of maternal or fetal distress. As with sinus tachycardia, determining the underlying cause is the most important aspect of the diagnosis.[28]

Sonographic Criteria

Analysis of fetal cardiac rhythm is based on the ability to record atrial and ventricular activity simultaneously. M-mode imaging was one of the first echocardiographic modalities used in assessing arrhythmias. Because of the high temporal resolution, it remains an important part of arrhythmia assessment. Electrical events are inferred from the motion of the cardiac chambers.[38] M-mode imaging is performed by aligning the cursor through one of the atrial and one of the ventricular walls from a four-chamber view (Fig. 21–3) or with the cursor between the left atrium and aorta from a short-axis view of the great vessels (Fig. 21–4).

Atrial extrasystoles, the most common form of arrhythmia, can be readily assessed by M-mode imaging. The premature atrial beats may be conducted to the ventricle or blocked in the atrioventricular node. If the PAC is conducted, it is followed by ventricular contraction and then a pause during which the sinus rate is reset (Fig. 21–5). If the PAC is blocked within the atrioventricular node, no ventricular contraction occurs (Fig. 21–6). M-mode imaging can help differentiate blocked PACs from

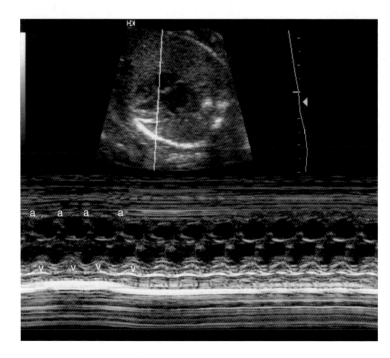

Figure 21–3 Normal M-mode tracing using a subcostal four-chamber view to demonstrate both atrial and ventricular contractility. The M-mode cursor traverses the right atrial and left ventricular walls. Ventricular contraction (*v*) follows each atrial contraction (*a*).

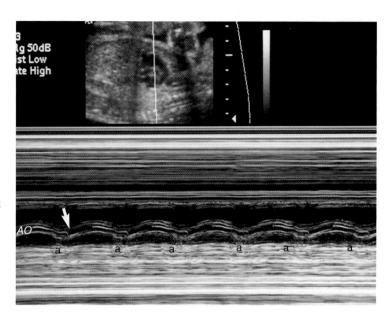

Figure 21–4 Normal M-mode tracing using a short-axis view of the great vessels to assess both atrial and ventricular contractility. The M-mode cursor traverses both the aorta and left atrial wall. Ventricular contraction corresponds with the opening of the aortic valve *(arrow)*. *a,* Atrial contraction; *AO,* aorta.

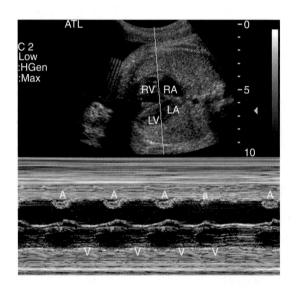

Figure 21–5 Conducted PAC. The M-mode cursor placed through the right atrium *(RA)* and left ventricular *(LV)* walls. Normal atrial contractions *(A)* are seen, followed by normal ventricular contractions *(V)*. When the premature atrial beat occurs *(a)*, it is conducted to the ventricle and thus followed by a premature ventricular beat *(v)*. *LA,* Left atrium; *RV,* right ventricle.

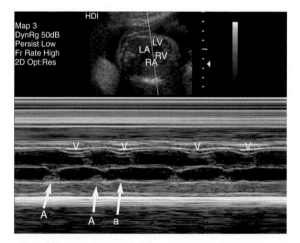

Figure 21–6 Blocked PAC. Two normal atrial beats *(A with arrow)* are followed by normal ventricular beats *(V)*. A PAC *(a with arrow)* then occurs that is not conducted to the ventricle; therefore no ventricular contraction follows. *LA,* Left atrium; *LV,* left ventricle; *RA,* right atrium; *RV,* right ventricle.

pathological causes of bradycardia, such as complete heart block. In atrial bigeminy with block, every other atrial contraction is premature and not conducted to the ventricle; the atrial rate appears irregular (Fig. 21–7). The atrial rate in complete heart block by contrast is very regular (Fig. 21–8).

In the setting of tachycardia, the 1:1 atrioventricular relationship seen in SVT is well demonstrated by M-mode imaging (Fig. 21–9); however, this must be distinguished from atrial flutter with 1:1 conduction. With SVT, the heart rate is maintained between 180 and 300 beats per minute. With atrial flutter, the atrial rate will be between 300 and 400 beats per minute, permitting the differentiation (Fig. 21–10). Atrial fibrillation is defined as an atrial rate greater than 400 beats per minute; however, it is rarely seen in the fetus.

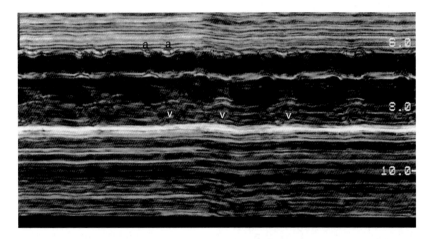

Figure 21–7 Atrial bigeminy with block. Every other atrial contraction is premature and not conducted to the ventricle. This results in a slow (94 beats/min) ventricular rate. *a,* Atrial contraction; *v,* ventricular contraction.

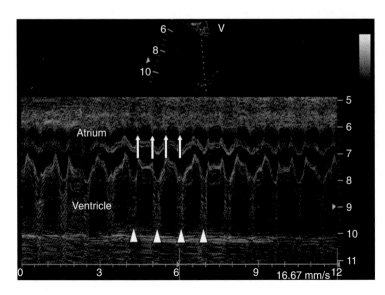

Figure 21–8 Complete heart block. The atrial contractions are shown by the arrows and occur at a regular and normal rate. The ventricular contractions shown by arrowheads occur at a slower rate and are dissociated from the atrial contractions.

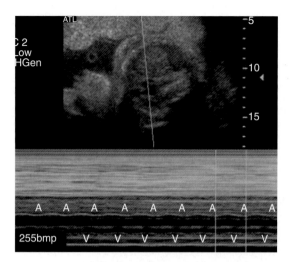

Figure 21–9 SVT. A one-to-one relationship exists between the atrial *(A)* and ventricular *(V)* contraction at an abnormally fast heart rate of 255 beats/min.

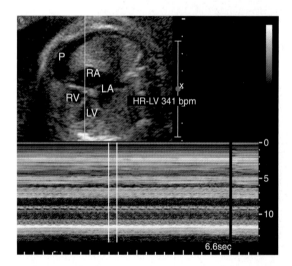

Figure 21–10 Atrial flutter. The atrial rate is rapid at 341 beats/min. A pleural effusion is also noted *(P)*. *LA,* Left atrium; *LV,* left ventricle; *RA,* right atrium; *RV,* right ventricle.

Despite the high temporal resolution, M-mode imaging is dependent on favorable fetal position and good image quality. Defining intracardiac time intervals by fetal M-mode imaging is limited by loss of clear markers of atrial and ventricular contractions in the hydropic fetus with hypocontractile myocardium and also by poor image resolution as a result of maternal body habitus, fetal position, and polyhydramnios or oligohydramnios.[39]

Pulsed-wave Doppler imaging (PWD) provides an important adjunct to M-mode imaging in assessing fetal arrhythmias because it is relatively independent of fetal position and image quality. Conventionally, PWD sampling has been performed in the left ventricular outflow tract area between the mitral and aortic valves.

By using a relatively large sample volume, inflow and outflow of the ventricle can be assessed simultaneously from an apical five-chamber view (Fig. 21–11) or from a long-axis view of the aorta (Fig. 21–12). PWD is very helpful in defining PACs because the filling pattern of the PAC is different from that of a sinus beat. When the PAC is conducted, the aortic ejection signal is smaller. The beat following the premature beat may demonstrate prolonged atrial filling (Fig. 21–13). When the PAC is blocked, no aortic ejection signal is present (Fig. 21–14). In the less common case of PVCs, the ventricular ejection signal is reduced in comparison with the sinus beats (Fig. 21–15).

Simultaneous PWD interrogation of venous and arterial flow in an adjacent vein and artery is a recent advancement in the evaluation of fetal arrhythmias. It is especially useful in defining intracardiac time intervals in the assessment of tachycardia. This method is most commonly performed with the cursor in the superior vena cava and adjacent ascending aorta (SVC/AA method); alternatively, the pulmonary vein and branch pulmonary artery[40] or inferior vena cava and descending aorta[41] can be assessed. The primary advantage to this method over using PWD in the left ventricular outflow tract area is that, at heart rates exceeding 160 beats per minute, overlap of the mitral E and A waves often occurs, limiting precise measurements of the intracardiac intervals.[7] In contrast, intracardiac intervals can be measured regardless of the heart rate with the SVC/AA method.[14]

The SVC/AA Doppler trace is obtained by rotating the transducer 90 degrees from a standard

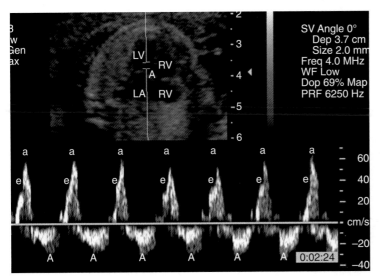

Figure 21-11 Normal pulsed Doppler image using an apical five-chamber view with the sample volume positioned in the left ventricle to obtain both ventricular inflow and outflow. The flow above the baseline is normal mitral flow with an e-point (e) and a-point (a). The e-point represents peak opening of the anterior valve leaflet. The a-point represents atrial contraction. The flow below the baseline represents left ventricular outflow through the aorta (A). LA, Left atrium; LV, left ventricle; RA, right atrium; RV, right ventricle.

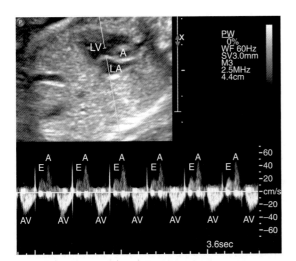

Figure 21-12 Normal pulsed Doppler image using a long-axis view of the aorta with the sample volume positioned in the left ventricle to obtain both ventricular inflow and outflow. The flow above the baseline is normal inflow of the mitral valve with an e-point (E) and an a-point (A). The flow below the baseline (AV) represents left ventricular outflow through the aorta. A, Aorta; LA, left atrium; LV, left ventricle.

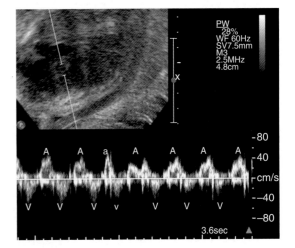

Figure 21-13 Pulsed Doppler image showing a conducted PAC. The sample volume is placed in a short-axis view of the great vessels to show normal mitral inflow from the atrium (A) and ventricular outflow (V) through the aorta. When the premature atrial beat (a) does occur, it is conducted to the ventricle; therefore a premature ventricular beat (v) follows.

four-chamber view in the vertical position to provide a sagittal view of the two vena cavae entering the right atrium. The sample volume is increased to include both flow signals, allowing the temporal relationship between atrial and ventricular contraction to be determined. Ven-

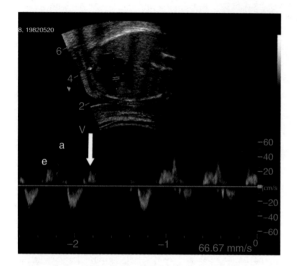

Figure 21–14 Blocked PAC seen by pulsed Doppler imaging. The PAC is denoted by the large arrow. There is no ventricular ejection after the premature beat, causing an irregular ventricular rate. The next beat has abnormal atrial filling, but sinus rhythm resumes with the following beat. *a,* a point; *e,* e point.

tricular systole is marked by antegrade flow in the ascending aorta, and atrial contraction is noted by transient flow reversal in the superior vena cava. The mechanical atrioventricular and ventriculoarterial intervals are thus measured. The atrioventricular interval serves as a surrogate for the PR interval on the ECG.[42,43] The relationship between the atrioventricular and ventriculoarterial intervals provides key insight into the mechanism of tachycardia.[14,39,44] With use of PWD at the SVC/AA site, the atrioventricular interval is measured from the beginning of atrial contraction (the "a" wave) in the superior vena cava trace to the beginning of ventricular systole (the "v" wave) in the ascending aorta. The ventriculoarterial interval is measured from the beginning of "v" wave to the beginning of the "a" wave (Fig. 21–16). When the ventriculoarterial interval is shorter than the atrioventricular interval (i.e., short ventriculoarterial tachycardia), a re-entrant mechanism through an accessory pathway is most likely present. This type of tachycardia is called atrioventricular re-entrant tachycardia, and it is the most common mechanism of fetal SVT, accounting for greater than 90% of cases of fetal SVT.[21] The accessory connection is located along the atrioventricular groove and electrically connects the atrium and ventricle, allowing the re-entrant circuit to be established. Because of the rapid conduction through the retrograde limb, atrial contraction occurs when the atrioventricular valve is closed, leading to the

Figure 21–15 Pulsed Doppler imaging showing a PVC. The flow above the baseline represents ventricular ejection as reflected through the aorta. A PVC is present *(arrow).*

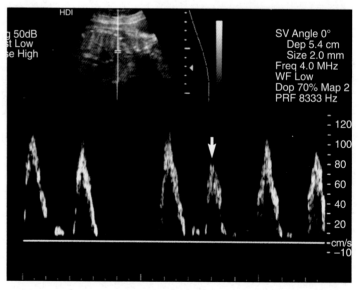

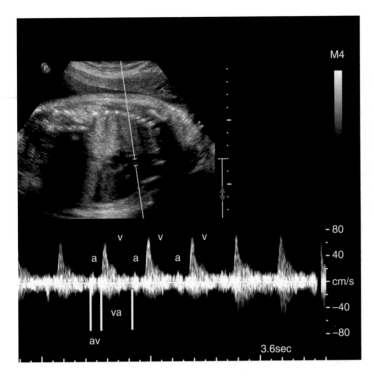

Figure 21–16 Pulsed Doppler tracing obtained using the SVC/AA method in a fetus in sinus rhythm. The sample volume is placed between the superior vena cava and ascending aorta with sufficient width to encompass both signals. Aortic ejection is noted above the baseline, while antegrade venous flow in the superior vena cava is demonstrated below the baseline. Atrial contraction is noted by small reverse "a" waves prior to each aortic ejection. The interval between atrial contraction ("a" wave) and the beginning of aortic ejection ("v" wave) is the atrioventricular *(av)* interval. The ventriculoarterial *(va)* interval is measured from the beginning of aortic ejection ("v" wave) to the "a" wave.

presence of tall "a" waves superimposed on the aortic ejection signal (Fig. 21–17).

Less commonly, when conduction through the retrograde limb is slow, the ventriculoarterial interval is longer than the atrioventricular interval (i.e., long ventriculoarterial tachycardia). The "a" waves are of normal amplitude in long ventriculoarterial tachycardia (Fig. 21–18). Examples of long ventriculoarterial tachycardia include atrial ectopic tachycardia and the permanent form of reciprocating junctional tachycardia, both of which tend to be incessant and unresponsive to most antiarrhythmic agents.[45] Concomitant onset of atrial and ventricular contraction can be seen in the setting of junctional ectopic tachycardia (Fig. 21–19).[46] Atrial flutter can be diagnosed by the appearance of the flutter waves on the superior vena cava tracing (Fig. 21–20). Use of the SVC/AA method to measure the atrioventricular and ventriculoarterial time intervals to define the tachycardia mechanism therefore is important in predicting prognosis and guiding medical therapy. The SVC/AA Doppler method can be useful in demonstrating dissociation between the atrial and ventricular rate as in complete heart block.

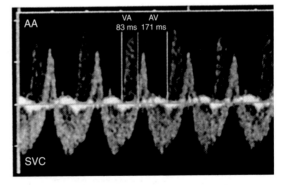

Figure 21–17 Doppler tracing obtained with the SVC/AA method in a fetus with tachycardia. The ventriculoarterial *(VA)* interval is significantly shorter than the atrioventricular *(AV)* interval, suggesting a short ventriculoarterial tachycardia. Tall (cannon) "a" waves are superimposed on the aortic ejection signal and are reflective of atrial contraction occurring against a closed atrioventricular valve. (From Fouron JC: Fetal arrhythmias: The Saint-Justine hospital experience. Prenat Diagn 2004; 24:1068–1080. Copyright John Wiley & Sons Limited. Reproduced with permission.)

Fetal Hemodynamics

Fetal echocardiography allows not only for diagnosis of arrhythmias but also for monitoring of the fetal circulatory system for possible signs of congestive heart failure. These include cardiomegaly (heart area/chest area >0.42), mitral or tricuspid regurgitation (not solely occurring with the premature beats), abnormal venous Doppler flow patterns, including reversal in the inferior vena cava or ductus venosus (Fig. 21–21) or pulsation of the umbilical vein, pericardial or pleural effusion, diminished function (shortening fraction <25%), and distended hepatic veins or umbilical vein (>6 mm).[1] Retrograde pulsations in the systemic and pulmonary veins are consistent with relative restriction to diastolic filling of the fetal ventricular myocardium, which has been exacerbated by inadequate duration of diastolic filling related to the fast heart rate.[21] Diastolic notching of the umbilical veins is a very poor prognostic sign that is associated with fetal hydrops.[47]

Assessment of fetal hemodynamics with venous Doppler imaging has become an important part of fetal arrhythmia evaluation. Accurate assessment of fetal cardiovascular status is important in fetuses with tachycardia or heart block, especially in the setting of hydrops, with the attendant risk of intrauterine death. Fetal cardiovascular status evaluation with venous Doppler imaging can reflect efficacy of therapy or facilitate management decisions regarding delivery. Abnormal pulsatility patterns consisting of increased velocity of blood flow reversal away from the heart during atrial contraction (a wave) may be a sign of increased end-diastolic pressure in the ventricles that occurs as a result of heart failure.[48] However, there are limitations of venous Doppler imaging, including inability to distinguish disturbances in venous flow from atrial ectopic beats, tachycardia, or fetal heart block. Flow reversal in the ductus venosus, for example, can be seen in atrial ectopic beats or complete heart block. Thus changes in venous Doppler imaging may actually reflect the

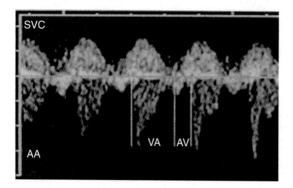

Figure 21–18 Doppler tracing obtained with the SVC/AA method in a fetus with tachycardia. The ventriculoarterial *(VA)* interval is longer than the atrioventricular *(AV)* interval, consistent with a long ventriculoarterial tachycardia. The "a" waves are of normal amplitude. (From Fouron JC: Fetal arrhythmias: The Saint-Justine hospital experience. Prenat Diagn 2004; 24:1068–1080. Copyright John Wiley & Sons Limited. Reproduced with permission.)

Figure 21–19 Pulsed Doppler tracing in the superior vena cava and ascending aorta in a fetus with tachycardia. Concomitant onset of atrial contraction *(a)* and aortic ejection *(v)* suggests junctional ectopic tachycardia. The tall "a" waves represent atrial contraction against a closed atrioventricular valve.

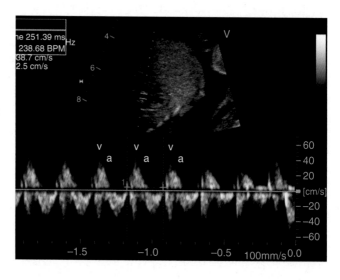

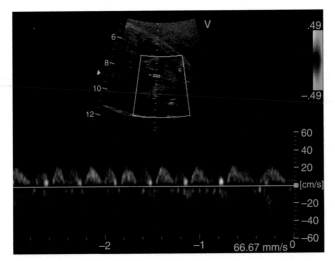

Figure 21-20 Pulsed Doppler imaging in the ascending aorta and superior vena cava in a fetus with atrial flutter. The flutter waves are seen above the baseline in the superior vena cava signal; aortic ejection signals are below the baseline. There is 2:1 atrioventricular block with two atrial contractions seen for every one ventricular ejection.

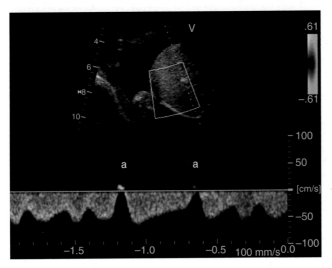

Figure 21-21 Pulsed-wave Doppler imaging in the ductus venosus in a fetus with PACs. Flow reversal is seen during atrial contraction in the presence of the premature atrial beats. *a,* Atrial contraction.

mechanism of the rhythm disturbance rather than the degree of cardiac dysfunction.

Fetal Magnetocardiography and Tissue Velocity Imaging

Fetal magnetocardiography (FMCG) provides actual cardiogram signals as opposed to the mechanical motion portrayed by M-mode and pulsed-wave Doppler imaging. FMCG can provide precise electrophysiological measurements such as atrioventricular and ventriculoarterial intervals, QRS duration, and QT interval, all of which are important in defining the mechanism of the tachycardia.[49] FMCG, however, is based on signal averaging, limiting efficacy in evaluating beat-to-beat variability as seen with irregular patterns such as premature beats. Tissue velocity imaging measures the motion of the myocardium and allows precise timing of atrial and ventricular events and measurements of diastolic function. Tissue Doppler imaging has the advantage of defining the mechanical relationship of atrial and ventricular wall motion,[50] thus permitting evaluation of beat-to-beat variability such as in the case of premature beats (Fig. 21–22) and in the setting of tachycardia (Figs. 21–23 and 21–24). In addition, tissue

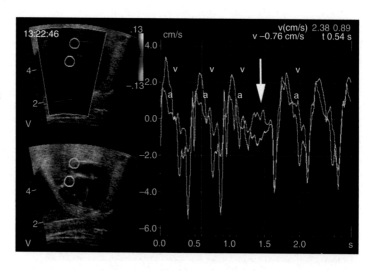

Figure 21–22 Tissue Doppler imaging in a fetus with a blocked PAC. The sample volume is placed in the atrial wall *(green line)* and ventricular wall *(yellow line).* The PAC *(arrow)* is blocked and therefore not followed by ventricular contraction. *a,* Atrial contraction; *v,* aortic ejection.

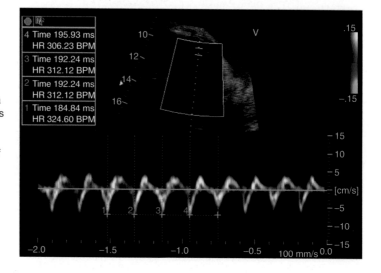

Figure 21–23 Tissue Doppler imaging in a fetus with atrial flutter; the sample volume is placed in the atrial wall. The rapid rate of atrial contraction is denoted by the signal below the baseline, indicating movement of the atrial wall away from the transducer.

velocity imaging provides a method of investigating the effects of antiarrhythmic agents on electrophysiological conduction in the fetal heart (Fig. 21–25).

Treatment

Fetal ectopy, including isolated PACs and PVCs, in general does not require antiarrhythmic therapy.[5] A complete fetal echocardiogram and Doppler assessment should be performed for every fetus with ectopy to rule out a congenital heart defect and assess the risk of progression to sustained tachycardia. The mother should be warned of

symptoms of fetal tachycardia, including decreased fetal movement and an increase in abdominal girth as a result of polyhydramnios. Any of these symptoms necessitate immediate referral for specific treatment of the arrhythmia. A logical risk/benefit analysis should be performed for each individual case, with consideration given to the potential benefits of attaining fetal sinus rhythm versus the potential dangers to the mother, including proarrhythmic and other adverse effects of antiarrhythmic agents. Serial maternal electrocardiograms, telemetry, and monitoring of drug concentrations are important components in guiding

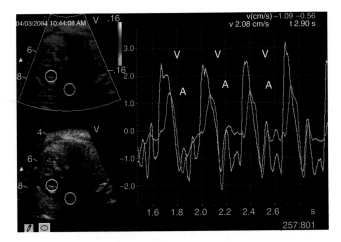

Figure 21–24 Tissue Doppler imaging in fetus with SVT. One cursor is placed in the atrial wall *(green line)* and one in the ventricular myocardium *(yellow line)*. Atrial and ventricular filling are denoted below the baseline as a result of movement of the atrial and ventricular walls away from the frame of reference during diastole. Atrial and ventricular contractions are seen above the baseline as the atrial and ventricular walls move toward the frame of reference during systole. The atrial contractions (A) occur after the ventricular contractions (V), suggesting the presence of retrograde conduction through an accessory pathway (atrioventricular re-entry tachycardia).

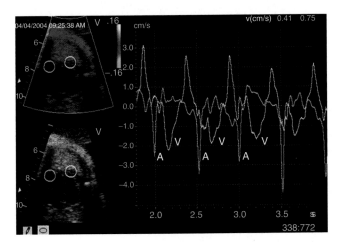

Figure 21–25 Tissue Doppler imaging in the same fetus after administration of digoxin with achievement of sinus rhythm. The atrial contractions (A) precede the ventricular contractions (V).

therapy. Fetal SVT that is intermittent (less than 30% of 24-hour period documented during in-hospital monitoring) and not associated with signs of cardiac failure can be managed conservatively with very close observation, including weekly echocardiographic examinations.[51] Sustained SVT should prompt delivery if at term or, if preterm, initiation of antiarrhythmic therapy. In cases of SVT with cardiac failure, intravenous digoxin has been recommended as first-line therapy.[4,5] Digoxin as a single agent therapy has been associated with an 80% to 85% success rate in the treatment of fetal SVT.[52,53] In the presence of hydrops, however, transplacental passage of digoxin may be impaired and thus concomitant administration of fetal intramuscular digoxin can shorten time to conver-sion,[54] so addition of second-line therapies is often required.

Amiodarone is generally preferred for SVT in the extremely ill fetus; however, there is no con-sensus currently regarding optimal second-line antiarrhythmic agents.[5] Flecainide, sotalol, and procainamide have been reported with variable success.[55–57] Flecainide has proarrhythmia effects,[58] sotalol causes prolongation of the QT interval, and procainamide can cause uterine contractions.[59] Amiodarone has been associated with neonatal hypothyroidism and pulmonary fibrosis. Larmay and Strasburger[5] reported conversion to sinus rhythm with amiodarone ranging from 65% to 95% within a week if the fetus is hydropic and within 48 hours in the absence of hydrops.

Treatment of atrial flutter is similar to that for SVT with digoxin as the first-line therapy; however, the conversion rate is only 30% to 85% and second agents are often required.[57] Sotalol is considered the drug of choice for refractory atrial flutter.[60]

Measurement of the mechanical PR interval (measured as the atrioventricular interval by echocardiogram) can help identify first-degree heart block early in fetuses at high risk for developing immune-mediated complete heart block in the setting of maternal anti-Ro/La antibody placental transfer. This may prove beneficial in guiding treatment. Beta-sympathomimetic agents have been shown to increase the ventricular rate by up to 20%; however, their effect on the overall mortality rate is unclear.[61,62] Corticosteroids have been shown to improve ventricular function in cases of complete heart block associated with maternal lupus erythematosus and normal fetal cardiac structure; however, they may be ineffective in reversing complete heart block or preventing progression to complete block from first- or second-degree atrioventricular block. Therefore the long-term adverse effects may outweigh the benefits of long-term use.[57] Fetal sinus bradycardia may be a harbinger of fetal distress and may prompt delivery. Fetal bradycardia resulting from long QT syndrome is associated with a high risk of cardiac arrest after delivery if not appropriately treated. Pacemaker insertion should be considered in those infants with second-degree atrioventricular block caused by long QT syndrome, along with initiation of beta-blocker therapy with propranolol or mexilitine.[5]

Prognosis

Isolated fetal arrhythmias generally result in a favorable perinatal outcome, with a 95% likelihood of survival.[20] SVT is associated with structural heart disease in 5% to 10% of patients.[18] SVT in the setting of structural heart disease is associated with a poor prognosis.[63] However, fetal tachycardia can result in cardiac failure, fetal hydrops, and fetal death[23] and thus require urgent evaluation and management. The risk of developing fetal heart failure is highest among those with more incessant the SVT, earlier onset (<32 weeks' gestation), and association with structural heart disease.[64] Hydrops, a severe manifestation of fetal heart failure, is defined as the presence of fluid collections in at least two of the abdominal, pleural, or pericardial spaces and/or anasarca.[44,65]

SVT may lead to the development of hydrops when it persists for more than 12 hours.[5] Hydrops is present at presentation or develops in 40% to 50% of cases of fetuses with sustained SVT.[66]

The overall mortality rate from treatment of SVT with hydrops varies from 2% up to 30%.[4,60,67] After birth, approximately 50% of infants who had fetal tachycardia require no treatment, and others outgrow the tachycardia by approximately 1 year of age. A late recurrence risk of about 30% for SVT is seen during late childhood in those with SVT as infants. Fetal sinus bradycardia not associated with long QT syndrome or structural heart disease is thought to have a good outcome.[68]

Despite advances in perinatal supportive therapy, the prognosis for complete heart block in the setting of structural heart disease remains poor, with a mortality rate of 50% when diagnosed in utero.[69,70] The prognosis is especially poor in the presence of hydrops, low ventricular rate (<55 beats/minute), or prematurity.[71,72]

References

1. Respondek M, Wloch A, Kaczmarek P, et al: Diagnostic and perinatal management of fetal extrasystole. Pediatr Cardiol 1997; 18:361–366.
2. Simpson JM, Yates RW, Sharland GK: Irregular heart rate in the fetus—Not always benign. Cardiol Young 1996; 6:28–31.
3. Ferrer P: Fetal arrhythmias. In Deal B, Wolff GS, Gelband H (eds): Current Concepts in Diagnosis and Treatment of Arrhythmias in Infants and Children. Armonk, NY, Futura, 1998, pp 17–63.
4. Strasburger J: Fetal arrhythmias. Prog Pediatr Cardiol 2000; 11:1–17.
5. Larmay HJ, Strasburger JF: Differential diagnosis and management of the fetus and newborn with an irregular or abnormal heart rate. Pediatr Clin North Am 2004; 51:1033–1050.
6. Southall DP, Richard I, Hardwick RA, et al: Prospective study of fetal heart rate and rhythm patterns. Arch Dis Child 1980; 55:506–511.
7. Simpson JM: Fetal arrhythmias. Ultrasound Obstet Gynecol 2006; 27:599–606.
8. Ho SY, Anderson RH: Embryology and anatomy of the normal and abnormal conduction system. In: Gillette PC, Carson A (eds): Pediatric Arrhythmias: Electrophysiology and Pacing. Philadelphia, WB Saunders, 1990, pp 2–27.
9. James TN: Cardiac conduction system: Fetal and postnatal development. Am J Cardiol 1970; 25:213–226.
10. Shenker L, Astle C, Reed K, et al: Embryonic heart rates before the seventh week of pregnancy. J Reprod Med 1986; 31:333–335.

11. Robinson HP, Shaw-Dunn J: Fetal heart rates as determined by sonar in early pregnancy. J Obstet Gynaecol 1973; 80:805–809.

12. Case CL, Fyfe DA: Fetal dysrhythmias. In: Gillette PC, Garson A (eds): Pediatric Arrhythmias: Electrophysiology and Pacing. Philadelphia, WB Saunders, 1990, pp 637–647.

13. Wolfson RN, Sorokin Y, Rosen MG: Autonomic control of fetal cardiac activity. In: Elkayam U, Gleicher N (eds): Cardiac Problems in Pregnancy. New York, Alan R. Liss, 1982, pp 365–379.

14. Fouron JC: Fetal arrhythmias: The Saint-Justine hospital experience. Prenat Diagn 2004; 24:1068–1080.

15. Copel JA, Liang RI, Demasia K, et al: The clinical significance of irregular fetal heart rhythm. Am J Obstet Gynecol 2000; 182:813–819.

16. Toro L, Weintraub R, Shiota T, et al: Relation between persistent atrial arrhythmias and redundant septum primum flap (atrial septal aneurysm) in fetuses. Am J Cariol 1994; 73:711–713.

17. Nyberg DA, Emerson DS: Cardiac malformations. In: Nyberg Da, Mahony BS, Pretorius DH (eds): Diagnostic Ultrasound of Fetal Anomalies: Text and Atlas. Chicago, Year Book Medical, 1990, pp 300–341.

18. Reed KL: Fetal arrhythmias: Etiology, diagnosis, pathophysiology, and treatment. Semin Perinatol 1989; 114:539–544.

19. Simpson, LL, Marx GR: Diagnosis and treatment of structural cardiac abnormality and dysrhythmia. Semin Perinatol 1994; 18:215–227.

20. Eronen M: Outcome of fetuses with heart disease diagnosed in utero. Arch Dis Child Fetal Neonat Ed 1997; 77:41–46.

21. Kleinman CS, Nehgme RA: Cardiac arrhythmia in the human fetus. Pediatr Cardiol 2004; 25:234–251.

22. Simpson LL: Fetal supraventricular tachycardias: Diagnosis and management. Semin Perinatol 2000; 24:360–372.

23. Vergani P, Mariani E, Ciriello E. et al: Fetal arrhythmias: natural history and management. Ultrasound Med Biol 2005; 31:1–6.

24. Fish F, Benson DJ: Disorders of cardiac rhythm and conduction. In Allen HD, Gutgesell H, Clark EB, et al (eds): Heart Disease in Infants, Children, and Adolescents, 6th ed. Philadelphia, Lippincott, 2001, pp 482–533.

25. Friedman WF: The intrinsic physiologic properties of the developing heart. In: Friedman WF, Lesch M, Sonnenblick EH (eds): Neonatal Heart Disease. Grune & Stratton, New York, 1993, pp 87–111.

26. Mahony L: Calcium homeostasis and control of contractility in the developing heart. Semin Perinatol 1996; 20:510–519.

27. Van Engelen AD, Weitjens O, Brenner JI, et al: Management outcome and follow up of fetal tachycardia. J Am Coll Cardiol 1994; 24:1371–1375.

28. Shenker L: Fetal cardiac arrhythmias. Obstet Gynecol Surv 1979; 34:561–572.

29. Wren C: Cardiac arrhythmias in the fetus and newborn. Semin Fetal Neonat Med 2006; 11:182–190.

30. Menendez T, Achenbach S, Hofbeck M, et al: Prenatal diagnosis of QT prolongation by magnetocardiography. PACE 2000; 23:105–107.

31. Cuneo BF, Ovadia M, Strasburger JF, et al: Prenatal diagnosis and in utero treatment of torsades de pointes associated with congenital long QT syndrome. Am J Cardiol 2003; 91:1395–1398.

32. Duke C, Stuart G, Simpson JM: Ventricular tachycardia secondary to prolongation of the QT interval in a fetus with autoimmune mediated congenital heart block. Cardiol Young 2005; 15:319–321.

33. Lin MT, Hsieh FJ, Shyu MK, et al: Postnatal outcome of fetal bradycardia without significant cardiac abnormalities. Am Heart J 2004; 147:540–544.

34. Baschat AA, Gembruch U, Knoplfe G, et al: First-trimester fetal heart block: A marker for cardiac anomaly. Ultrasound Obstet Gynecol 1999: 14:311–314

35. Jaeggi ET, Hornberger LK, Smallhorn JF, et al: Prenatal diagnosis of complete atrioventricular block associated with structural heart disease: Combined experience of two tertiary care centers and review of the literature. Ultrasound Obstet Gynecol 2005; 26:16–21.

36. Berg C, Geipel A, Kohl T, et al: Atrioventricular block detected in fetal life: Associated anomalies and potential prognostic markers. Ultrasound Obstet Gynecol 2005; 26:4–15.

37. Sharland G, Tingay R, Jones A, et al: Atrioventricular and ventriculo-arterial discordance (congenitally corrected transposition of the great arteries): Echocardiographic features, associations and outcome in 34 fetuses. Heart 2005; 91:1453–1458.

38. Simpson J, Silverman N: Diagnosis of cardiac arrhythmias during fetal life. In Gembruch U (ed): Fetal Cardiology. Martin Dunitz, London, 2003, pp 333–344.

39. Fouron JC, Fournier A, Proulx F, et al: Brassard. management of fetal tachyarrhythmia based on superior vena cava/aorta Doppler flow recordings. Heart 2003; 89:1211–1216.

40. Carvalho JS, Prefumo F, Ciardelli V, et al: Evaluation of fetal arrhythmias from simultaneous pulsed wave Doppler in pulmonary artery and vein. Heart 2007; 93:1448–1453. E-pub 2006 Dec 12.

41. Chan FY, Wao SK, Chlosk A, et al: Prenatal diagnosis of congenital fetal arrhythmias by simultaneous pulsed Doppler velocimetry of the fetal abdominal aorta and inferior vena cava. Obstet Gynecol 1990; 76:2000–2005.

42. Glickstein J, Buyon J, Kim M, et al: The fetal Doppler mechanical PR interval: A validation study. Fetal Diagn Ther 2004; 19:31–34.

43. Van Bergen AH, Cuneo BF, Davis N: Prospective echocardiographic evaluation of atrioventricular conduction in fetuses with maternal Sjögren's antibodies. Am J Obstet Gynecol 2004; 191:1014–1018.

44. Jaeggi E, Fouron JC, van Doesburg N, et al: Ventriculoarterial-atrial time interval on M-mode echocardiography: A determining element in diagnosis, treatment, and prognosis of fetal supraventricular tachycardia. Heart 1998; 79:582–587.

45. Ludomirsky A, Garson A: Supraventricular tachycardia. In: Gillete PC, Garson A (eds): Pediatric Arrhythmias: Electrophysiology and Pacing. WB Saunders, Philadelphia, 1990, pp 380–426.

46. Dubin AM, Cuneo BF, Strasburger JF, et al: Congenital junctional ectopic tachycardia and congenital complete atrioventricular block: A shared etiology? Heart Rhythm J 2005; 2:313–315.

47. Reed KL, Appleton CP, Anderson CF, et al: Doppler studies of vena cava flows in human fetuses. Insights into normal and abnormal cardiac physiology. Circulation 1990; 81:498–505.

48. Huhta JC: Guidelines for evaluation of heart failure in the fetus with or without hydrops. Pediatr Cardiol 2004; 25:274–286.

49. Wakai RT, Strasburger JF, Li Z, et al: Magnetocardiographic rhythm patterns at initiation and termination of fetal supraventricular tachycardia. Circulation 2003; 107:307–312.

50. Rein AJ, O'Donnell C, Geva T, et al: Use of tissue velocity imaging in the diagnosis of fetal cardiac arrhythmias. Circulation 2002; 106:1827–1833.

51. Cuneo BF, Strasburger JF: Management strategies for fetal tachycardia. Obstet Gynecol 2000; 96:575–581.

52. Wren C: Mechanisms of fetal tachycardia [editorial]. Heart 1998; 79:536–537.

53. Simpson JM, Sharland G: Fetal tachycardias: Management and outcome of 127 cases. Heart 1998; 79:576–581.

54. Parilla B. Strasburger J, Socol M: Fetal supraventricular tachycardia complicated by hydrops fetalis: A role for direct fetal intramuscular therapy. Am J Perinatol 1996; 13:483–486.

55. Cuneo B, Strasburger JF: Management strategies for fetal tachycardia. Obstet Gynecol 2000; 96:575–581.

56. Krapp M. Baschat AA, Gembruch U, et al: Flecainide in the in utero treatment of fetal supraventricular tachycardia. Ultrasound Obstet Gynecol 2002; 19:158–164.

57. Sorensson SE: Treatment of fetal arrhythmias. Conference Proceedings. Association of European Pediatric Cardiologists. Amsterdam, The Netherlands, 2003.

58. Echt DS, Liebson PR, Mitchell LB, et al. Mortality and morbidity in patients receiving encainide, flecainide, or placebo: The Cardiac Arrhythmia Suppression Trial. N Engl J Med 1991; 324:781–788.

59. Strasburger JF: Prenatal diagnosis of fetal arrhythmias [review]. Clin Perinatol 2005; 32:891–912.

60. Oudijk MA, Michon MM, Kleinman CS, et al: Sotolol in the treatment of fetal dysrrhythmias. Circulation 2000; 101:2721–2726.

61. Groves A, Allan LD, Rosenthal E: Therapeutic trial of sympathomimetics in three cases of complete atrioventricular block in the fetus. Circulation 1995; 92:3394–3396.

62. Copel J, Buyon J, Kleinman C: Successful in utero therapy of fetal heart block. Am J Obstet Gynecol 1995; 173:1384–1390.

63. Bergmans MG, Jonker GJ, Kock HC: Fetal supraventricular tachycardia: Review of the literature. Obstet Gynecol Surv 1985; 40:61–68.

64. Naheed ZJ, Strasburger JF, Beal BJ, et al: Fetal tachycardia mechanisms and predictors of hydrops fetalis. J Am Coll Cardiol 1996; 27:1736–1740.

65. Skoll MA, Sharland GK, Allan LD: Is the ultrasound definition of fluid collections in non-immune hydrops fetalis helpful in defining the underlying cause or predicting outcome? Ultrasound Obstet Gynecol 1991; 1:309–312.

66. Hornberger K, Sahn DJ: Rhythm abnormalities of the fetus. Heart 2007; 93:1294–1300.

67. Jouannic JM, Delahaye S, Fermont L, et al: Fetal supraventricular tachycardia: A role for amiodarone as second-line therapy? Prenat Diagn 2003; 23:152–156.

68. Maeno Y, Rikitake N, Toyoda O, et al: Prenatal diagnosis of sustained bradycardia with 1:1 atrioventricular conduction. Ultrasound Obstet Gynecol 2003: 21:234–238.

69. Gladman G, Silverman ED, Yuk-Law O, et al: Fetal echocardiographic screening of pregnancies of mothers with anti-Ro and/or anti-La antibodies. Am J Perinatol 2002; 19:73–80.
70. Eronen M, Siren MK, Ekblad H, et al: Short and long-term outcome of children with congenital complete heart block diagnosed in utero or as a newborn. Pediatrics 2000; 106:86–91.
71. Schmidt KG, Ulmer HE, Silverman NH, et al: Perinatal outcome of fetal complete atrioventricular block: A multicenter experience. J Am Coll Cardiol 1991; 17:1360–1366.
72. Jaeggi ET, Hamilton RM, Silverman ED, et al: Outcome of children with fetal, neonatal, or childhood diagnosis of isolated congenital atrioventricular block: A single institution's experience of 30 years. J Am Coll Cardiol 2002; 39:130–137.

CHAPTER 22

First-Trimester Fetal Echocardiography

Marsha Wheeler

OUTLINE

Timing
Accuracy
Indications
Technique

Congenital heart disease is a common condition that accounts for approximately half of perinatal deaths resulting from congenital abnormalities and the majority of neonatal deaths.[1] The goal of prenatal diagnosis of congenital heart disease is to optimize prenatal and neonatal care. Preoperative morbidity and mortality rates are lower for prenatally diagnosed cardiac lesions because delivery can be arranged in a center with adequate neonatal resuscitation and surgical expertise.[2]

The diagnosis of abnormalities of the fetal heart also allows for comprehensive counseling, so parents may make an informed decision about continuing the pregnancy, consider medical therapies, make preparations for potential cardiac surgery, and entertain the possibility of invasive intrauterine intervention if appropriate.[3] Last, prenatal diagnosis allows the providers who care for these infants in the delivery room and nurseries to be prepared for problems that might develop after birth.

Fetal echocardiograms performed between 18 and 22 weeks' gestation remain the gold standard for diagnosis of congenital cardiac anomalies.[4] It is during this time frame that the fetus is thought to be large enough to allow a thorough evaluation of the heart but not far enough in gestation to encounter factors that can impede an adequate evaluation. These include acoustic shadowing from fetal bone, fetal position, and decreased amniotic fluid. Eighteen to 22 weeks' gestation also affords the opportunity to consider in utero intervention or termination when warranted.

Recently, advances in ultrasound equipment functionality and image resolution, and introduction of first-trimester aneuploidy screening, have contributed to an interest in first-trimester fetal echocardiography.[5] Earlier fetal echocardiography has known potential benefits, including earlier confirmation of a cardiac abnormality in high-risk patients, allowing for safer termination of pregnancy, longer time frame for fetal karyotyping and genetic counseling, and in some cases earlier initiation of in utero therapy.[6]

However, first-trimester fetal echocardiography does have limitations and should be considered an adjunct to the second-trimester fetal echocardiogram, not a replacement. The fetal heart is a very small structure at any time in gestation. This is particularly true in the first trimester. Even with the advent of high-resolution transvaginal transducers, identification of all cardiac structures necessary to constitute a complete examination is not possible. Additionally, it is well established that some congenital cardiac lesions, particularly left-sided abnormalities such as hypoplastic left heart syndrome, can be progressive abnormalities, with alterations in myocardial thickening and size of the great vessels occurring later in pregnancy.[7] Therefore a normal first-trimester fetal echocardiogram does not exclude congenital heart disease.

Timing

Development of the fetal cardiovascular system occurs by 3 to 6 weeks after conception.[1] By 10 weeks' gestation a four-chambered structure is established.[6] Current literature reports considerable variability regarding when fetal cardiac anatomy can be adequately visualized by ultrasonography. Haak et al[8] reported cardiac anatomy being adequately evaluated in 20% of cases at 11 weeks' gestation and 95% of cases at 14 weeks' gestation. Yagel et al[6] reported cardiac anatomy fully discernible in 95% of cases at 11 to 12 weeks' gestation and in 100% at 13 to 15 weeks' gestation transvaginally. Lederer et al[9] were able to obtain a four-chamber view of the heart in the first trimester in 75 of 130 (57%) cases and outflow tracts in 87 of 130 (59%) cases. Vimpelli et al[10] were able to visualize standard views of the fetal heart 58% of the time between 11 weeks and 13 weeks 6 days. Factors influencing visualization include operator experience, equipment capabilities, maternal body habitus, and fetal position.[11] Publications reporting experience with early fetal echocardiography suggest that the ideal gestational age to perform the study ranges between 11 and 16 weeks' gestation.[1,5,6,12,13]

However, it should be borne in mind that it is not prudent to use pulsed Doppler imaging, which is an essential part of a complete fetal echocardiogram, on a fetus at less than 12 weeks' gestation.

Accuracy

Yagel et al[14] summarized 6000 cases that had a transvaginal fetal echocardiogram at 13 to 16 weeks compared with 15,000 patients scanned only at mid second trimester. The sensitivity of the two approaches was compared. A total of 42 malformations were identified in the group that underwent early echocardiography. Of these, 64% were detected at the first transvaginal scan, with an additional 17% detected in the mid second trimester. Another 4% were detected in the third trimester. Fifteen percent were only diagnosed

postnatally. This compared with 80 malformations identified in the group that were only scanned in the mid second trimester. Seventy-eight percent of these abnormalities were diagnosed at the initial echocardiogram and 7% in the third trimester. Six cases were only diagnosed postnatally. In both groups the prenatal detection rate was 85%. The lesions that were missed were thought to be progressive congenital heart defects. This study demonstrates the utility of repeated scans.

Smrcek et al[15] reported 2165 cases scanned between 11 and 14 weeks' gestation. Twenty cardiac anomalies were diagnosed on an early fetal echocardiogram, with an additional nine defects detected in the second trimester and two in the third trimester. This gave an 87% detection rate prenatally.

In contrast, other studies have reported poorer results. Westin et al[12] randomized 39,000 women to either a 12-week or 18-week anatomy scan with fetal echocardiography when indicated. They had an 11% detection rate in the 12-week scan group and 15% in the 18-week group.

Delayed or missed diagnoses fall into four categories:

- Inability to visualize the anatomy because of technological limits of resolution. An example of this would be missed diagnosis of ventricular septal defects, which are the most commonly missed lesions on fetal echocardiogram at any gestational age.
- Fetal size and position, which can complicate and compromise the examination, particularly with the limited range of motion of transvaginal transducers.
- Progression of cardiac lesions in utero.
- Operator error. A high level of expertise is necessary to accurately perform any fetal echocardiogram. This may be particularly true when a fetal echocardiogram is attempted in the first trimester.

Intuitively, the more severe the cardiac abnormality, the higher the likelihood it will be diagnosed on first-trimester fetal echocardiography.[5]

Indications

Because of the lower accuracy of first-trimester fetal echocardiography, equipment requirements, and the operator expertise required, early echocardiography should be restricted to the high-risk fetus.[5] Another concern in today's health care arena is the restrictions implemented by some insurance carriers regarding the number of ultrasound examinations covered during pregnancy.

Indications that would define a patient as being at high risk are similar to those suggested for performance of a fetal echocardiogram in the second trimester (see Chapter 2). These include family history, maternal disease, abnormal karyotype, and the presence of extracardiac abnormalities. One of the driving forces of first-trimester fetal echocardiography has been the implementation of first-trimester nuchal translucency screening. This involves a first-trimester ultrasound examination to assess the size of the nuchal translucency combined with first- and second-trimester blood tests.[16]

Fetuses found to have an increased nuchal translucency, and those with positive sequential screens, were discovered to be at increased risk for aneuploidy and congenital heart defects.[17] For example, trisomy 21 is associated with a 40% to 50% occurrence of a congenital cardiac defect.[18-21] Trisomy 13 and trisomy 18 carry an association with congenital heart abnormalities of almost 100%.[20] As an isolated finding, an increased nuchal translucency carries a risk of an associated heart defect of approximately 2% to 5%.[22-26] This risk increases exponentially with an increase in nuchal translucency thickness.[26] Many, although not all,

congenital heart defects found in chromosomally normal fetuses with an increased nuchal translucency are left-sided defects such as hypoplastic left heart syndrome, coarctation of the aorta, aortic stenosis, or aortic atresia. Pathological examination of the heart and great vessels in these fetuses after termination of pregnancy has shown a greater degree of narrowing of the aortic isthmus than is seen in normal fetuses. It is hypothesized that this narrowing could result in greater perfusion of the head and neck, which in turn results in a transient increase in subcutaneous neck edema, thus the increased nuchal translucency. However, it should be kept in mind that a variety of heart defects are seen in the setting of increased nuchal translucency with normal chromosomes, so this does not explain this finding in all affected fetuses.[23] Ironically, these left-sided lesions are the most likely to be progressive, thus not apparent on early echocardiography. The caveat, however, is that if a lesion such as valvular stenosis is diagnosed early in pregnancy, it could theoretically allow earlier intervention, such as in utero balloon dilation, that in turn might alter the natural progression of the lesion.

Technique

First-trimester fetal echocardiography can be attempted with a transabdominal transducer (Fig. 22–1). However, the small size of the fetal heart at this stage, and technical factors that impede transabdominal ultrasonography, make this approach inadequate in most cases.

Transvaginal ultrasonography provides a higher frequency transducer and a decreased probe-to-target distance, both of which increase image resolution (Fig. 22–2). Despite this, transvaginal ultrasonography does have its limitations. Specifically, imaging planes are limited by a narrow focal range, and angles of insonation are limited. Spatial orientation compared with transabdominal sonography is also more difficult.[5] Ideally, all views of the heart recommended for a fetal echocardiogram performed in the second trimester should also be used in a first trimester fetal echocardiogram. Because of the limitations mentioned previously, this is not feasible.

An attempt to acquire as much information as possible should be made.

Cardiac position and axis should be identified. Visualization of the four cardiac chambers and outflow tracts is usually possible (Figs. 22–3 and

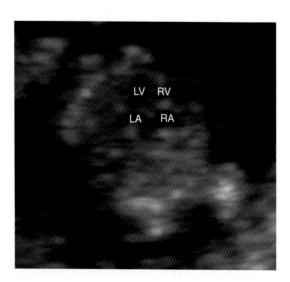

Figure 22–1 Transabdominal apical four-chamber view in a first-trimester fetus. *LA,* Left atrium; *LV,* left ventricle; *RA,* right atrium; *RV,* right ventricle.

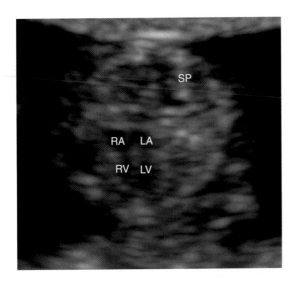

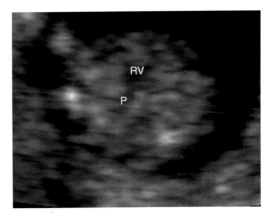

Figure 22–4 Transabdominal long-axis view of the pulmonary artery. *P*, Pulmonary artery; *RV*, right ventricle.

Figure 22–2 Transvaginal apical four-chamber view in a first-trimester fetus. *LA*, Left atrium; *LV*, left ventricle; *RA*, right atrium; *RV*, right ventricle; *SP*, spine.

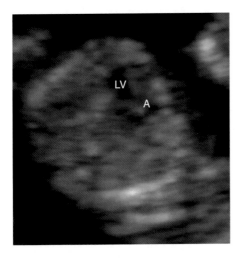

Figure 22–3 Transabdominal long-axis view of the aorta. *A*, Aorta; *LV*, left ventricle.

22–4). However, normal great artery relationship or overriding of a great vessel may be difficult to appreciate. Assessment of systemic veins, pulmonary veins, and the aortic and ductal arches may be limited by image resolution.[11] Assessment of cardiac size at this early gestational age is usually of little value.

The use of color or power Doppler imaging may allow some assessment of cardiac connections and

valve function.[23] Yagel advocates early fetal echocardiography with use of five transverse planes (Fig. 22–5).[27] With this protocol, the examination begins from a transverse image of the fetal upper abdomen showing the spine, stomach, and inferior vena cava. This plane establishes fetal orientation and situs. The transducer is then moved cephalad on the fetus to the level of the four-chamber view. At this level the presence and size of all four chambers should be evaluated. A continuation of this cephalad movement results in the third plane, often referred to as the five-chamber view.

The five-chamber view allows assessment of the relationship between the ascending aorta and the left ventricle. Aortic size and possible override may be visualized in this plane.

A fourth plane, still continuing on a cephalad path, results in visualization of the bifurcation of the pulmonary arteries. Similar to the aorta, this level provides information regarding vessel orientation and relationship to the ventricle. The fifth and final level is the three-vessel and trachea view. It is obtained by continuing the cephalad movement of the transducer and obliquing the plane slightly. As reviewed in Chapter 2, this view allows visualization of the main pulmonary artery/ductus arteriosus confluence, the transverse aortic arch, and the superior vena cava. Confirmation of vessel presence and a comparison in size can be made in this view. Additionally, correct location of both great vessels to the left of the trachea can be

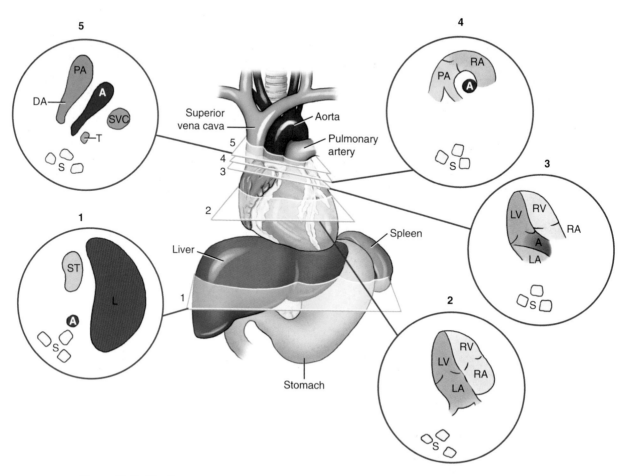

Figure 22–5 The five transverse planes advocated by Yagel et al[27] to assess the fetal heart in the first trimester. *1*, Transverse view of the fetal abdomen used to identify abdominal situs. *2*, Apical four-chamber view used to confirm the presence of four chambers. *3*, Apical five-chamber view used to confirm orientation of the aorta and continuity with the left ventricle. *4*, Pulmonary artery bifurcation view used to confirm orientation of the pulmonary artery and continuity with the right ventricle. *5*, Three-vessel trachea view used to confirm presence, size, and orientation of the great vessels. Both should be leftward of the trachea in the normal heart. *A*, Aorta; *L*, liver; *LA*, left atrium; *LV*, left ventricle; *PA*, pulmonary artery; *RA*, right atrium; *RV*, right ventricle; *S*, spine; *SVC*, superior vena cava.

confirmed. M-mode imaging is also important in a first-trimester fetal echocardiogram to assess the fetal heart rate (Figs. 22–6 and 22–7). Abnormal heart rates (slow, fast, or irregular), especially in the setting of an increased nuchal translucency, raises the suspicion of congenital heart disease. It may also increase the risk of spontaneous abortion. Early detection of fetal tachycardias can provide the possibility of earlier in utero intervention.[24]

In summary, first-trimester fetal echocardiography is feasible and may be advantageous in a high-risk population. However, it requires high-resolution ultrasound equipment and significant operator expertise. Severe congenital heart disease may be identified on first-trimester fetal echocardiography, but more subtle lesions and progressive anomalies will be missed. Therefore it should be used as an adjunct to second-trimester fetal echocardiography and not a replacement.

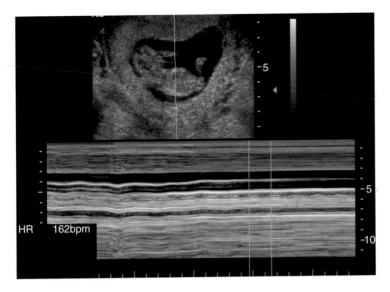

Figure 22–6 Transabdominal image of a first-trimester fetus with M-mode imaging to determine fetal heart rate.

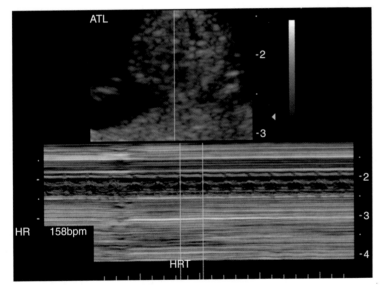

Figure 22–7 Transvaginal image of a first-trimester fetus with M-mode imaging to determine fetal heart rate.

References

1. Johnson B, Simpson L: Screening for congenital heart disease: A move toward earlier echocardiography. Am J Perinatol 2007; 24:449–456.
2. Jaeffi ET, Sholler GF, Jones OD, et al: Comparative analysis of pattern, management and outcome of pre- versus postnatally diagnosed major congenital heart disease: A population-based study. Ultrasound Obstet Gynecol 2001; 17:380–385.
3. Allan L: Screening the fetal heart. Ultrasound Obstet Gynecol 2006; 28:5–7.
4. Lee W: Performance of the fetal cardiac ultrasound examination. J Ultrasound Med 1998; 17:601–607.
5. Gabriel CC, Galindo A, Martinez JM, et al: Early prenatal diagnosis of major cardiac anomalies in a

high-risk population. Prenat Diagn 2002; 22:586–593.

6. Yagel S, Cohen SM, Messing B: First and early second trimester fetal heart screening. Curr Opin Obstet Gynecol 2007; 19:183–190.

7. Fliedner R, Kreiselmaier P, Schwarze A, et al: Development of hypoplastic left heart syndrome after diagnosis of aortic stenosis in the first trimester by early echocardiography. Ultrasound Obstet Gynecol 2006; 28:106–109.

8. Haak MC, Twisk JWR, van Vugt JM: How successful is fetal echocardiographic examination in the first trimester of pregnancy? Ultrasound Obstet Gynecol 2002; 20:9–13.

9. Lederer A, Hasenohrl G, Gruber R, et al: Feasibility of fetal echocardiography at 11–14 weeks scan. Ultraschall Med 2006; 27:563–567.

10. Vimpelli T, Huhtala H, Acharya G: Fetal echocardiography during routine first-trimester screening: A feasibility study in an unselected population. Prenat Diagn 2006; 26:475–482.

11. McAuliffe FM, Trines J, Nield LE, et al: Early fetal echocardiography—A reliable prenatal diagnosis tool. Am J Obstet Gynecol 2005; 193:1253–1259.

12. Westin M, Saltvedt S, Bergman G, et al: Routine ultrasound examination at 12 or 18 gestational weeks for prenatal detection of major congenital heart malformations? A randomized controlled trial comprising 36,299 fetuses. BJOG 2006; 113:675–682.

13. Lopes LM, Brizot ML, Lopes MAB, et al: Structural and functional cardiac abnormalities identified prior to 16 weeks' gestation in fetuses with increased nuchal translucency. Ultrasound Obstet Gynecol 2003; 22:470–478.

14. Yagel S, Weissman A, Rotstein Z, et al: Congenital heart defects: Natural course and in utero development. Circulation 1997; 96:550–555.

15. Smrcek JM, Berg C, Geipel A, et al: Detection rate of early fetal echocardiography and in utero development of congenital heart defects. J Ultrasound Med 2006; 25:187–196.

16. Nicolaides KH, Azar G, Byrne D, et al: Fetal nuchal translucency: ultrasound screening for chromosomal defects in first trimester of pregnancy. BMJ 1992; 304:867–869.

17. Makrydimas G, Sotiriadis A, Huggon IC, et al: Nuchal translucency and fetal cardiac defects: A pooled analysis of major fetal echocardiography centers. Am J Obstet Gynecol 2005; 192:89–95.

18. Ferencz C, Neill CA: Cardiovascular malformations: Prevalence at livebirth. In: Freedom RM, Benson LN, Smallhorn JF (eds): Neonatal Heart Disease. London, Springer-Verlag, 1992, pp 19–29.

19. Stewart PA, Wladimiroff JW, Reuss A, et al: Fetal echocardiography: A review of six years experience. Fetal Ther 1987; 2:222–231.

20. Nicolaides K, Shawwa L, Brizot M, et al: Ultrasonographically detectable markers of fetal chromosomal defects. Ultrasound Obstet Gynecol 1993; 3:56–59.

21. Cleves MA, Hobbs CA, Cleves PA, et al: Congenital defects among liveborn infants with Down syndrome. Birth Defects Research (Part A) 2007; 79:657–663.

22. Friedberg MK, Silverman NH: Changing indications for fetal echocardiography in a university center population. Prenat Diagn 2004; 24:781–786.

23. McAuliffe FM, Hornberger LK, Winsor S, et al: Fetal cardiac defects and increased nuchal translucency thickness: A prospective study. Am J Obstet Gynecol 2004; 191:1486–1490.

24. Westin M, Saltvedt S, Bergman G, et al: Is measurement of nuchal translucency thickness a useful screening tool for heart defects? A study of 16,383 fetuses. Ultrasound Obstet Gynecol 2006; 27:632–639.

25. Muller MA, Clur SA, Timmerman E, et al: Nuchal translucency measurement and congenital heart defects: Modest association in low-risk pregnancies. Prenat Diagn 2007; 27:164–169.

26. Atzei A, Gajewska K, Huggon IC, et al: Relationship between nuchal translucency thickness and prevalence of major cardiac defects in fetuses with normal karyotype. Ultrasound Obstet Gynecol 2005; 26:154–157.

27. Yagel S, Cohen SM, Achiron R: Examination of the fetal heart by five short-axis views: A proposed screening a method for comprehensive cardiac evaluation. Ultrasound Obstet Gynecol 2001; 17:367–369.

CHAPTER 23

Three-Dimensional Fetal Echocardiography

Julia A. Drose

Ultrasound technology has improved significantly over the last few decades. As three-dimensional (3-D) and four-dimensional (4-D) technologies have improved, so has the interest in applying them to fetal echocardiography. Two primary reasons drive this interest. First, the technology is now readily available on most ultrasound systems. Second, standard two-dimensional (2-D) fetal echocardiography requires considerable expertise to perform and interpret correctly. It can also be very time consuming. Major drawbacks to applying 3-D/4-D technologies to the heart have been acquisition time and the need for cardiac gating. Recent improvements in technology allow for near real-time examination.[1]

3-D ultrasonography requires a volume of sonographic data to be acquired and stored. Once this is accomplished, the data can be manipulated in different ways to display a variety of scan planes. This offers an advantage in the fetal heart because a fetus cannot cooperate with positioning, making certain scan planes unobtainable with standard 2-D imaging.

Volume acquisition requires specialized transducers that are equipped with an electromagnetic position sensor to supply spatial position and orientation data. The transducer is held stationary over the area of interest while an electronic "sweep" is made, acquiring numerous slices of information. These volumes are stored in the systems computer and can then be manipulated either on the ultrasound system itself or on a separate workstation to generate surface images or 2-D sections.

4-D ultrasonography refers to the real-time display of 3-D images. In other words, it consists of three dimensions plus time.

Techniques

Several different techniques for acquiring 3-D data have recently emerged. These include spatiotemporal image correlation (STIC), multiplanar reconstruction, spatiotemporal image correlation with tomographic ultrasound imaging (TUI-STIC), tissue Doppler gating (TDOG), matrix array real-time 3-D, and inversion mode (IM).

Spatiotemporal Image Correlation

STIC is an automated volume acquisition technique.[2] It is based on a transducer sweep that acquires a large volume set. The volume set is usually acquired over a period of 7.5 to 30 seconds, at a sweep angle of 20 degree to 40 degrees and a frame rate of 150 frames per second.[1,3]

The ultrasound system then applies mathematical algorithms to process the volume set. Image gating is accomplished by peak systole signals being automatically detected from the underlying images. The B-mode images are then correlated with the heart rate, and a complete heart cycle is displayed. This 4-D loop can be manipulated to display any acquired scanning plane at any point of the cardiac cycle.[4] The advantage of STIC technology is that reconstruction takes place immediately. It can also be combined with other applications such as B-flow, color Doppler imaging, power Doppler imaging, and tissue Doppler imaging.

Multiplanar Reconstruction

Multiplanar reconstruction displays the X, Y, and Z axes of an acquired volume set, all on one panel. The operator is then able to manipulate the volume to display any plane within it. The fourth image on the panel will then display a surface rendering of the desired structure or level (Fig. 23–1).[1]

Spatiotemporal Image Correlation with Tomographic Ultrasound Imaging

TUI-STIC uses STIC technology, which allows the acquisition of cardiac volumes combined with tomographic ultrasound imaging. This allows a variable number (up to nine) of reconstructed 2-D sections to be displayed on a single panel.[5,6] With TUI-STIC, an acquisition is performed orthogonal to the fetal body (i.e., from an apical or subcostal four-chamber view). If the volume is large enough, all consecutive slices through the fetal heart will be displayed. This results in being able to view most cardiovascular connections necessary to thoroughly evaluate the fetal heart at the same time. Visualizing all views on a single panel may increase the ability to determine whether a heart is normal or aid in understanding the abnormality at hand. TUI-STIC can also be combined with color Doppler imaging, which may provide functional information.

The major limitation of TUI-STIC technology is that a large volume of images is necessary to display planes throughout the entire fetal heart. This corresponds to files that range in size from 4 to 8 megabytes for a second-trimester fetal heart, to 20 to 30 megabytes for a third-trimester fetal heart. Another issue encountered with fetuses later in gestation is increased mineralization of fetal bone, which can impede the ability to acquire images in sequence.[5]

Tissue Doppler Gating

TDOG is a technique applied to 3-D ultrasound imaging that uses tissue Doppler data to calculate a gating signal.[7] Velocity of tissue is measured on each point in a sector or linear grid. These data are acquired simultaneously with the 2-D image, and the images are then correlated with different points of the cardiac cycle. Reconstruction is then required to convert the B-mode scan lines into a sequence of voxel data sets. 3-D or 4-D display is then possible.

Matrix Array Real-Time Three-Dimensional Imaging

Matrix transducers are biplane probes that allow the display of two simultaneous orthogonal imaging planes without having to move the transducer (Fig. 23–2).[8] From these planes, a real-time 3-D image (4-D) can be displayed (Fig. 23–3). This is accomplished without any transfer or postprocessing of data. Additionally, cardiac gating is not required. Advantages of this method are that either a biplane or a 3-D image can be immediately displayed and evaluated. A limitation is that the size capabilities of the 3-D volume may not be able to contain the entire fetal heart. Also, currently available matrix transducers are of frequencies (2–4 MHz) that are more applicable to pediatric or adult echocardiography. However, technological advances should allow this technology to be applied to higher frequency transducers in the near future.

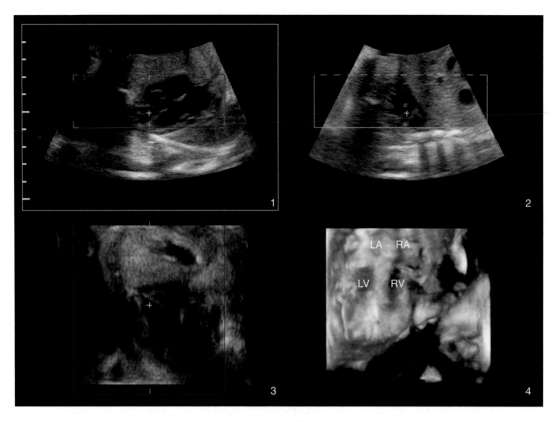

Figure 23–1 Multiplanar reconstruction of the fetal heart showing a four-chamber view *(4)*. A cursor is placed on the X *(1)*, Y *(2)*, and Z *(3)* planes to identify the desired area of reconstruction. A surface rendering of that specified area is then displayed in the lower right hand corner. *LA,* Left atrium; *LV,* left ventricle; *RA,* right atrium; *RV,* right ventricle.

Inversion Mode

IM is a form of postprocessing static 3-D or STIC images that inverts the gray scale of tissue and fluid-filled spaces. This results in fluid-filled spaces such as the cardiac chambers to be displayed as white, whereas tissue such as myocardium essentially disappears. This technique has potential for aiding in quantifying ventricular volumes. Yagel et al[1] used IM combined with STIC acquisition to derive nomograms for fetal stroke volume and cardiac ejection fraction.

Benefits and Limitations of Three-Dimensional and Four-Dimensional Fetal Echocardiography

Two-dimensional evaluation of the fetal heart is still the gold standard for assessing the presence or absence of congenital heart disease.[9] It can,

however, be a time-intensive examination that requires a considerable amount of expertise both to acquire and interpret images correctly.[10,11] Examiners must also be able to mentally recreate a 3-D image from 2-D picture.

3-D and 4-D imaging may aid in diagnosis of fetal cardiac abnormalities by using computer reconstruction to display intracardiac connections that may be abnormal in the setting of congenital heart disease in a variety of different planes. Other potential advantages of 3-D and 4-D fetal echocardiography include the following:

- Standardization and ease of imaging that could reduce operator dependency[10]
- 4-D display allows an examiner to dynamically visualize the heart in orthogonal planes at the same time, potentially aiding in identification of congenital heart disease.

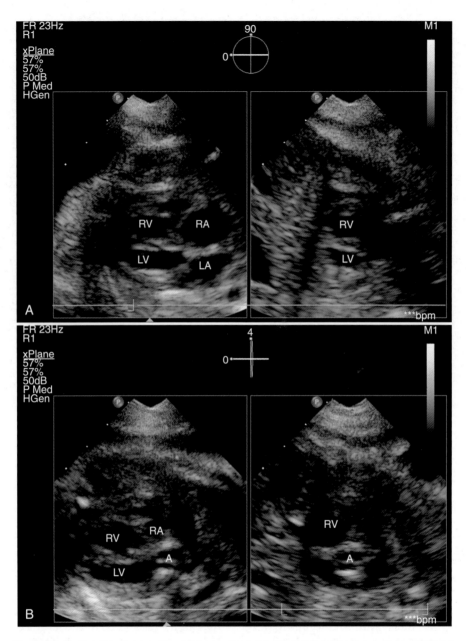

Figure 23–2 X-matrix images allowing two orthogonal planes of a structure to be evaluated in real-time simultaneously. **A,** Imaging a four-chamber view and short-axis view of the ventricles simultaneously. **B,** Imaging long-axis and short-axis views of the aorta *(A)* simultaneously. *LA,* Left atrium; *LV,* left ventricle; *RA,* right atrium; *RV,* right ventricle.

- Planes can be obtained with off-line image rendering that may not be possible to obtain during a 2-D examination because of fetal position.[11]
- Some technologies such as STIC may decrease evaluation time.[8]
- Provides the examiner with an unlimited number of images for review.[8]
- Data volumes can be stored and reviewed off-line by the examiner at any time or can be sent electronically to a remote site if a fetal echocardiography specialist is not available on site.[8]
- Available software allows postprocessing of 3-D volumes with the ability to prioritize display of hyperechoic or anechoic areas within a volume.[8]

Current limitations to 3-D and 4-D fetal echocardiography include the following:

- Acquisition artifacts resulting from fetal or maternal motion. These are being minimized with a variety of gating methods available on current technologies and decreasing acquisition periods.[10,12]
- Early gestational age, fetal position, and increased maternal body habitus may limit the ability to acquire sequential images or images with sufficient image resolution to aid in diagnosis. Many of these factors are also inherent with 2-D imaging.
- Fetal arrhythmias may interfere with image gating methods, causing misregistration of information.[3]
- Quality of the 3-D or 4-D image is highly dependent on the quality of the 2-D image.[12]
- Depending on the piece of equipment used to obtain 3-D or 4-D acquisitions, operator controls can be complicated.[5]

Accuracy

Accuracy is dependent on the method of image acquisition used. Herberg et al[12] used a freehand 3-D acquisition with a concurrent Doppler signal to provide gating. They reported that not all fetal cardiac anomalies seen on 2-D imaging could be identified on 3-D acquisition.

Goncalves et al[6] used TUI-STIC technology and reported visualization rates of the four-chamber, five-chamber, and three-vessel views of 97.4%, 88.2%, and 79.5%, respectively. They also reported

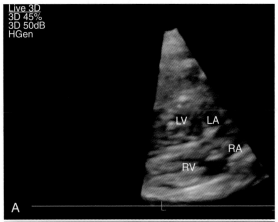

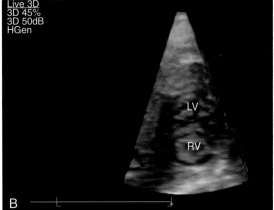

Figure 23–3 3-D real-time (4-D) images obtained from the x-matrix planes, showing a subcostal four-chamber view **(A)** and short-axis view of the ventricles **(B)**. *LA*, Left atrium; *LV*, left ventricle; *RA*, right ventricle; *RV*, right ventricle.

a 73.3% correlation between abnormalities suspected on 3-D fetal echocardiography and postnatal diagnosis. Paladini et al[5] reported acceptable image quality in 67.8% of cases attempted. Chaoui et al[3] evaluated 62 fetuses with STIC technology and color Doppler imaging. Diagnostic image quality was obtained in 88% of cases. Acar et al[8] used 3-D matrix technology and reported successful image acquisition in 93% of cases.

Finally, it should be borne in mind that 3-D rendering creates virtual images.[1] Application of algorithms designed to smooth images may lead to loss of data from the original sweep. Therefore

3-D fetal echocardiography should always be used as a correlative to standard 2-D ultrasound imaging.

In summary, 3-D and 4-D ultrasonography are common adjuncts to standard obstetrical imaging. The application of these technologies to fetal echocardiography is not as straightforward. No large studies have been performed to quantify the ability of 3-D or 4-D ultrasound imaging to improve the accuracy of the detection of congenital cardiac abnormalities in the fetus. Information obtained from 3-D or 4-D imaging may be useful in making a cardiac diagnosis, but currently it is only an adjunct to 2-D imaging and not required to make an accurate diagnosis.

References

1. Yagel S, Cohen SM, Shapiro I, et al: 3D and 4D ultrasound in fetal cardiac scanning: A new look at the fetal heart. Ultrasound Obstet Gynecol 2007; 29:81–95.
2. Devore GR, Falkensammer P, Sklansky MS, et al: Spatio-temporal image correlation (STIC): New technology for evaluation of the fetal heart. Ultrasound Obstet Gynecol 2003; 22:380–387.
3. Chaoui R, Hoffmann J, Heling KS: Three-dimensional (3D) and 4D color Doppler fetal echocardiography using spatio-temporal image correlation (STIC). Ultrasound Obstet Gynecol 2004; 23:535–545.
4. Gonçalves LF, Lee W, Espinoza J, et al: Examination of the fetal heart by four-dimensional (4D) ultrasound with spatio-temporal image correlation (STIC). Ultrasound Obstet Gynecol 2006; 27:336–348.
5. Paladini D, Vassallo M, Sglavo G, et al: The role of spatio-temporal image correlation (STIC) with tomographic ultrasound imaging (TUI) in the sequential analysis of fetal congenital heart disease. Ultrasound Obstet Gynecol 2006; 27:555–561.
6. Gonçalves LF, Espinoza J, Romero R, et al: Four-dimensional ultrasonography of the fetal heart using a novel tomographic ultrasound imaging display. J Perinat Med 2006; 34:39–55.
7. Brekke S, Tegnander E, Torp HG, et al: Tissue Doppler gated (TDOG) dynamic three-dimensional ultrasound imaging of the fetal heart. Ultrasound Obstet Gynecol 2004; 24:192–198.
8. Acar P, Dulac Y, Taktak A, et al: Real-time three-dimensional fetal echocardiography using matrix probe. Prenatal Diagn 2005; 25:370–375.
9. Volpe P, Campobasso G, DeRobertis V, et al: Two- and four-dimensional echocardiography with B-flow imaging and spatiotemporal image correlation in prenatal diagnosis of isolated total anomalous pulmonary venous connection. Ultrasound Obstet Gynecol 2007; 30:830–837.
10. Gonçalves LF, Lee W, Chaiworapongsa T, et al: Four-dimensional ultrasonography of the fetal heart with spatiotemporal image correlation. Am J Obstet Gynecol 2003; 189:1792–1802.
11. Vinals F, Pacheco V, Giuliano A: Fetal atrioventricular valve junction in normal fetuses and in fetuses with complete atrioventricular septal defect assessed by 4D volume rendering. Ultrasound Obstet Gynecol 2006; 28:26–31.
12. Herberg U, Goldberg H, Breuer J: Three-and four-dimensional freehand fetal echocardiography: A feasibility study using a hand-held Doppler probe for cardiac gating. Ultrasound Obstet Gynecol 2005; 25:362–371.

CHAPTER 24

Prenatal Intervention in the Fetus with Cardiac Disease

Adel K. Younoszai

Modern-day treatment of congenital heart disease has been redefined by the success of neonatal surgery to address complex structural disorders. Conditions that were palliated or lethal are now routinely addressed within the first days of life. Tetralogy of Fallot, historically not repaired until early childhood, is routinely corrected by 3 to 4 months of age to promote normal development of the right ventricle and pulmonary arteries.[1-4] In addition, for complex cardiac lesions that remain unrepairable, such as hypoplastic left heart syndrome, successful palliative operations have been developed with remarkably good outcomes. Many centers now report survival rates for the Norwood palliative approach for hypoplastic left heart syndrome as high as 80% to 90% at 5 years of life.[5,6]

Fetal intervention for cardiac lesions is not a new concept. It was tried with limited technical success 15 to 20 years ago, but with no evidence of overall improvement in cardiac performance, it was not aggressively pursued.[7-9] The advent of improved ultrasound equipment and interventional technology led to renewed interest in prenatal intervention. The concept was aggressively revisited just after the turn of the millennium, with published reports of technical success and safety in 2004.[10,11]

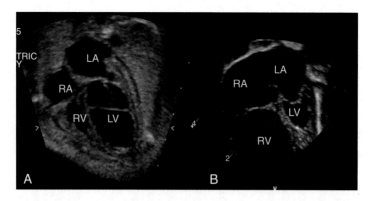

Figure 24–1 Fetal critical aortic stenosis and postnatal hypoplastic left heart syndrome. **A,** Prenatal echocardiogram showing dilation of the left ventricle *(LV)* in the setting of a severely stenotic aortic valve. **B,** Postnatal echocardiogram reveals a small, non-apex-forming left ventricle. *LA,* Left atrium; *RA,* right atrium; *RV,* right ventricle.

Candidate Lesions

To be considered for fetal intervention, a lesion should meet the following criteria. First, it should have a poor prognosis with standard therapy. In other words, there should be significant potential to improve the outcome. Also, the fetal cardiac abnormality should be progressive such that an intervention may alter this progression in a beneficial way.

Critical Aortic Stenosis

Critical aortic stenosis has, perhaps, been the lesion generating the most interest in fetal intervention. Although mild disease may be well tolerated in a fetus and only require postnatal balloon valvuloplasty, severe obstruction typically presents in the second trimester with left ventricular enlargement and dysfunction. Studies have shown the natural history of this lesion is to develop progressive dysfunction and endocardial fibroelastosis with disproportionate growth, resulting in functional hypoplastic left heart syndrome (Fig. 24–1).[12] In hypoplastic left heart syndrome, the left heart is severely underdeveloped and dysfunctional and therefore cannot support a normal stroke volume and cardiac output. The postnatal palliative approach to address this inadequacy is the Norwood palliation, which subjects the child to a series of surgeries designed to utilize the single functional right ventricle to support both the pulmonary and systemic circulations. Despite the remarkable advances in surgical techniques and

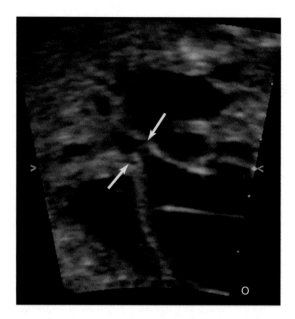

Figure 24–2 Aortic valve in fetal critical aortic stenosis. *Arrows* indicate a thickened and doming aortic valve.

perioperative care with improved early survival, the long-term prognosis for these patients remains guarded at best.

Sonographically, several features can be evaluated to help determine the severity of the aortic valve disease and therefore the risk of progression to hypoplastic left heart syndrome. Typically, the aortic valve is small with thickened, severely immobile leaflets (Fig. 24–2) and only a tiny jet of antegrade flow into the ascending aorta by color or pulsed Doppler imaging. The papillary muscles and endocardium of the left ventricle are often echogenic, suggesting the presence of scar tissue or endocardial fibroelastosis. Flow across the foramen ovale is reversed as a result of left ventricular dysfunction and resultant high filling pressure in the left atrium. Finally, as the cardiac output decreases because of valve obstruction and left ventricular dysfunction, the flow through the aortic arch reverses, with the right ventricular output coursing across the ductus arteriosus and retrograde through the arch to perfuse the upper body in the absence of adequate forward flow. The Doppler gradient across the aortic valve is not typically useful to estimate the severity of disease because this may only be a sign of poor ventricular function. In rare cases the left heart can enlarge so severely that it compromises the right ventricular cardiac performance, causing fetal hydrops and death.

The objective of fetal intervention is to balloon the aortic valve, relieving the obstruction to the left ventricle and allowing it to recover function and grow as the fetus develops, preventing progression to hypoplastic left heart syndrome.

Hypoplastic Left Heart Syndrome with Intact Atrial Septum

Another lesion potentially amenable to fetal intervention is the atrial septum when it is restrictive or intact in the setting of hypoplastic left heart syndrome. Although, as previously mentioned, the survival rates for hypoplastic left heart syndrome are considerably higher than they used to be, in 5% to 10% of cases the foramen ovale can become severely restrictive or close completely. After delivery this results in an inability to adequately drain the pulmonary vascular bed as a result of distal obstruction and the inability to decompress across the foramen ovale (Fig. 24–3). Historically, the prognosis for these infants has been extremely poor, with mortality rates as high at 90% with death typically occurring immediately after birth. Despite new aggressive therapy, including delivery in the operating room or catheterization laboratory for immediate intervention, the mortality rate remains at 60% to 70% at best. One explanation for these continued poor outcomes may be the period of time in utero during which the pulmonary venous system cannot adequately drain, causing damage to the pulmonary venous system. Examination of the postmortem

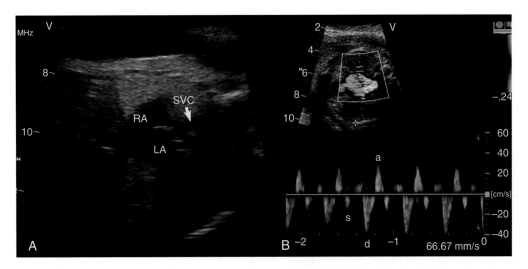

Figure 24–3 Fetal hypoplastic left heart syndrome with intact atrial septum. **A,** Fetal echocardiogram in the sagittal plane showing the bowing of the atrial septum into the right atrium *(RA)* because of high left atrial pressure. **B,** Doppler tracing of a pulmonary vein in the same patient. There is prominence of the atrial reversal wave *(a)*, indicating a significant amount of reversed flow into the pulmonary veins with atrial contraction because the left atrium *(LA)* is otherwise obstructed. *d,* Diastole; *s,* systole; *SVC,* superior vena cava.

lungs reveals arterialization of the pulmonary veins, which likely contributes to the persistent pulmonary edema and high vascular resistance that occurs despite adequate decompression of the left atrium through a newly created atrial septal communication.[13]

Fetal intervention to open the atrial septum hopes to decompress the left atrium and lungs, allowing for normal pulmonary venous development, a stable neonate, and improved prognosis for the palliative approach to hypoplastic left heart syndrome.

Pulmonary Atresia with Intact Ventricular Septum

Similar to the left side, when there is severe obstruction of the right heart without a communication between the two ventricles, the right ventricle and tricuspid valve become hypoplastic (Fig. 24–4). In patients where the tricuspid valve appears of adequate size, postnatal ballooning of the pulmonary valve can lead to remodeling and growth of the right ventricle with a functionally normal right side. However, when the tricuspid valve or the right ventricle are severely underdeveloped to the point where they cannot sustain a normal cardiac output, the result is hypoplastic right heart syndrome with reliance on the left ventricle as the single circulating pump. The outcome for this disease is similar to that of hypoplastic left heart syndrome. Although the single left ventricle is better able to handle the workload than is a single right ventricle, the significant incidence of right ventricle–to–coronary artery fistulas and coronary artery stenosis results in relatively high mortality rates, with a 5-year survival rate of approximately 65%.[14-16]

The goal of fetal intervention would be to balloon open the pulmonary valve, increasing flow across the right heart and therefore promoting its normal growth and development in utero.

Technical Aspects

The techniques for fetal intervention have been discussed in several excellent review articles on fetal intervention.[17-20] Performance of cardiac intervention in the fetus is complex, requiring multispecialty coordination and communication because there are two patients, the mother and the fetus, to monitor, treat, and care for.

Program Development

Before a fetal intervention can be performed, a well-organized team must be formed. The basic components of the team should include a perinatologist with the ability to assess the fetal heart, a sonologist who can guide placement of the needle into the correct orientation within the heart, and a pediatric cardiac interventionalist who will manipulate the wires and catheters that enter the heart for the procedure. The skills, handoffs, and communication must be practiced ahead of time to make the procedure as quick and efficient as possible. In addition to the team that performs the procedure, there must be an anesthesiologist dedicated to monitoring the health and status of the mother, and it is recommended to also have a pediatric anesthesiologist available who can monitor the status of the fetus. For the obstetrical and interventional procedures, often nursing and other medical assistance is needed to manipulate the equipment. Because there is limited experience with fetal intervention, it is also important to enlist institutional support. Depending on the institution, this may come in the form of preprocedure submittal to the institutional review board to approve fetal intervention as an innovative practice or research protocol.

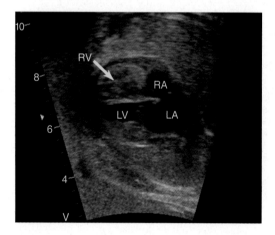

Figure 24–4 Fetal pulmonary atresia with intact ventricular septum. The right ventricle *(RV) (arrow)* has the typical appearance, with severe hypertrophy and diminished chamber size. *LA*, Left atrium; *LV*, left ventricle; *RA*, right atrium.

Counseling and Consent

It cannot be overstated that the potential risk to both the mother and fetus is a serious consideration in pursuing a treatment option that remains relatively novel. With that in mind, any mother who is considering the procedure should be fully counseled by both the obstetrician and fetal cardiologist involved in the procedure. In addition, involvement of a bioethics committee in development of the program and counseling of the patient may help to ensure that informed consent is obtained.

Timing

In theory, the earlier that an intervention can be performed, the more potential impact there is for normal development. In practice, the diagnosis of a candidate lesion is not made until 18 to 24 weeks' gestation. In addition, the technical feasibility of performing interventions on the basis of the size of the equipment places a lower limit of approximately 22 weeks' gestation in general. It is likely that intervening later in gestation has a lower procedural risk; however, that must be balanced against a theoretical decrease in potential benefit.

Techniques

Three approaches to intervention in the fetus are possible: percutaneous, transuterine, and open fetal surgery.

Percutaneous. The most commonly used technique is the percutaneous approach, which has the advantage of minimizing the invasive nature of the procedure for the mother. With this approach the mother is monitored but typically is awake for the procedure. The fetal position is checked by ultrasonography and optimized, if needed, by external manipulation. In some cases, maternal general anesthesia is used to help relax the uterus for improved manipulation. Although the fetus may be somewhat anesthetized by transplacental administration of maternal anesthesia, for optimal control during the procedure the fetus is typically given an intramuscular injection of medications; typically a combination of paralytic, narcotic, and atropine to preemptively address any fetal bradycardia that may occur during the procedure.

Under sonographic guidance, a hollow needle with a stylet is introduced across the skin, through the uterine wall, into the amniotic sac, and then across the fetal chest or abdominal wall, depending on the desired orientation, and into the heart (Fig. 24–5). With the needle in good position, the

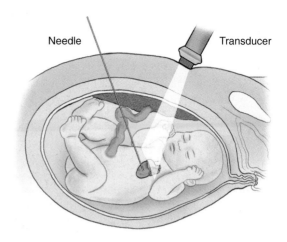

Figure 24–5 The percutaneous approach to access the fetal heart. Ultrasound is used to guide the trochar through the uterine wall and fetal chest wall, into the fetal heart.

stylet is removed and a wire advanced into the desired location. A balloon catheter is then advanced over the wire and the balloon inflated, typically several times, until the desired effect is achieved (Fig. 24–6). The balloon and wire are then removed, the stylet replaced in the needle, and the entire system withdrawn from the fetus and maternal abdomen.

Although ultrasound is typically used to visualize the cardiac structures, the use of a fiberoptic cardioscope for direct visualization of the aortic valve has been described as well.[21] If significant bradycardia or fetal instability is noted during the examination, medications such as epinephrine can be administered to the fetus by direct intracardiac or alternatively intramuscular injection, depending on the location of the needle at the time. Also, if a pericardial effusion is noted, the needle can be placed in the pericardial space and the effusion evacuated.

For ballooning of the aortic valve, the cannula is introduced through the apex of the left ventricle and oriented anteriorly, pointing up toward the left ventricular outflow tract with advancement of the guidewire across the aortic valve and into the ascending aorta. In the case of an atrial septostomy, the needle is introduced through the chest wall and right atrium and advanced at a perpendicular angle to the septum. Several methods have been described to cross the atrial septum,

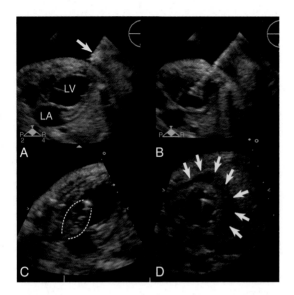

Figure 24–6 Fetal intervention for critical aortic stenosis. **A,** Placement of a trocar *(arrow)* into the amniotic sac just outside the fetal chest wall positioned at the apex of the left ventricle *(LV)*. *LA,* Left atrium. **B,** Advancement of the trocar into the left ventricle with the tip directed toward the outflow tract. **C,** Inflation of the balloon (outlined by *dashed line*) across the aortic valve. **D,** Pericardial effusion (outlined by *arrows*) noted after a second attempt at ballooning. The needle was withdrawn into the pericardial space and the fluid evacuated without reaccumulation.

including use of the introduction catheter to create a defect, puncture of the septum with a small stiff wire, radiofrequency ablation, and even photofulguration of the septal tissue with a neodymium: yttrium-aluminum-garnet laser fiber.[22]

Transuterine.   Although the percutaneous approach minimizes risk to the mother, the manipulation of the fetus and imaging of the heart can be very limited, especially in the case of a large maternal habitus with a significant amount of subcutaneous fat interposed between the skin and uterus. Because optimal orientation of the fetus during the procedure is essential for success, some institutions have performed a limited laparotomy to access the uterine wall directly. After the laparotomy is performed and the fetus well positioned, the procedure is performed as previously outlined, directly through the uterine wall. This approach necessitates the use of general anesthesia in the mother, which, as previously mentioned, can also relax the uterus, so typically the fetus can be

placed in a good position with relative ease. An added benefit to this procedure is the ability to place the ultrasound transducer directly on the uterus through a sterile sleeve, resulting in very clear imaging of the cardiac structures and physiological features.

Fetal surgery.   A third potential approach is to incise the uterus and expose the fetus with direct access of the vasculature by cannulation of the carotid artery or a systemic vein. Although this approach yields the most direct access, the significantly increased risk to the fetus and pregnancy compared with the other options has precluded its use thus far. As fetal surgery progresses and becomes safer in other settings, further evaluation of cardiac intervention through this approach is likely to be entertained in the future.

Equipment

Fetal imaging is performed by use of standard echocardiographic equipment and the highest frequency transducer that yields a clear picture of the anatomical structures. The introducer should be a small as possible to allow the entry of the balloon catheter. Typically, a 19-gauge cannula with a solid tip, 10 to 15 cm in length, is used depending on the depth needed. The catheters used have traditionally been adult coronary balloon catheters; however, shorter catheters specifically designed for fetal use have also been developed. The balloon size used should be one to one and a half times the size of the valve annulus. Most commonly, balloon diameters range from 2.5 to 4 mm and track over small, floppy-tipped guidewires for optimal placement across the targeted valve or atrial septum.

Outcomes

The recently published review on fetal intervention by Matsui and Gardiner[18] outlines the published data very well.

Critical Aortic Stenosis

The most experience with fetal intervention has been with critical aortic stenosis. The published experience worldwide is approximately 65 to 70 cases and has been performed in a number of institutions, with the largest experience reported by Tworetzky et al[10] at Boston Children's Hospital with approximately 40 cases. Overall, approximately 75% have been technically successful, with that percentage significantly higher over the last several years as the techniques have been practiced and improved. There is a significant fetal and neonatal mortality rate specifically from the earliest reports with small numbers. The data from the published series of Tworetzky et al is more optimistic, with approximately 90% survival to delivery. From the same series, approximately 30% of patients with a technically successful procedure have gone on to a biventricular repair. In the case of the technically unsuccessful procedures, all the fetuses that survived went on to a single ventricle palliation.

The same group has reported improvement in left ventricular hemodynamics after intervention with improved left ventricular ejection fraction, increased incidence of forward flow through the aortic arch, and in some cases right to left flow across the atrial septum. In addition, there was less significant mitral regurgitation and typically a change in the mitral inflow to a more normal biphasic pattern. [23]

It is important to point out that a biventricular outcome is not synonymous with a normal heart.

After delivery, these patients continue to have severe aortic valve disease, abnormal left ventricles, and typically mitral valve disease as well. In changing the natural history by fetal intervention of progression of critical aortic stenosis to hypoplasia of the left ventricle, a new form of heart disease has been created. The hope is that with two functional, if not normal, ventricles the outcomes for these children will be improved; however, that conclusion will have to wait until there are greater numbers of aortic valvuloplasties performed and long-term survival and development can be assessed.

Hypoplastic Left Heart Syndrome with Intact Atrial Septum

There are fewer cases of ballooning of the atrial septum in utero. Of the 18 cases that have been reported, all but one have been technically successful. The majority were performed by the percutaneous approach with one case performed by the transuterine approach.[24] Despite the technical success of the procedure, the postnatal results remain poor, with only half the infants surviving past infancy. Of note, in the largest series reported, there were very abnormal pulmonary venous Doppler patterns that are typically seen in this disease process at baseline. After the atrial septum

was ballooned and flow was established, the Doppler flow patterns did not improve.[11] That finding has led to speculation that once an atrial communication has been obtained, it may need to be stented open for adequate decompression of the left atrium. Of interest, in the case report in which the transuterine approach was used, the septum was ballooned with a 4-mm balloon, and significant improvement in the pulmonary venous Doppler pattern was seen immediately after the procedure (Fig. 24–7). That child went on to have all three stages of the Norwood procedure and is alive at 3 years of age.

In summary, although initial results have not shown significant improvement over aggressive neonatal management, anecdotal reports suggest that there may be promise for improved results as techniques improve.

Pulmonary Atresia with Intact Atrial Septum

At this point very little is known about fetal intervention for pulmonary atresia with intact atrial septum. The procedure has been successful in just over half the cases attempted; however, there are no data on postnatal or long-term outcomes.

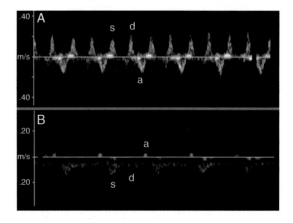

Figure 24–7 Pulmonary venous tracings in a patient with hypoplastic left heart syndrome and intact atrial septum. **A,** Preintervention the typical pattern of pulmonary venous drainage is seen with small amounts of forward flow in systole *(s)* and diastole *(d)* and prominent reversal of flow with atrial contraction *(a)*. **B,** Postballooning of the atrial septum in the same patient; the normal pattern of pulmonary venous drainage is immediately seen with good egress of flow in systole and diastole with only minimal reversal during atrial contraction.

Complications

The health and reproductive future of the mother during this procedure remains of utmost importance. Women with significant heath problems that place them at risk for wound healing or general anesthesia may not be candidates given the limited data on the benefit of the procedure.

Maternal complications that may occur include problems with anesthesia, pain, and wound healing. In addition, if the fetus becomes ill, premature labor may be induced, resulting in delivery of a premature infant with significant heart disease, which is typically a lethal combination. In the limited published data, there have been no maternal deaths and relatively limited morbidity.

Fetal complications are more common and may be related to the amount of manipulation required to perform the procedure. In general, the fewer attempts to access the heart and the least amount of time spent with the needle in the cardiac chambers the lower the chance of problems. The most common complications reported are fetal bradycardia, which occurs frequently with transventricular puncture, and pericardial effusions.

Fetal bradycardia is typically responsive to treatment with intracardiac epinephrine. Pericardial effusions can typically be drained during the procedure, but at least one fetal death has been attributed to massive hemopericardium.[23] Other reported deaths related to fetal intervention have typically occurred when the procedure was technically difficult and prolonged, or in fetuses that were hydropic and in extremis before the intervention.

It is too early to speculate on the success and future of fetal intervention. More data and experience are required to obtain confidence in this approach. It is possible that the combined maternal and fetal risk will preclude the benefits, which appear limited at present.

However, there is hope that as our experience grows, new technology will be developed and maternal risk minimized. If well-controlled long-term studies reveal benefit, then extension of these techniques to other lesions may be considered. Instead of salvaging patients with high mortality rates, it is conceivable that future fetal intervention may be applied with a focus of improving the outcomes in children with other cardiac lesions that currently survive after birth but require a lifetime of treatment and reoperation.

References

1. Hirsch JC, Mosca RS, Bove EL: Complete repair of tetralogy of Fallot in the neonate: Results in the modern era. Ann Surg 2000; 232:508–514.
2. Seliem MA, Wu YT, Glenwright K: Relation between age at surgery and regression of right ventricular hypertrophy in tetralogy of Fallot. Pediatr Cardiol 1995; 16:53–55.
3. Reddy VM, Liddicoat JR, McElhinney DB, et al: Routine primary repair of tetralogy of Fallot in neonates and infants less than three months of age. Ann Thorac Surg 1995; 60(6 Suppl):S592–596.
4. Di Donato RM, Jonas RA, Mayer JE, et al: Neonatal repair of Fallot's tetralogy with and without pulmonary atresia. Nippon Kyobu Geka Gakkai Zasshi 1989; 37(Suppl):97.
5. Pigula FA, Vida V, Del Nido P, et al: Contemporary results and current strategies in the management of hypoplastic left heart syndrome. Semin Thorac Cardiovasc Surg 2007; 19:238–244.
6. Tweddell JS, Hoffman GM, Mussatto KA, et al: Improved survival of patients undergoing palliation of hypoplastic left heart syndrome: Lessons learned from 115 consecutive patients. Circulation 2002; 106(12 Suppl):I82–I89.
7. Kohl T, Sharland G, Allan LD, et al: World experience of percutaneous ultrasound-guided balloon valvuloplasty in human fetuses with severe aortic valve obstruction. Am J Cardiol 2000; 85:1230–1233.
8. Allan LD, Maxwell DJ, Carminati M, et al: Survival after fetal aortic balloon valvoplasty. Ultrasound Obstet Gynecol 1995; 5:90–91.
9. Maxwell D, Allan L, Tynan MJ: Balloon dilatation of the aortic valve in the fetus: A report of two cases. Br Heart J 1991; 65:256–258.
10. Tworetzky W, Wilkins-Haug L, Jennings RW, et al: Balloon dilation of severe aortic stenosis in the fetus: Potential for prevention of hypoplastic left heart syndrome: Candidate selection, technique, and results of successful intervention. Circulation 2004; 110:2125–2131.
11. Marshall AC, van der Velde ME, Tworetzky W, et al: Creation of an atrial septal defect in utero for fetuses with hypoplastic left heart syndrome and intact or highly restrictive atrial septum. Circulation 2004; 110:253–258.
12. Hornberger LK, Need L, Benacerraf BR: Development of significant left and right ventricular hypoplasia in the second and third trimester fetus. J Ultrasound Med 1996; 15:655–659.
13. Rychik J, Rome JJ, Collins MH, et al: The hypoplastic left heart syndrome with intact atrial septum: atrial morphology, pulmonary vascular

histopathology and outcome. J Am Coll Cardiol 1999; 34:554–560.

14. Dyamenahalli U, McCrindle BW, McDonald C, et al: Pulmonary atresia with intact ventricular septum: Management of, and outcomes for, a cohort of 210 consecutive patients. Cardiol Young 2004; 14:299–308.

15. Daubeney PE, Sharland GK, Cook AC, et al: Pulmonary atresia with intact ventricular septum: Impact of fetal echocardiography on incidence at birth and postnatal outcome. UK and Eire Collaborative Study of Pulmonary Atresia with Intact Ventricular Septum. Circulation 1998; 98:562–566.

16. Hanley FL, Sade RM, Blackstone EH, et al: Outcomes in neonatal pulmonary atresia with intact ventricular septum: A multiinstitutional study. J Thorac Cardiovasc Surg 1993; 105:406–427.

17. Huhta J, Quintero RA, Suh E, et al: Advances in fetal cardiac intervention. Curr Opin Pediatr 2004; 16:487–493.

18. Matsui H, Gardiner H: Fetal intervention for cardiac disease: the cutting edge of perinatal care. Semin Fetal Neonatal Med 2007; 12:482–489.

19. Tworetzky W, Marshall AC: Balloon valvuloplasty for congenital heart disease in the fetus. Clin Perinatol 2003; 30:541–550.

20. Tworetzky W, Marshall AC: Fetal interventions for cardiac defects. Pediatr Clin North Am 2004; 51:1503–1513, vii.

21. Suh E, Quintessenza J, Huhta J, et al: How to grow a heart: Fiber optic guided fetal aortic valvotomy. Cardiol Young 2006; 16(1 Suppl): 43–46.

22. Quintero RA, Huhta J, Suh E, et al: In utero cardiac fetal surgery: Laser atrial septotomy in the treatment of hypoplastic left heart syndrome with intact atrial septum. Am J Obstet Gynecol 2005; 193:1424–1428.

23. Mizrahi-Arnaud A, Tworetzky W, Bulich LA, et al: Pathophysiology, management, and outcomes of fetal hemodynamic instability during prenatal cardiac intervention. Pediatr Res 2007; 62:325–330.

24. Von Bergen NH, Burkhart HM, Latson LA, et al: Complete cavopulmonary shunt completion after in utero balloon atrial septoplasty for hypoplastic left heart syndrome. J Thorac Cardiovasc Surg 2007; 134:1355–1356.

Index

Page numbers followed by f indicate
figure(s); t, table(s); b, box(es).

Perfect your skills—and prepare for the certification exam—with the interactive resources on the enclosed CD!

The **Companion CD** included with this textbook is your key to enhanced understanding of the fetal echo techniques you need to know for effective clinical practice!

Prepare for professional success with...

• **Brief video clips** of scanning procedures covered in the textbook to help you master techniques that cannot be easily conveyed with still images.

• **More than 250 review questions**, sortable by chapter, that test your knowledge and help you study for the certification exam.

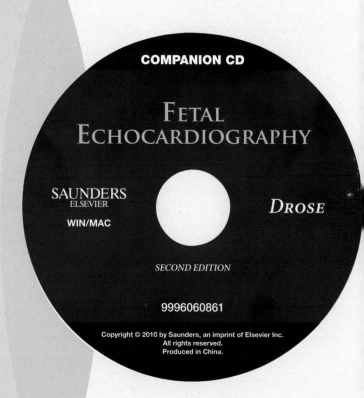

COMPANION CD

FETAL ECHOCARDIOGRAPHY

SAUNDERS
ELSEVIER

WIN/MAC

DROSE

SECOND EDITION

9996060861

Master the latest fetal echocardiography techniques—start using your companion CD now!